The Fragrant Mind

Also by
Valerie Ann Worwood

THE COMPLETE BOOK OF
ESSENTIAL OILS & AROMATHERAPY

AROMANTICS

The Fragrant Mind

Aromatherapy for Personality, Mind, Mood, and Emotion

Valerie Ann Worwood

NEW WORLD LIBRARY
NOVATO, CALIFORNIA

New World Library
14 Pamaron Way
Novato, California 94949

© 1996 Valerie Ann Worwood

Editorial: Becky Benenate and Jason Gardner
Cover illustration: Chantal Saperstein
Black & white drawings: Edwina Hannam
Text design: Linda Corwin

Library of Congress Cataloging-in-Publication Data

Worwood, Valerie Ann, 1945-
The fragrant mind : aromatherapy for personality,
mind, mood, and emotion / Valerie Ann Worwood.
Includes bibliographical references and index
ISBN 1-880032-91-0 (pbk. : alk. paper)
1. Aromatherapy. I. Title
RM666.A68W68 1996   96-6316
615'.321--dc20   CIP

Printed in Canada on acid-free paper
ISBN 1-880032-91-0

Distributed to the trade by Publishers Group West

10 9

Dedication

For my Dad, who read me Omar Khayyám, told me stories about his Fairy and the Tiger, and gave me gifts of dreams and imagination.

Acknowledgments

A sincere thank you goes to Julia Stonehouse for her invaluable assistance, encouragement, and humor and to my daughter, Emma, for giving me precious space and time to write.

Thanks also go to the following tutors and practitioners who gave up precious personal time to send me their thoughts on favorite essential oils for part three: Susan Worwood, Vivienne Lunny, Norma Gilbert, Elizabeth Jones, Teddy Fearnhamm, Nicole Perez, Maureen Farrell, Anne Marie Joyeux, Olive Beachamp, Shirley Price, Rodolphe Balz, Dietrich Gumbel, Jan Kusmirek.

Over the last two decades many people have contributed directly and indirectly to the concept of *The Fragrant Mind*, including my patients and students, fellow practitioners and lecturers, as well as researchers and scientists exploring the universal mind. To these, and the unseen hands that guide me, I give thanks.

Contents

Part Four

The material in this book is not meant to take place of diagnosis and treatment by a qualified medical practitioner. Because the actual use of essential oils by others is beyond the author's and publisher's control, no expressed or implied guarantee as to the effects of their use can be given nor liability taken. Any application of the recommendations set forth in the following pages is at the reader's sole risk. Essential oils are to be used at the reader's own discretion. The author and publisher disclaim any liability arising directly or indirectly from the use of this book and assume no responsibility for any actions taken.

Introduction

"I planted the seed, and Apollo watered it.
But God made it grow."
– Corinthians, 3:6

The Alternative Service Book

Welcome to *The Fragrant Mind* — a new approach to emotional well-being. The subject of this book is essential oils — highly concentrated aromatic plant essences that are used in aromatherapy — and their application to enhance mind, mood, and emotion. This is not a new subject, of course, and plant essences have in various ways been used for thousands of years to cheer people up, calm them down, and make them feel good about themselves. This book, for the first time, presents a comprehensive guide to this subject of natural mind enhancement with essential oils.

Over recent years there has been a significant growth of interest in aromatherapy. What has made it so successful is the fact that people gain tremendous benefit from essential oils in terms of emotional well-being. Indeed, when most people think about aromatherapy, they think about it being able to alleviate stress and tension. However, this is just the tip of the iceberg, so to speak, because, in fact, essential oils provide a complete materia medica for mind, mood and emotion.

You do not have to be ill to use essential oils for the mind. Indeed, essential oils are all about potential — not only the potential of the body to be healed, a medical system, but about the potential of the mind to work at optimum emotional harmony, a system of aroma-tology — well-being of the mind. A huge spectrum of possibility presents itself.

The Fragrant Mind is presented in three parts. The first, *Pathways to the Mind*, explains how essential oils appear to work on the brain, and the many diverse ways in which they can be used, both by the layperson and the professional. Part Two, *Emotional Healing and Aromatherapy*, gives detailed suggestions relevant to a very wide variety of emotional conditions. This includes blends for happiness and other positive states, as well as an essential oil guide for an A-Z of negative emotional problems. Part Three, *Aroma-Genera: Human Characteristics and Personalities of Essential Oils*, explains the typology of essential oils, and acts as a guide for choosing the right oils for your personality.

This last section, *Aroma-Genera*, is used in the field of aroma-psychology — a brand new branch of aromatherapy. It is about using essential oils in a positive way to enhance personality. The groups that essential oils fall into are known as the typology, and these are described here for the first time as Florals, Fruities, Herbies, Leafies, Resinies, Rooties, Seedies, Spicies, and Woodies. These classifications act as a guide to positive and negative personality traits, and help indicate which particular essential oils would suit a particular person. In addition to this, each essential oil has its own unique personality, and forty-five essential oils are described here.

Not only can essential oils be used for anxiety, doubt, or fear, they can also be used to make a person more assertive, confident, or creative. Aromatherapy is not just about "stress and tension," although of course it is tremendously beneficial in these areas. It goes very deeply into the psyche on all levels of human experience. Essential oils are nature's pharmacopoeia, fully able to deal with the mind in all its aspects, a fabulous gift for us all.

This book has been many years in the making and the material on these pages is a synthesis of practical application and knowledge, experienced by real-life people who have benefited from essential oil use. The information here presented is not based on some ancient texts which may have had relevance many hundreds of years ago, but on many years of experience as a clinical aromatherapist, in contact with others in my profession.

Today, all over the world, for different reasons, researchers are increasingly becoming interested in the fact that these precious concentrated substances actually work, and are more than the sum of their component parts. Pictures produced by sophisticated technology can now be taken showing aroma molecules working on the brain. We are talking here about powerful aromatic substances which, through the olfactory bulb, gain immediate access to our mind, mood, and emotions. Aromatherapy may be an ancient art but it is also increasingly being seen as a hugely interesting field of future research and development.

Essential oils allow you to take control of your emotional well-being. These are not unknown quantities but substances that have been used by millions of people over thousands of years and continue to be used today in a wide variety of ways — some of which you will be familiar with. For example, some of the essential oils mentioned in this book are used in perfumery and cosmetics, others are ingredients in food and drink products and, of course, essential oils are used as medicines.

Essential oils are distilled from certain varieties of certain species of plants. Some coming from petals, others from stems, twigs, leaves, roots, trees, grasses, or fruits. These exquisite aromatic substances provide a rich treasury for human beings, in all their aspects of mind, body, and spirit. Well-being is a difficult thing to quantify, but essential oils can certainly help us discover it. My aim with *The Fragrant Mind* is to pass on some of the information I have acquired in an easy-to-use form, so that others can walk on Mother Nature's pathway to a fragrant mind.

———

Part 1

Pathways to the Mind

"The most beautiful and deepest experience a man can have is the sense of the mysterious.
It is the underlying principle of religion as well as all serious endeavor in art and science."

– ALBERT EINSTEIN
In a speech delivered at the German
League of Human Rights, 1932

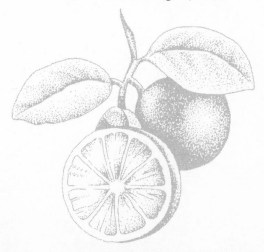

CHAPTER 1

THE HISTORY OF DRUGS

I wonder what's around the bend? said the explorer
I wonder what that plant is? said the collector
I wonder what's in it? said the chemist
I wonder what activity it has? said the pharmacologist
I wonder if it'll work in this case? said the physician
I hope she lives! said the father
Please God! said the mother
I think she'll be all right in the morning, said the nurse

– MARGARET KREIG
Green Medicine

Ever since human beings first walked this earth they have searched for materials that would ease their suffering. As time went on they came to know which plants would feed their hunger, which would poison, and which would heal. In the ancient Sumerian town of Nippur, prescriptions were written on clay tablets and from these we know that over 4,000 years ago people used flowers, seeds, leaves, fruits, roots, and barks in their medicines. Among the plants they used were thyme, myrrh, and pine — which are still used today in the form of essential oils — and willow, the source of aspirin.

Aspirin is another name for acetylsalicylic acid, a synthetic first produced in 1899 and derived from salicin, the active ingredient, named after salix — a family of willow tree. For thousands of years resins and juices from the bark and leaves of the willow have been used to treat rheumatism, neuralgia, and other ailments. The scientific history of the willow is traced to an 18th century clergyman, Edmund Stone, who had by recommendation or accident acquired the habit of chewing the bark. Interestingly, salicin is also a drug for the tree itself — conferring "systematic acquired resistance" on it, according to scientists at the Agricultural Biotechnology Research Unit of Ciba-Geigy, the multinational chemical company. Apparently, the willow trees use it to ward off infections, which they are prone to because they often grow by stagnant water.

Malaria has killed more people in this world than any other disease. The first drug treatment was quinine, which continues to be used against strains of the disease that are resistant to newer antimalarials, and is more commonly prescribed to prevent painful leg cramps at night. The source of this drug is the bark of a flowering evergreen, *Cinchona*, which grows on the Andean slopes of South America. The bark, first imported to Europe in 1645, was widely used as an antimalarial although its mysteries were not uncovered until 1819 when pharmaceutical chemists extracted one of the alkaloids and named it quinine after the Peruvian Indian word *quina-quina*, the "bark of barks."

As people explored their natural environment, they inevitably came across those plants that have an effect on the mind. So it was in India and Africa where for hundreds and perhaps thousands of years people used the root of related species of rauwolfia as a tranquilizer and treatment for "moon madness" — lunacy. In 1925 an eminent Nigerian living in London became psychotic but the doctors treating him couldn't help. The witchdoctor was summoned and arrived with his rauwolfia root — which did the trick. The active substances in rauwolfia (named after Leonhard Rauwolf, the 16th century physician and plant explorer) were isolated in the late 1940s by Indian scientists and after more work by the Swiss drug company, Ciba-Geigy, the first mind or mood altering drug based on rauwolfia alkaloids, reserpine, hit the market. And what a market it was — $80 million by the mid 1970s.

Not all alkaloids are so easy to reproduce chemically because they have large compounds which are difficult to synthesize. An example of this is the Madagascan Periwinkle, the source of vincristine sulfate, an essential drug in any pharmacy dealing with childhood leukemia and certain lymphomas. It still takes 12 tons of crushed leaves to produce one ounce of the drug — also the source of Vinblastine, used to treat Hodgkin's disease. Over the years untold suffering has been alleviated by this innocent-looking pink and white ornamental, *Catharanthus roseus*, which gardeners appropriately call "bright eyes." Cancer treatment would be a harder task today without the 70% of antitumor drugs derived from native medicines.

Originally, all drugs were natural. The Ayurvedic system of medicine, thought to be at least 5,000 years old, is still extensively used in the Indian subcontinent and is studied by many Western medics as well. The text books mention 8,000 different natural medicines, using plant, animal, and mineral materials. Chinese herbal medicine is also becoming popular in the West, and of course continues to be of central importance in the materia medica of China. The first drug directory that we know of is the 2800 B.C. *Pen Ts'ao*, written by herbalist Shen Nung. In the Western tradition, credit for establishing medical botany as an applied science is given to the Greek physician Pedanios Dioscorides who in 78 A.D. published his *Materia Medica,* which detailed the properties of about 600 medicinal plants, as well as the medicinal value of certain animal products. Books such as these, recording the properties of natural products, were the mainstay of western medicine for about 1,400 years. The concept of medicinal chemistry was introduced in the 1520s by Paracelsus, a Swiss pharmacist-physician whose "real" name was Theophrastus Bombastus von Hohenheim. Paracelsus advocated the use of mineral salts and acids and experimented with various chemical processes including distillation. It would be another three hundred years before medical chemistry really took off, however, inspired by the German apothecary's assistant Friedrich Serturner, who in 1806 isolated the first active alkaloid of a natural drug — raw opium from the poppy *Papaver somniferum*. Serturner named it morphine after Morpheus, the Greek god of Dreams. Codeine is a derivative of morphine.

The history of drugs clearly shows the source of inspiration — nature. However, nature has its disadvantages. Imagine yourself the manager of a drug company looking at your storehouse full of bags of herbs, barks, roots, leaves, and flowers imported from all over the world. You start thinking about what could go wrong with your supplies. Natural products are vulnerable to adverse weather conditions, including flood and drought, as well as to pest catastrophes. But if just one of these raw materials fails to make it to the factory, drugs cannot be made and people die. Also, natural raw materials are unpredictable in terms of the quantity of active ingredients they contain, and huge quantities of the stuff have to be processed to produce small quantities of the required drug. On top of that, the raw material has to be purified and quantified — all of which is more effort. You can see why chemists tried to find a way of creating the active ingredients of medicinal plants by more easily controlled, chemical means.

Over the years we have seen a major shift of emphasis. To begin with, natural products were either the raw material of drugs, or the inspiration for chemical copies. As chemists became more confident, they made cocktails using more and more compounds — some natural, some not. Nowadays, scientists create chemical cocktails that have little to do with nature as we know it. What effect these will have on the population is still little understood because long-term studies cannot yet be made. Unlike natural drugs, these chemical cocktails have new molecular arrangements that haven't been on trial for thousands of years. Indeed, their trials are of necessity rather short because a company has to register the 30-year patent for the new drug before it can carry out trials. That patent is liable to run out if the company doesn't get its act together quickly and produce the evidence of efficacy and safety required to get a product license. The quicker a trial can be done, the more time there is left on the patent in which the company can exclusively exploit their invention.

Chemical companies are still interested in nature. In the deepest jungles and the most far-off corners of the earth, representatives from drug companies continue to scour the landscape looking for new varieties of nature to exploit. They are not intending, however, to manage huge fields of these natural products, and extract from them the drug required. They are simply going to try to isolate the active substances and replicate them in the laboratory. In their dreams, scientists imagine a future biotechnology when the physiological and psychoactive substances in plants can be produced cheaply and easily using microbes or whatever.

Biotechnology is here, however. Take Hirudin, for example, the latest potential drug from Ciba-Geigy, which is at the human trials stage. The leech *Hirudo medicinalis* was used for centuries to draw blood from patients. The saliva of the leech is now known to contain substances which act as a powerful and highly predictable anticoagulant, which may be very useful in the prevention of thrombosis, stroke and heart attack — the western world's largest killer disease. The problem is, it takes the saliva from 10,000 leeches to make a single human treatment and, I imagine, extracting it is quite a job! Biotechnology, however, gets around the problem by taking the appropriate gene from the leech and putting it in yeast cells, which produce Hirudin molecules.

New discoveries continue to be made. In a recent article in the *Lancet*, co-authored by Nobel Laureate B.S. Blumberg, clinical research was presented which proved that the hepatitis B virus was eliminated from the bodies of 59% of people treated for thirty days with dried and powdered *Phyllanthus amarus*, a plant used for over 2,000 years in Ayurvedic medicine to treat liver disease, including jaundice. The plant has also been used in China, the Philippines, Cuba, Nigeria, Guam, East and West Africa, the Caribbean, and Central and South America. Despite the fact that the plant is used so extensively, and the fact that it has now been studied for over ten years, and has shown no toxic or side effects in animals or humans, it will probably never reach the marketplace in Britain or America. *Phyllanthus* needs more than the keen advocacy of the eminent Blumberg, who got his Nobel prize for discovering the hepatitis B virus and developing the blood test to detect it. *Phyllanthus* needs tens of millions of dollars to go through clinical testing, and chemical companies aren't going to support that work because, to date, they have no intention of selling herbs. They may well look at *Phyllanthus*, and try to copy its active constituents, but that is another matter.

In the land of the BMW, Germany,

things are different. The laws allow natural medicines to be sold, but as food supplements without any indication of use on the label. Even so, everyone knows what they are for. For example, we see *ginkgo biloba* extract, taken from the plant much used in herbalism, becoming a best-selling prescription drug in Germany — where it is used to stimulate cerebral circulation in the elderly. [1]

I don't understand why chemical companies don't switch their attention to producing extracts or essential oils from natural plants. It may have something to do with the difficulty in patenting remedies that have been known for centuries. But it is possible to quite easily extract the active constituents of plants, and it's much easier than trying to replicate their extraordinarily complex powers in chemistry. Lavender is the classic case in point. It is the treatment *par excellence* for burns. Put on badly burnt skin, lavender nothing short of miraculously returns the burnt skin to normal, and very, very quickly. But, for all the work on it, lavender will not easily give up her secrets. Chemists can make a liquid that *smells* like lavender, and they can even break it apart and label a certain number of its constituents, but they cannot make a substance that is like lavender that heals burns. As systems of analysis get better, more molecular and other secrets will be revealed. Meanwhile, in burn departments in hospitals, people suffer.

Of course science has made great strides in the field of medicine, and we all have reason to be grateful, but let us not forget the relationship between science and nature. Science looks to nature in amazement, tries to break it apart and copy it. Nature makes cells and gets them to interact in unbelievably complex ways, while the whole of science and technology cannot between them make a single cell — plant, animal, or human. Looking at nature and science, we must ask ourselves which is the most clever?

The Shamans

Consciousness is at the core of humanity. Deprived of sight, hearing, touch, taste, and smell, we still have consciousness. It is, if you like, the essence of being, but throughout time people have strived to enlarge their consciousness or to change it so that other dimensions of being are reached. Substances which alter perception are used to put people in touch with the spirits of dead ancestors; or to seek union with the god-head; or by traditional healers who want to gain a more profound insight into the nature of a patient's disease — often perceived as the result of outside, nonmaterial, forces.

The Matse are a small, seminomadic tribe of hunter-gatherers who live in the rainforest on the Peru/Brazil border. Their pharmacopoeia includes a drug, *nu-nu*, which hunters use to induce visions of the future movements of animals. They see the animal situated in a particular place, and from clues in the vision, they estimate the time of day. Armed with this information, they lie in wait and make the kill. Peter Gorman may be the only westerner who has tried *nu-nu*, which is blown into the nostrils down a hollow reed tube, and this is his description of the experience:

"When the nu-nu hit, it seemed to explode inside my face. It burnt my nose and I began to choke up wretched green phlegm. But the pain quickly subsided and I closed my eyes. Out of the blackness I began to have visions of animals — tapir, monkey, and wild boar — that I saw more clearly than my limited experience with them should have allowed. Then suddenly the boars stampeded in front of me."[2]

Gorman told the Matses what he had seen, and from the clues in his vision, the time and place of the stampede was determined. The next morning Gorman and several Indians set off for the place seen in the vision. He writes: "As we neared it, I was astounded to hear the thunderous roar of dozens of boars charging across the river in front of us. We jumped out of the boat and chased them." They returned to the village with seven boars — "enough meat for the entire village for four days."

Gorman also took another Matse drug, *sapo*, which is made from the secretions of a frog, *dow-kiet!* or *phyllomedusa bicolor*. The immediate physical effects of ingesting this drug were horrendous, according to Gorman's account, but the results were worth it. His hearing was greatly improved, and more besides:

"My vision, my sense of smell, everything about me felt larger than life, and my body felt immensely strong... During the next few days,
my feeling of strength didn't diminish; I could go whole days without being hungry or thirsty and move through the jungle for hours without tiring. Every sense I possessed was heightened and in tune with the environment, as though the sapo put the rhythm of the jungle into my blood."[3]

The Matses use huge quantities of the drug *sapo* to do nothing less than project their animas, their spirit, into the form of an animal, which they use as a lure for real animals. Gorman's informant, Pablo, set a trap in the forest then returned to the village where he took the *sapo* for two days. The next morning he woke Gorman up before dawn and, with the rest of the village, rushed to the place where the trap had been set. Just as the people arrived, a tapir was approaching the trap — and was duly caught. On analysis, it turns out that *sapo* contains seven bioactive peptides, triggers which cause chemical reactions in the body. However, why *sapo* should give a person the ability to project their animas remains a mystery!

People living in the depths of nature seem to have an extraordinary sensitivity. One thinks about the reports of people back at camp whooping and shouting at the precise moment the hunting party, many miles away, makes a kill. How did they know? These are mysteries of communication we can only guess at. On top of this degree of "extrasensory" perception, native peoples seek to go further. With a little help from nature, they project themselves into the very form of animals, they see the future, they communicate with dead relatives, they speak to nature spirits, they get outside their conscious selves and into another, equally real, dimension.

In our culture, such concepts are difficult to grasp, but we too experiment with consciousness-raising drugs, seeking our own understanding of the universe. Over the past three decades, LSD, mescaline, and psilocybin have been widely used in this way and, interestingly, all these drugs resemble human brain chemicals in their chemical structure. The alkaloid mescaline comes from the Peyote cactus and is closely related to noradrenaline, a neurotransmitter (which acts in the chemical transmission of impulses between nerves in the brain). Mescaline and the neurotransmitter noradrenaline (norepinephrine) have the same basic chemical structure and both are derived from phenylethylamine, another derivative of which is phenylalanine, an essential amino acid found extensively in humans. Psilocybin and psilocine are the active principles of the Mexican mushroom, *teonanacatl*, and, like the brain hormone serotonin, are derived from tryptamine — as are the hallucinogenic properties of Morning Glory, *Ololuiqui*, the inspiration of the semi-synthetic LSD. Chemically, LSD is extremely close to lysergic acid amide and lysergic acid hydroxyethylamide, the hallucinogenic principles of *Ololuiqui*.

In the excellent *Plants of the Gods*, Dr. Richard Schultes and Dr. Albert Hofmann (the man who discovered LSD) explain the psychotropic potency of these hallucinogenics:

"Having the same basic structure, these hallucinogens may act at the same sites in the nervous system as the above-mentioned brain hormones, like similar keys fitting the same lock. As a result, the psychophysiological functions associated with those brain sites are altered, suppressed, stimulated, or otherwise modified." [4]

But it isn't just about chemistry. According to Schultes and Hofmann:

"The ability of hallucinogens to provide changes in brain function is due not only to their having a particular chemical composition, but also to the peculiar spacial arrangement of the atoms in their molecules." [5]

LSD is a case in point. The semi-synthetic hallucinogen LSD differs from the semi-synthetic compound iso-LSD only in the spacial arrangement of the diethylamide group, but the iso-LSD has practically no hallucinogenic effect.

Life teaches us that the mind is a very strange thing. Speed alters in an emergency. It goes in slow motion as we helplessly watch our car smash into another. For one friend, time stood still when, walking in the wilderness, she inadvertently stepped into a mud pool like quicksand — in which she could quite easily have disappeared without trace. With the mud more liquid below her feet, and her companions walking on ahead, she knew she was on the fence between life and death. Time stood still, she tells me, and to this day she doesn't know whether she was there for five minutes, five hours or five centuries!

The mind is clearly capable of playing tricks on us, and there is probably some self-preservation reason at root. The point, however, is that this Pandora's box of perceptual tricks can be stimulated by outside means — life experiences which provoke exceptional chemical phenomena, synthetic hallucinogenics, and natural plant and animal materials.

There are essential oils that have narcotic or mind-altering principles, but I shall not list them here, you won't find them in other aromatherapy books, and they are not discussed in aromatherapy schools. Indeed, it is a matter of professional responsibility to ensure that no potentially harmful substances are used. In *The Fragrant Mind* I promote the use of subtle and gentle substances which allow you to seek your own visions or understandings — a vision quest in which you have the control. Essential oils are the non-toxic and harmless way to allow your mind free will to explore its untapped potential.

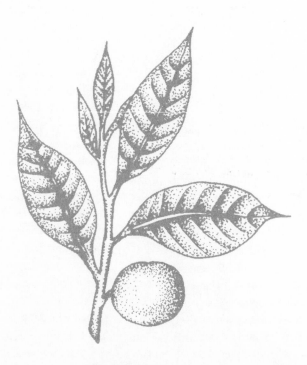

Petitgrain

CHAPTER 2

ESSENTIAL OILS AND THE MIND

Essential oils and human beings have a great deal in common. We are both alive — chemically, electrically, and in terms of infrared radiation. Essential oils come from plants, while we ourselves rely totally on plants for our sustenance. We eat plants, and animals which eat plants, and breathe air made possible by plants. Human beings and plants are related because all living organisms are descended from the same single-cell line.[1] The chemical composition of DNA in plants and people is virtually the same.[2] Neurobiologist Donald Kennedy has done a detailed study of the difference between plants and animals and has come to the conclusion that there is very little difference! He took tissue from a spruce tree and compared it to that from a moose. Cells from both the spruce and moose have walls, both contain little organs called *organelles,* and both have a nucleus, with its own membrane, and genetic material DNA — the chemical composition of which is identical between spruce and moose.[3]

Plants and humans both depend on a chelating chemical, which in humans is red *heme* and transports the oxygen released from plants in the blood, while in plants it's chlorophyll. Chemically, the only difference between the two is that a magnesium atom replaces an iron atom.[4] The similar chemical composition of plants and humans may explain why essential oils — distillations of certain parts of certain plants — seem to act like keys to our physical and mental mechanisms.

It's becoming increasingly clear that there is still much to learn about plants. Trees might look helpless, locked to one spot in the ground, but we now know, using chemistry, that they talk to each other, defend themselves against animal invaders, and attack plant species to protect resources. Genetically, trees are very resourceful, adapting over one generation to deal with many generations of short-lived but highly adaptive insects. An old oak tree, for example, could have ten branches carrying ten different genetic messages. This evolutionary advantage may help explain why some trees, like *Pinus aristata,* can live for over 2,000 years!

Chemically, trees are very active. When under attack from a predator they can produce extra chemicals called tannins, which deter and even kill the predator, and then distribute this chemical to the leaves. In Africa, Professor Wouter van Hoven tested a variety of trees to see how much extra tannin the trees produced. He had his students thrash the trees with sticks and belts, replicating the harsh treatment trees get from browsing deer and the like, and then he tested the increase. After 15 minutes, *Acacia caffra* had increased its tannin production by 94% while *Rhus leptodictya's* went up by 76%. After an hour, the off-putting tannins had increased in the leaves of wattle by 256% and in the acacia by 282%. Other species show similar reactions. It took the trees between 24 and 100 hours after the attack to return to their normal chemical state. And, the trees had somehow transmitted the news of "predators about" to nearby trees, which also started to produce extra tannins. Because the message was relayed to trees not connected by their root systems, as Dr. David Rhoads of the University of Washington has suggested with red alder and sitka willow, what we may have at work here are "airborne pheromonal substances" — chemical

messengers or hormones. In another piece of chemical wizardry, to protect their personal space, trees produce allelochemicals which insects ingest and, through their droppings, deposit on the ground around the tree. These allelochemicals prevent other plants from growing nearby, thus conserving resources for the tree.

There is a whole chemical way of life for plants, which we are only just beginning to discover — speaking from a laboratory perspective, at least. People have for countless millennia been interacting with plants and a knowledge has built up about the chemical movements within plants so they can be harvested at their peak. An essential oil could be distilled from a jasmine flower that is not one day old, or a sandalwood tree that is not less than thirty years old. Some plants are harvested in the morning, some at night. And, of course, there are seasons. People have learned to pick the plants at the optimum moment, even though they haven't understood why the particular required chemicals should be in that particular part of the plant, at that particular time. But there is more to life than chemistry, as we shall later see, and the beauty of essential oils is that whatever way you look at them, they seem to be in perfect harmony with the human organism.

What Are Essential Oils?

For as long as we know, people have been distilling and otherwise processing certain plant materials to extract their powerful healing essences. The word *chemistry* comes from the Greek word *chemia*, meaning plant juice. In turn, according to some scholars, *chemia* may derive from the Persian word *kimiya*, which referred to a group of Chinese tonic herbs. In Medieval Latin, Paracelsus referred to the oils he distilled from medicinal plants as the *quinta essentia* — the quintessence of the plant — and that is where the term "essential oil" comes from.

Essential oils are distilled or otherwise processed from very specific parts of particular species of plants. Vascular plants such as flowering species and conifers contain special tissues or vessels for the circulation of fluids. In the case of lavender, the oil is distilled from the flowers, in the case of ginger it's the root, and in patchouli it's the leaves. Essential oils are made from flowers, leaves, barks, roots, fruits, seeds, grasses, and resins. They're produced in practically every country of the world. Oil of spearmint comes from America, oil of chamomile from England, bergamot from Italy, Rose from Bulgaria, Frankincense from Somalia, pine and cypress from Bhutan, and so on. Oils come from specific species of plant groups. For example, there are over three hundred varieties of tea tree in Australia, but only a few produce oil with medicinal properties.

There are an estimated half-million species of flora in the world, of which about 300 produce an essential oil which is used in modern aromatherapy. Of course, traditional medicine and shamanism throughout the world utilizes many

more, whose properties we do not yet know. Essential oils are examined in various ways, particularly in terms of chemistry by gas chromatography and the mass spectrograph. Although over 3,000 compounds have been found in essential oils, there are many other compounds that have yet to be isolated, named, and understood. These unknown compounds tend to be "disappeared" by the literature, which concentrates on what we *do* know. Long lists of components in oils may look very impressive but what science doesn't tell us is that if all the known chemicals were mixed together in a pot, they would not make the essential oil they were trying to copy. Something vital is missing. The question is, "what?"

Reductionism doesn't work with essential oils. Tea tree oil is powerfully antimicrobial, but its two main components — terpinen-4-ol (40% volume) and gamma terpinene (28%) are much less so. It is the *synergistic* effect of *all* the components that makes an essential oil what it is. This is why there isn't a chemist in the world who can tell you *how* essential oils work. In a rose oil, for example, there may be over 1,000 compounds, some known and some not, and figuring out how they all work as an integrated unit is not at all easy. Essential oils are complex chemical structures, still beyond the powers of scientific analysis.

As individual oils are so mysterious, imagine the difficulty in analyzing *mixtures* of oils. But blends of different oils are used every day by millions of people all over the world. Indeed, complex blending has been a feature of herbal life for as long as we know, and for the medicine men and women and shamans working to help the people around them know, it is not only individual plants that are interesting, but the synergistic effect of them when combined.

Absolutes

In the general term "essential oils," some could be more accurately called "absolutes" because they have been through a particular form of extraction which brings into the "oil" more components than essential oils produced by steam distillation. The process of distillation releases only the lighter aromatic molecules, which are subsequently separated and packaged, while absolutes contain both the lighter and the heavier molecules. The absolutes include jasmine, tuberose, rose maroc, narcissus, cistus, and hyacinth, among others, and are made from the most fragrant and delicate of flowers.

It is an ironic yet poetic fact of nature that the most fragrant flowers are the most difficult from which to extract the fragrance. You might simply pass a rose in the garden but the aroma wafts towards you and stays with you for half a day. One jasmine plant can perfume an entire garden. Capturing this power is phenomenally difficult with many millions of petals being required to fill one small bottle of jasmine essential oil.

It is not an easy job to coax the powerful aroma from the delicate flowers from which absolutes are made. Distillation is too harsh, so over the years other methods have been employed. Our ancestors used fat-extraction, a method which has been continued during the following many centuries in the form of maceration or enfleurage, but today we have CO_2 (carbon dioxide) extraction to obtain the aromatic material. This produces an "essential oil" or, if you want to be exact, "an absolute," that smells exactly like the flower it came from. The same cannot be said for steam-distilled essential oils, which often differ somewhat in aroma from the plant itself.

Absolutes contain in them more components of the plant from which they came, including waxes, color pigments, fatty acids, vitamins, and minerals. These tend to give the absolute a more three-dimensional aroma, much appreciated by the perfume industry. The very name "absolute" does, in fact, describe this class of oils very well because they are absolutely complete in their aromatic complexity.

There has been a long debate in the aromatherapy field about these absolutes, with some people saying that the extraction methods bring into the "oil" residues of solvents and particles of the plant which are not therapeutic. It has now been shown that absolutes do not necessarily contain residues of solvents that can be organic substances. Also, the newer method of CO_2 extraction eliminates the question of solvents.

The growing appreciation of absolutes has generated the new practice of extracting absolutes from plants usually distilled by steam distillation. We are discovering that chamomile absolute, as distinct from chamomile essential oil, smells different than it, and may have properties different than it as well. The difference between essential oils and absolutes could be said to be a degree of dimension. The absolutes are, as their name implies, more absolute, i.e., complete or entire. In essential oil terms, this means they extend, perhaps more than some essential oils, from their medicinal therapeutic value into aroma-psychology and the dimension of emotional and even spiritual value.

Chemistry

On average, an essential oil is made up of over a hundred components. Some are ten times more complex than this. The main categories of compounds are terpenes, alcohols, esters, aldehydes, ketones, and phenols. At the present time it is known that up to 50% of the essential oil of *Lavendula officinalis* is made up of alcohols including lavandulol, borneol, terpineol, geraniol, and linalol — in esterified form, linalyl acetate. Between 48-52% is comprised of esters derived from the alcohols: lavandylyl acetate, linalyl acetate, bornyl acetate. Oxides account for between 2-3%, like 1,8 cineole, linalyl oxide and caryophyllene oxide. There are also minuscule but vital other components such as coumarin: herniarine, umbelliferone, santonine. Terpenes such as myrcene, limonene, and ocimene can account for up to 5%, while the sesquiterpene, caryophyllene, is about 3%. There is also

ketone camphor, methyl heptyl ketone, lactones, and aldehydes. The trouble is, if you were to put together a stew of chemical ingredients, following the above formula, you would not get a lavender oil capable of healing burns. There are still undiscovered compounds in essential oils, or perhaps other forces, which may one day explain their extraordinary healing powers.

Current methods of analysis depend very much upon the sensitivity of the machine and the operator. Different chromatography machines give different readings so an operator needs to be familiar with his or her machine. The operator doesn't exactly *read* the data so much as *interpret* it. For this reason, accurate analysis of essential oils may have to wait until technology has built the tools which can interpret nature.

Electro-magnetism

The word electron was adopted from the Greek by William Herbert, physician to Queen Elizabeth I of England, in the 16th century. Gilbert demonstrated the electron factor by applying friction to amber (a plant resin), which attracts light objects, like feathers, to it. But electricity and magnetism are more impressive than this. In the 1960s Wilderanck showed that if an electric field was applied to cells in a fluid suspension they would join up to make strings or chains which would orientate along the lines of magnetic force. When the field was turned off, the cells returned to their individual unconnected state.

All life has electric properties. The ion channels in cell membranes cause a voltage difference across the membrane of nearly one tenth of a volt. If you put 20 neurons together in the correct way you could get a charge of 1.5 volts — enough to run a small flashlight. Chains of molecules (polymers) are polarized like the DNA helix, which has a positively charged end and a negatively charged end — just like a magnet. Human beings react to sunspots happening 93,000 miles away like receivers of energy. Doctors apply electrical impulses to broken limbs that have proved difficult to mend, and they heal. Electrical osteogenesis is just one aspect of the new branch of science, electrical medicine, which continues to develop.

Essential oils have electrical properties that are defined in terms of positive-negative and polarity. Thus an aroma molecule might be negative and polar, negative and nonpolar, positive and polar, or positive and nonpolar. Even the electrical properties of individual components in essential oils can be measured. We know, for example, that aldehydes have an electro-negative character, while mono terpene hydro carbons have moderately electro-positive molecules. Phenols are electro-positive while turpene alcohols are for the most part mildly electro-positive. Esters are electrically neutral, aldehydes have a distinct electro-negative character and phenols have an electron deficiency. [5] The electrical cocktail going on in essential oils is similar to the electrical cocktail going on in the human body — positives and negatives all firing at different times, yet in synchrinicity. According to essential oil researchers, Pierre Francomme and Daniel Penoel, essential oils are carriers of negative or positive energy depending on whether they have an excess or lack of electrons, whether donors or acceptors of electrons. This makes essential oils very dynamic, and a good set of therapeutic tools to work with.

Infrared Radiation

The aroma molecules which rise up from a corn field can be detected by moths flying between 500-2,000 feet above. This remarkable perception was once attributed entirely to the moth's sense of smell, but it's now thought moths also recognize the infrared radiation produced by the aroma molecules. The scientific field of infrared spectrophotometry was discovered by the nineteenth century Irish genius, John Tyndall, who, aside from discovering why the sky is blue, found that infrared radiation is absorbed by the essential oils of patchouli, sandalwood, cloves, lavender, rose, lemon, thyme, rosemary, spikenard and aniseed, among others.

What significance this infrared factor has vis-à-vis humans is not known, but humans are themselves surrounded by an aura of infrared emanation. [6] According to Tompkins and Bird in Secrets of The Soil, "the subtle molecular odors that surround human bodies are stimulated to radiation by this infrared emission."

When I was working in Europe over twenty years ago it was usual for therapists to leave the client under an infrared lamp for five minutes before starting the treatment because it was thought this helped the absorption of essential oils. This may well be so because infrared improves circulation, opens blood vessels, and brings blood to the surface, so the essential oil can be absorbed better. On the infrared question then, we have several factors to consider: aroma molecules may produce infrared radiation; they also absorb it; human beings are surrounded by infrared emissions; and circulation is helped when they are exposed to more of it. Clearly, there are interactions between essential oils and human beings on the infrared level, interactions that need further investigation, which may one day help to explain their efficacy.

How Do Essential Oils Get into the Body?

There are several ways of taking essential oils into the body. One of the most effective ways is through percutaneous absorption — through the skin. As aroma molecules, essential oils set off reactions in receptor cells in the nose, leading to enzyme activity and electrical impulses to the olfaction bulb — which is actually an extension of the brain. Some people, under very particular circumstances also take essential oils orally, but generally, this is their least effective means of absorption because they end up in the digestive tract with all sorts of other materials, with which they will react (this is also the case

with chemical drugs). Because of the high absorption of essential oils by the mucous membranes of the respiratory tract, they can be inhaled as airborne particles. In France, essential oils are delivered in suppositories and pessaries. The state of acidity in the delicate mucous membranes allows them to very effectively absorb materials into the body. There is a particularly absorbent area under the tongue, which is now being utilized in the delivery of "sublinguals," usually vitamin supplements — the latest medicinal craze. But also, the nose has many surface capillaries, through which molecules can go straight into the bloodstream. For this reason, you can now buy vitamin supplements like B_{12}, for example, which are packaged in gels that you squirt up the nose. Cocaine and the South American drug *nu-nu* are other substances that may gain entry to the bloodstream via this route.

When you have essential oils in your environment, they could have an effect on you via many routes. As airborne particles in a diffuser, for example, their effect would be very subtle — affecting the mind via receptor cells in the nose and the olfaction bulb, and getting into the blood stream when absorbed through mucous membrane of the nose, mouth, and respiratory tract. In the bath, essential oils work both percutaneously and through airborne manners, as they do during massage, which generally gives much higher concentrations. With essential oils more is not always best. Sometimes, less is best. The different methods of use all have their advantages, depending on the circumstances.

In a later section I discuss how essential oils work on the brain, but here it is just worth noting that essential oils manage to do what no other known substance can do — they move through the body with great ease, passing through the interstitial fluid with no problem. The ease with which essential oils pass through the body makes them a perfect drug delivery system, a fact fully appreciated by manufacturers looking to develop "the magic bullet" — a drug which will go directly to the place in the body where it's required.

The Sense of Smell

According to Dr. Alan Hirsch of the Smell and Taste Research Foundation in Chicago, by the year 2000 many of us will be living in houses that have aroma-air-conditioning systems. Ten minutes before we want to wake up they'll start to pump a stimulating aroma into the air. Our eyes will open. When we go into a cafe for breakfast we're induced by prepackaged aromas to eat more (or less). At work, aromas will be designed to cut the error rate, while in the gym they'll be designed to invigorate. When you come

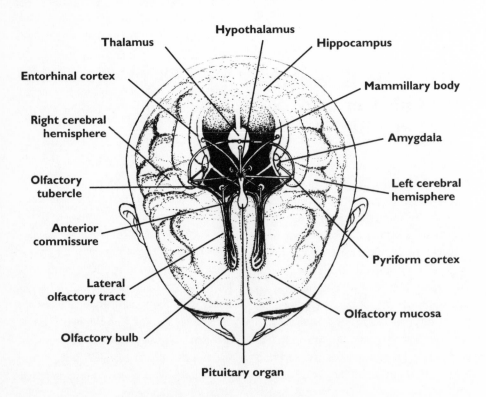

Hypothalamus
Thalamus
Hippocampus
Entorhinal cortex
Mammillary body
Right cerebral hemisphere
Amygdala
Olfactory tubercle
Left cerebral hemisphere
Anterior commissure
Pyriform cortex
Lateral olfactory tract
Olfactory mucosa
Olfactory bulb
Pituitary organ

OLFACTORY NERVOUS PATHWAYS

home, there will be a relaxing aroma in the house, and when you go to bed, a soporific or amorous one, depending on your choice. Dr. Hirsch and his team have carried out forty-six research studies including one involving 12,000 people which looked at the effect of olfaction on learning. Among other things, Dr. Hirsch has discovered that people will judge a product a better value when bought from a shop where there is a pleasant aroma. In another trial he found that when a mixed floral aroma was suffused throughout a room of calculus students, they increased their speed of learning by 230%. When gambling machines in Las Vegas were "aromatized" with a certain aroma number 1, Dr. Hirsch discovered that the players spent 45% more cash! These and other recent discoveries are leading us into an aromatic future — whether we know it or not. Next time you go into an office to make a furious complaint, and come out unplacated but subdued, consider the possibility that the waiting room was suffused with an aroma to make clients calm down. It is possible, and it gets more probable every day.

Science is catching up with what aromatherapists have been saying for years: aromas can improve performance and capacity to remember, they can make you alert, or relaxed, and change your mood. Aromatherapy uses natural aromas which have, of course, been used for similar purposes throughout the centuries. While it is nice to have one's work confirmed, we now have the situation where even more man-made, synthetic, nonbiodegradable chemicals will be pumped into the atmos-

phere. Do we really need them when naturals will do as well, if not better?

The reason aroma has such a direct action on the brain is that aroma molecules connect with receptor cells in the cilia extending from the two olfaction bulbs, which are themselves actually extensions of, and part of, the brain. Olfaction is thus the most direct interface between the brain and the outside world. Through our sense of smell, aroma molecules set off a cascade of reactions involving proteins, enzymes, cell depolarization, and second messengers — all leading to an electrical impulse being sent to the brain. The part of the brain most directly involved is the limbic system, evolutionarily the oldest part of the brain, and home of our emotions.

The olfaction bulbs are extraordinary organs, looking like two small upside-down spoons. Directly under the small match-head-sized bulbs is the cribiform plate, made of thin bone. The olfactory neurons pass through this plate and end in protein-rich cilia, inside the nose. Here the receptor cells and ion channels convert an odor, eventually, into an electrical impulse to the brain. That's the theory anyway; it's not been proved. The cilia are embedded in a layer of mucous about the size of two shirt buttons, on the top and either side of the nasal cavity. Aroma molecules must pass through this before reaching the receptor cells on the cilia.

In 1991, Linda Buck and Richard Axel identified a family of 7-transmembrane domain receptors, which are thought to be the first known olfaction receptors. They appear to be likely candidates because they are found only in the nose and resemble other neurotransmitter receptors in structure. Attempts, however, to replicate the function of the receptors have so far failed.

Because we have not yet definitely identified the receptors that odor molecules interact with, it is impossible to say *how* an aroma molecule translates into smell. The crucial factor may be related to the chemistry of the aroma molecule, or its shape, whether it is laevorotatory or dextrorotatory, electrically positive or negative, polar or apolar, or some combination of these. As human beings can distinguish between 10,000 aromas, it is thought by some that there are, among the 50 million receptors on the cilia, 10,000 types of receptor. Others think there are just a thousand or even a mere hundred types of receptors that in some way adapt

or amplify (or both) the aroma molecule, thus giving the system its extreme subtlety. For example, the same aroma molecule might smell like one thing if the connection with the receptor is strong but like another thing if it is weak.

Olfaction is a very complex business. For example, the compound carvone is molecularly identical whether L-carvone or D-carvone, but the L-type smells like spearmint and the D-type smells like caraway. These two are stereo-isomers — which means they are copies of each other except that a hydrogen atom sits either to the left or to the right. This difference causes the plane of polarization of light to rotate either to the left or right, giving the definitions "L" for laevorotatory (to the left) and "D" for dextrorotatory (to the right). When identical aroma molecules differing only in their laevorotatory or dextrorotatory

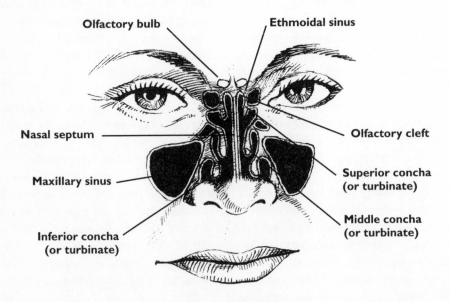

Olfactory bulb   **Ethmoidal sinus**

Nasal septum   **Olfactory cleft**

Maxillary sinus   **Superior concha (or turbinate)**

                                                   Middle concha (or turbinate)

Inferior concha (or turbinate)

NASAL PASSAGE

characteristics are perceived as two completely different smells — spearmint and caraway — you can begin to see how complex the problem of olfaction is.

Discoveries are being made all the time, however. Researchers are currently working on a group of enzymes known as the P450s. These have been found in the nasal mucus and are thought to chemically change odorants, perhaps disintegrating them and facilitating their expulsion from the body. It has been suggested that an absence of these enzymes may be the reason some people have lost their smell sensitivity and as there are about 2 million anosmic people in America alone, any further research in this area would be welcome.

The machinery used to analyze odors by gas-liquid chromatography and mass spectrometry is less sensitive than a healthy human nose. Olfactory neurons are physiologically remarkable in that they are in a state of continuous regeneration. This seems to indicate their importance for our survival, perhaps not so much now as a few thousand years ago. The system remains, however, and it connects directly with the oldest part of the brain, the limbic system. In the old days, aromas would come to us and depending on them, we would approach, attack, make love, or run, and although today we may be less aware of it, aroma still plays a crucial role in our emotions and reactions. The limbic system is made up of the hippocampus, amygdala, the septal area, and several regions of the cerebral cortex. The hippocampus is believed to be involved in memory and learning. The connection between aroma and memory is well-

known, but the connection between aroma and learning is only now being scientifically appreciated.

Olfaction research involves chemistry, stereochemistry (the shape of the molecule), vibrational frequency, electrochemical factors, enzymes and proteins, and a whole lot more besides. It is multidimensional in a way sight and hearing are not. This makes the sense of smell a very difficult mystery to unlock. In the meantime, olfaction research is becoming more interesting to biologists, psychologists, teachers, sales managers, people managers, and even defense departments. Olfaction is no longer the forgotten sense.

Most of the research currently being done on smell is by people who want to bombard you with it for commercial reasons, as we shall later see. In the labs, subjects are exposed to fragrance and wired up to equipment that measure electrical skin response, skin temperature, muscle tension, heart rate, respiration, and blood pressure. Pictures of the brain can be seen changing under the influence of aroma. According to Dr. Craig Warren and Dr. Stephen Warrenburg at International Flavors and Fragrances, New Jersey, "pleasant odors tended to enhance creative performance, generate more positive evaluations of words and pictures of people, and elicit more happy memories."[7] It is this aspect of olfaction that big business wants to harness, but we can harness it too — the natural way.

Percutaneous Absorption

Applying essential oils, in a base oil,

directly onto the skin is central to aromatherapy and many trials have shown that essential oils, or components of them, show up in the blood or urine shortly after being applied through massage. Meanwhile, their absorption through the skin during baths is less of a mystery since Dr. Peter Slynko at the Kiev Institute of Physiology (Ukrainian Academy of Science) proved that, for several minutes after sweating, the pores remain open and suck in whatever happens to be on the surface of the skin, which later shows up in blood and the lymph.

Clearly the essential oils pass through the skin. The questions are, how many of the components in essential oils pass through, and how do they do it? The first question is raised by the fact that the skin, the largest organ of the human body, is a site of metabolism — a place where chemicals in the body alter molecules, to incorporate them into the body, to use them as fuel, or to expel them more easily. Esterase enzymes, for example, are involved in these functions. The skin is also a place where one of the body's most efficient metabolic alterants are at work in the form of P450 enzymes. These enzymes are found in high concentrations in the liver — the ultimate de-toxification machine and, as we have seen, in the olfactory mucous. As the purpose of the P450s is to prevent toxins from damaging the body, this may help to explain the remarkably safe history of percutaneous essential oil use. It could be that the P450s either alter any harmful molecules or immobilize them, leaving them in the upper, dead layer of skin, ready to be expelled.

The excellent skin permeability of essential oils is usually attributed to their high lipophilicity. Once through the epidermal (outer) layer of skin, the molecules are transported by the capillary blood and by interstitial fluid. Heat tends to favor their absorption — by having the room warm, the massaging hands warm, and by warming the oil in the hands before applying to the skin. Absorption is also helped by covering the areas of skin to which oil has just been applied, with a towel for example, thus preventing evaporation. The great advantage of percutaneous absorption is that essential oils can be applied directly to the area where they are required — to treat pain or inflammation, and it is also an excellent way to get essential oils into the bloodstream, and from there, into all areas of the human body, including the brain.

Their Exit

Essential oils have different routes of exit, depending on their variety. It's thought that eucalyptus is exhaled through breath, sandalwood leaves in the urine, patchouli in the feces, and rose oil via perspiration through the whole skin. After a massage with 2% lavender oil, the main constituents — linalol and linalyl acetate — can be detected in the blood after just five minutes. After 20 minutes there is a maximum concentration, while after 90 minutes most of the linalol and linalyl acetatel had been eliminated from the blood. This isn't to say that the effect of the lavender doesn't linger on — lavender and the other oils set off all kinds of chemical reactions in the body. The keys are turned in the locks, their jobs are done, and they can leave. It should also be said that while some of the more detectable components exit the body, the smaller compounds may be left behind in the body for a longer time, to finish their job perhaps and, as we shall later see, there may be other factors at work.

The Mind

Philosophers throughout the millennia have spent much effort in trying to define "the mind" and even today, it's not at all clear what exactly it is. Some would say the mind is the seat of the soul and others that it is nothing more that the sum total of one's experiences, which could also be called "consciousness." For the sake of simplicity, I am calling "mind" here all that can be said to be primarily experienced in the head — personality, thinking process, intellectual capacity, moods, as in feeling "up" or "down," and emotions such as love and fear.

Ironically perhaps for the "seat of feeling," the brain has no pain receptors so after cutting through the skull with local anesthetic, brain surgery can be done without anesthetic and the patient conscious. The brain seems a well-defined organ but some of the nerves within it are over a meter long. So where does the brain end and the body begin? One could say the brain ends at our fingertips because, working on a computer terminal for example, that's how far the brain's messages go (bio-

logically, at least). Technically, the brain is about three pounds of pink and gray wet matter, 90% water. From an engineering and computational point of view, the brain is the most complex structure known. It has 100 billion cells and 100 trillion possible connections.

With training, people with a certain aptitude can perform remarkable mathematical feats, as in the case quoted in Lyall Watson's *Supernature II,* of A.C. Aitken who, when asked to turn 4/47 into a decimal he replied in four seconds with "Point 0851063829787234042553191 4," then he paused for breath and continued, "89361702127659574468 — and that's the repeating point. It starts again then at 085." Aitken, who was professor of mathematics at the University of Edinburgh, is obviously a smart guy, but to accomplish these feats he had to train his memory, which everyone can do. As far as can be guessed, good memory was evolutionarily advantageous in the days when we needed to communicate survival information, history, and custom from generation to generation, but had no writing with which to do it. The memorizers were the libraries. Then, as now, the brain constantly modifies itself, learning more each day, using and reusing connections, finding new ways to do things. As we know, if children are started early enough with intense teaching, they can absorb a phenomenal amount of information by their teens. Why we have this huge mental capacity and whatever its evolutionary past may be, it is a delight for humans to exercise and test our brains. We take pride in being able to fix the car, finish the crossword, win an argument, put across our political point, pass an exam, etc. But the brain is more than our most valued tool, it is our friend, our confidant, our security, and our home.

We more than remember and compute, we *feel*. Tears pop out of our eyes; rage turns our face red. All this may be an evolution advantage — if we didn't feel angry when someone stole our last fish, we wouldn't fight to get it back and maybe we would starve; and if we didn't feel love, who would take care of the babies? Emotions may not seem so great when you're sitting on the sofa, tears rolling down the cheeks because your partner just moved out, but it's a mechanism, feeling loss, which accentuates its other side — feeling great together, which is the glue that keeps us in evolutionarily favorable pair-bonding and social groups. Working in small or large teams, whether specialist or not, means we can get more done, more easily. That's one reason why we are where we are — in control of the world.

These days the brain is under tremendous pressure. Was it designed, I wonder, to do what a typical day in a modern city requires of it? We all wake up to the news — which is usually bad, if not horrifying and depressing, then the mail arrives, with bills we can't pay. The drive to work is a nightmare of split-second life-or-death decisions, or a torture of being packed with too many people in a subway train or on a bus. Breathing in polluted air, commands come at us — "walk" or "don't walk" the signals say. The com-

mands continue when we get to the work place — in which we have to watch our mouths and our moves or we might get laid off. Whatever politics and unpleasantness is thrown at us, we have to get on with our work, or there's no money on payday. Flicking through magazines on our ten-minute coffee break, we read articles telling us to be better mothers, fathers, lovers, go on diets, be better dressers, lookers, and achievers. We start feeling guilty. On the way home from work, we stop at the supermarket. More decisions. We pick up an apple. Is it fresh enough? Has it been waxed, irradiated, or sprayed with chemicals? We pick up a yogurt — has the date indicating freshness ticket expired? What's in it? We look in the freezer — will one of these products be acceptable to all members of the family or is someone going to say, "I don't eat that?" Temptation looms at the checkout, then the bill arrives. We go home and watch TV. We cry at a sad old movie, then watch horrified at the news pictures of a plane crash. Half an hour later we're sitting on the edge of our seats, cheering our team on in football. Then the ads come on and scream, "buy me! buy me!" We think about tomorrow, put a load of wash in the machine and iron a couple of shirts. By the time we get into bed, we're exhausted — mentally as much as physically. Was the mind designed for all this, or was it meant to look out over a clear night sky and ponder the nature of the universe?

It would be convenient for scientists if all brains were the same because it would be much easier to establish a "normal" brain from which others could be judged. But it's not that simple — every brain is different. Nevertheless, the measuring goes on. Not only do we have static computerized axial tomography (CAT) scan photos, we've got moving living images through positron-emission tomography (PET), magnetic resonance imaging (MRI), and superconducting quantum interference devices (SQUIDS).

A great deal has been heard this past couple of decades about neurotransmitters or brain chemicals. You hear the words seratonin, noradrenaline, etc., tossed around as if they were everyday things we knew everything about, especially as many modern drugs are intended to mimic them in some way. In fact the only synapse in the mammalian central nervous system where scientists are *certain* what the transmitter is is in the case of the acetylcholine (ACh) synapses between the motor neuron axon collaterals and interneurons.[8] Except in this case, scientists have been unable to make pure cultures of other synapses and although the action of ACh is understood at neuromuscular junctions, how the ACh circuits in the brain work is still not known. Books on the brain are full of words like presumably, probably, and may, and expressions like "one must be very careful about drawing conclusions." This isn't out of misplaced lack of confidence, but actual fact — we don't know how the brain's chemicals work.

According to Richard Thompson in *The Brain*, "we are only beginning to understand the functional circuitry of the brain."[9] Apparently, "the most is known about the least common transmitters in the brain,"[10] dopamine and norepinephrine, and the neurons that contain them — but they account for only a few percent of total neurotransmitters in the brain. Aside from transmitters, many neuron terminals also contain peptides — which could act as transmitters, but not a great deal is known about their function.[11] Although human beings have been building a library of information on opium for at least five thousand years, science discovered only relatively recently that the brain produces opiates in the neurons and the pituitary, which, like morphine, alleviate pain and produce pleasurable sensations. We know there are several opiate receptors on neurons in the brain but Thompson admits "little is really known about the possible differential functions of the different brain opioids and the different opiod receptors."[12] What little we know about opiates has been highlighted by the very recent discovery, by Dr. Goldstein at Stanford University, of dynorphin, which is over 200 times more potent than morphine. The mind boggles!

Scientifically, there's a world of difference between knowing *that* a certain chemical can effect a certain change, and knowing *how* it does it. Brain science is at the stage of recognizing that certain brain chemicals elicit a certain response, and mostly they seek to inhibit or encourage the flow of these chemicals. However, let us not overestimate what is known or how well-understood modern drugs are. According to Thompson, on the drug used to treat manic depression, for example, "the reasons for Lithium's effectiveness are still largely obscure."

How Essential Oils Work on the Brain

Essential oils have an effect on the brain via two routes: olfaction and essential oil absorption. The olfactory bulb, which is just above the top of the nose and is actually a part of the brain, extends from the "limbic system." The name comes from Latin, limbus, meaning border because, comprising of several structures, it forms a ring-like base to the cerebral cortex. It is the home of our emotions, sexual feelings, memory, and learning, and with olfaction these can be evoked — even subconsciously. The limbic system is a link between the voluntary and involuntary nervous centers, and a link between left and right brain. Essential oils connect directly into this system through the olfactory bulb. As for the science of olfaction, it's like a huge jigsaw made up of many pieces, a few of which we have. These tell us something, but not how olfaction works.

One thing we know is that benzodiazepene receptors are located all through the human brain, and it is on these receptors that drugs such as valium and librium work. But these receptors were in the brain long before chemists invented drugs, presumably because there are substances in nature that do the same thing. We also now know that benzodiazepene receptors are found in large quantity on the olfactory bulb of rats and, it is

thought, humans. Perhaps we were designed to receive tranquilizers through the nose — in the form of aroma molecules from plants.

The circulatory system has devised structures that prevent large molecules passing into the brain. This is "the blood-brain barrier." Presumably because of the small size of certain essential oil molecules and their lipophilic nature, they pass the blood-brain barrier and thus enter the brain, as do many chemical drugs. Essential oils get into the bloodstream in many different ways — through the capillary system at the top of the nose, through the delicate mucous membrane of the mouth and respiratory tract, through the vagina and anus if given in pessary or suppository form, through the digestive system if given orally, and through the skin if applied through massage. Although the brain only accounts for 2% of our body weight, it gets 15% of the blood supply.

The simple answer to the question, "how do essential oils work on the brain?" is "we don't know." Because human beings rely so totally on plants for their sustenance and well-being, and because the chemistry of plants and humans is so similar, they might be thought of as a set of keys for turning on the body's mechanisms — whether this is thought of in terms of chemistry or stereochemistry (the shape of the molecule). There are many different ways drugs can affect brain chemicals — they can block the synthesis of a naturally occurring chemical, or block its transport down an axon, its formation into vesicles, its release into the synapse, its attachment to the receptor etc. — and science does not often exactly understand which mechanisms are at work. It seems unreasonable, therefore, to expect us to know how essential oils work.

However, the science of brain chemistry has introduced a new element into the discussion as to why certain essential oils should be "adaptogens." For example, lavender oil taken in small quantity is a sedative but when taken in larger quantity, becomes a stimulant. This apparent paradox has mystified students of essential oils, but we now know that even within our own brain chemical system such adaptogenic processes are going on — as with dopamine, for example, or acetylcholine, which inhibits the activity of cardiac muscle cells, yet excites the activity of skeletal muscle cells. Dr. Wagner and his team at the University of Munich, Germany, published a review of herbs used as "adaptogens." Their definition is: "substances meant to put the organism into a state of nonspecific heightened resistance in order to better resist stresses and adapt to extraordinary challenges." [13] That seems a pretty good definition to me!

Essential oils have many interesting features which may help explain how they work. They seem to affect the working of enzymes — a class of complex organic substances that cause chemical transformations in animals and plants. According to Dr. Gerhard Buchbauer, "...some monoterpene derivatives, such as frenchone or carvacrol, inhibit enzymes like the acetylcholinesterase, which inactivate the spasmogenic musculotropic inhibi-

tion mechanism." [14] He also says:

> *"The constituents of essential oils, the aroma chemicals, accumulate in the nerve cell membrane, thus causing a sterical blocking of embedded function proteins, which are the ion channels. This blocking causes a change in the physical properties of the membrane, especially a modification of its ion permeability."* [15]

If, as is thought, essential oils interact with certain membrane lipids causing a change in the calcium ion-channel functions, we are talking here about effecting change in a fundamental physiological process. Also, as we have seen, essential oils affect enzymes. Neurotransmitters are often made from substances that come from plant foods. For example, seratonin is made (via 5-HTP) from tryptophan (once sold as a natural anti-depressant) — a naturally occurring amino acid found in bananas and other vegetative materials. Add to this the fact that essential oils have electrical properties, polarity, are dextrorotatory or laevorotatory, and emit infrared radiation, and you have a cocktail of factors we are nowhere near understanding. Whether essential oils are seen as keys unlocking chemical reactions, as catalysts that cause chemical transformation, or as electrical moderators, they are basically *effectors* — bringing about a stimulation of the body's healing mechanisms.

My feeling is that the energetic state and medicinal value of most essential oils start to diminish after two years. They still smell good, but therapeutically they don't work nearly as well. Some oils defy this rule and retain their antiseptic value for many years — thyme, eucalyptus, and oregano being examples. Essential oils feel to different degrees "alive." That's not a very scientific explanation, I know, but some oils just don't have a vibrancy in them, a difficult thing to judge without experience or very sophisticated equipment.

The fact that essential oils leave the body by different routes — exhaled air, perspiration through the entire skin, via urine or feces, raises the question of why a particular oil should take a particular direction. Aromatherapists sometimes talk in terms of particular organs being "in resonance" with a particular oil while physicists might talk about it in terms of "selective synchronous vibration" (the opposite of gravity). Another curious fact is that people are often strongly attracted or repelled by certain aromas, and not simply because good or bad memories are evoked. Spikenard is an oil people seldom come across, for example, and when they first smell it, they react in different ways. Aromas are very personal, for reasons we do not know.

The Water Connection

There is a common misconception that essential oils and water do not mix. In fact, as a by-product of essential oil distillation, rose water and other hydrolats are routinely produced. The steam carrying the aromatic molecules of plants rises during the distillation process and, after cooling, separates into essential oil at the top and water, the hydrolat, at the bottom. Hydrolats are used most particularly in European phytotherapy, a form of herbal medicine, but rose water has been used for centuries in Europe for cooking. Although one might not see how, technically, any of the rose could be left in the water during the process of distillation, the fact is that the water is distinctly rose-scented, or scented with the particular plant being distilled. Even if you put, say, 6 drops of geranium essential oil in a bath, and can see that the essential oil floats on the top of the water, if you were to taste some of the water that seems untouched by the oil, the geranium is nevertheless evident. In some way, the aromatic molecule, or the vibration of the essential oil, has managed to become imprinted in the water.

I was, then, very interested to read in the scientific journal *Nature* (June 30th, 1988) a paper authored by thirteen scientists which showed that, even when antibodies were not technologically detectable in a highly diluted aqueous solution, the memory of them lingered on, making the solution still biologically active. Commenting on the paper, the deputy editor of *Nature*, Peter Newmark, said that if the results were confirmed to be true, "we will have to abandon two centuries of observation and rational thinking about biology because this can't be explained by ordinary physical laws." [16] The man at the center of this discovery, Dr. Jacques Benveniste, later appeared with his detractors on a three-hour television program, *After Dark*,[17] in which his work was debated. As the argument heated up, the viewer was shown an example of how a totally new scientific pathway is very difficult for unimaginative people to grasp. Dr. Benveniste was at the time of his discovery working for INSERM — the national medical research institution of France and was one of France's leading biologists and immunologists, the author of four previous *Nature* articles and over 200 other scientific articles — two are called citation classics. Before he could publish this particular piece of work, however, Benveniste was forced by *Nature* to have the work replicated by other labs — and this was successfully carried out in Israel, Canada, and Italy. Nevertheless, the controversy continues.

The implications of Benveniste's discovery are far-reaching — for allopathic and homeopathic medicine, and for aromatherapy and essential oil use (not to mention public water management). When an aromatic molecule enters water, the function of the molecule becomes imprinted throughout that water-body. To understand how this may work, we need to look at water itself.

Water is ubiquitous in that it is everywhere, including our bodies (65%) and brain (90%). Yet, according to Patrick Flanagan, MD (MA), who was listed at age 17 by *Life* magazine as one of America's top ten scientists, water is "one of the world's most mysteriously anomalous substances." [18] Flanagan became interested in water when he was a student of Dr. Henry Coanda, who discovered in the 1920s that a fluid flowing over any surface tends to cling to that surface — the Coander effect. Coander was interested in the profusion of colloidal (as opposed to ionic) minerals found in the water that the Hunza people, living on the Western edge of the Himalayan range, drink — who routinely live healthy lives to the age of 100 and over. The word "colloid" comes from the Greek word for glue and describes substances that are found throughout the human body, in plants, animals, and elsewhere in nature. (One of their functions in plants is to prevent damage to the cell from freezing). According to Flanagan, colloids in water take on the quality of tiny "seeds" of energy. In the human body, they are known to be crucial in all body processes because of their impact on electrical flow.

Water is an excellent conductor of electricity, which is an important point to keep in mind considering that the brain is 90% water. Water is fluid because the hydrogen atoms in it only have one electron to offer other atoms so when it links with oxygen, the link is tenuous. Water could be described as one long molecule, which would explain why an input at one end — an essential oil for example — can be detected at the other end. Next time you see essential oil floating on water, keep in mind that the entire body of water is imprinted with the properties of that essential oil. What implications this has for the watery mucous at the top of the nasal cavity, which receives aroma molecules and translates them into messages for the olfaction bulb, is yet to be discovered. It is known, however, that substances put into water enter the body by osmosis, and this is how the benefits of essential oils are taken in during baths, etc.

The Somatid Connection

One of the most interesting components of both living and nonliving matter are things called *somatids,* named as such by Gaston Naessens. Somatids are described as ultramicroscopic, subcellular, living and reproducing entities. They are remarkable in that they cannot be destroyed by ultraviolet radiation (routinely used to sterilize), or by 50,000 rems of nuclear radiation, or temperatures of over 200 degrees centigrade, and they are impossible to cut by diamond, and do not respond to any of the strongest antibacterial or antifungal chemical agents.

Gaston Naessens was able to see somatids because, working in the 1950s with artisans from the Lietz optical factory and the French military contractors Barbier-Bernard et Turenne, he constructed a microscope which could magnify *live* elements to enlargements of 30,000X, with a resolution of 150 Angstroms (1 Angstom = 100 millionth of a centimeter). The electron microscope can enlarge to the order of 400,000X, with a resolution of 30-50 angstroms but, as Naessens puts it, it "... necessitates manipulations that alter the physical aspects of objects being observed." To understand the somatids, or even identify them correctly, however, one has to be able to see the changes they go through. Consequently, when tiny bits and pieces were found in the blood they were called "dross" or crasse sanguine. Naessens has discovered that these small particles are in fact polymorphous (which means they occur in many or various forms) living things.

In 1990, I had the opportunity to see a film showing somatids, which look like short, sparkling, aquamarine worms, tiny in comparison to red blood corpuscles and far more numerous. In a healthy person, somatids go through a three-stage cycle (somatids, spores, double spores), and produce, it is thought, *trephone,* a hormone indispensable to cellular division. However, when the immune system is weakened or destabilized through stress or trauma, the somatid goes through another thirteen evolving forms (including bacteria, mycobacterial forms, yeast-like forms, ascopores, asci, and mycelial forms).

Somatids are found in all living organisms, including the sap in plants. According to Francoise Naessens, Gaston's wife and assistant, "... the 'tiny bodies' ... are fundamentally electrical in nature .... Somatids are actually tiny living condensers of energy, the smallest ever found." [19] To understand the significance of this discussion, consider the fact that if a cube of fresh meat is injected with an *in vitro* culture of somatids, placed in a vacuum sealed vessel and put in the sun, the meat will not only remain fresh, but will grow!

Gaston Naessens says, "... we have observed, in all biological liquids and particularly in the blood, an elementary particle endowed with a movement of electronegative repulsion, possessing a polymorphic nature." [20] Essential oils are a biological liquid and there is no reason not to suppose that somatids are not present in them. It may well be that as further research is carried out, we will discover that essential oils in some way transfer somatids, the little condensers of energy, or influence the *trephone* factor — either chemically, electrically, or energetically — and keep the somatids to a healthy (for us) three-stage cycle.

Not only has Naessens discovered an extraordinary and marvelous microscope, and discovered somatids, he has developed a product based on camphor and its derivative called 714-X which has arrested and reversed the progress of disease in over 1,000 cases of cancer as well as in several dozen cases of AIDS. Naessens writes, "...after having carried out numerous experiments on camphor and its derivative, we have discovered that this product is endowed with remarkable pharmaceutical properties ... it carries to the tumor cells all the nitrogen that it needs, suppressing by the same action the secretion that would paralyze the immune system." [21] Aromatherapists will find it interesting that he has chosen to work with camphor. Oil of Borneo Camphor (*Dryobalanops camphora*) is used in aromatherapy for depressive states, and acts as a tonic, among other things. Borneol is also found in small amounts in the essential oils of lavender, cinnnamon, rosemary, and certain types of hyssop.

Other Factors

Invisible forces are a fact of life. The air is full of invisible messages — from mobile phone conversations to satellite TV pictures. No biologist discusses physiological processes without talking about electricity, which you or I don't see. Physicists tell us that all life is basically vibration, and there are even reputable scientists saying that life is just a big hologram! [22] Com-

pared to this, talk about etheric emanations seems positively old hat and perhaps it's not so surprising that university professors are proving the existence of auric bodies and chakras. Preliminary studies are proving what aromatherapists have long known — that essential oils have an effect far beyond the physical body.

Summary

In the biological sciences there is still much to learn. To discuss essential oils solely in terms of chemical components is dismissive of other important factors in the nature of life. Aside from this, science has not yet identified all essential oil components. Life is *living*, that is the point! Nature has the capacity to retain life within it to a remarkable degree. In Denmark, *Spergula arvensis* seeds were germinated after 1,700 years, and in China seeds of a Manchurian lotus were found to be fertile after 1,000 years. While recognizing and acknowledging the importance of the therapeutic value of the known chemical components of essential oils, they are probably working in tandem with other factors, and synergistically with each other. The fact is that certain essential oils work in therapy in certain conditions, yet chemically their effects cannot be explained. Sitting on the shelf in bottles, essential oils might be regarded as nothing more than a chemical cocktail, but they are powerful, energetic, dynamic liquids. Despite the criticism of being vague, aromatherapists continue to say that essential oils contain a "life force," but it may be some time before science can prove them wrong!

Which Medicine?

Having worked in a clinical setting as an aromatherapist for many years, I find it immeasurably sad that there is a reluctance on the part of the medical professions to take advantage of the benefits offered by essential oils. A confrontational stance seems to have been adopted with "them" (natural therapies) on one side and "us" (doctors and chemical drugs manufacturers) on the other. Instead of scanning the various complementary therapies and asking, "what can you do for my patients?" doctors all too often dismiss complementary medicines, which they neither understand nor have experience of, as too weak, or too strong, just a placebo or unresearched, etc.

There are historic reasons behind this divide, having to do with the growth of the chemical drug industry and the protection of market interests, financial profit, in other words. The drug industry spends millions of dollars employing political lobbyists, public relations officers, and sales representatives who influence the decisionmakers, the public, and doctors against natural alternatives. In this market protectionism, however, the patient suffers.

One can forgive general practitioners who have little enough time to talk to their patients, yet alone read the actual research behind many of the drugs they are prescribing. But hospital specialists, who have a limited number of conditions to treat, should most certainly look into complementary therapies and see what is available. It is a great shame that essential oils are not further researched for use in mind-related conditions, and nor are the anti-viral essential oils investigated for the alleviation of earache, colds and flu, and other more serious viral conditions. One can understand that chemical drugs are used when they are available, but there are many conditions for which nothing is available in the "chemical medicine chest," but where natural options exist.

One criticism leveled against aromatherapy is that it is unscientifically tested — that we don't know how it works. On the face of it this might seem like a valid complaint until one realizes that the chemical drugs industry, who orchestrate the opposition to natural therapies for financial reasons, very often has little idea how its drugs work. For example, for many years doctors have been told that tricyclic drugs used to treat depression are effective because they work to change the natural levels of the neurotransmitters norepinephrine and seratonin. But, because of our limited knowledge about how neurotransmitters actually work in the brain, and the pathways they take, this is all just theory. The first problem with the theory is that testing urine for the level of these substances is an unreliable measure of how much is actually in the brain and there is, moreover, no convincing evidence that depressed individuals actually have lower levels of these naturally occurring chemicals. Also, and mysteriously, tricyclics act on norepinephrine and seratonin synapses within minutes, but it takes weeks for their beneficial effects on depression to develop. This time gap cannot be explained (as it cannot for the dopamine/schizophrenia theory). Drug experts are aware in a way the general public (and even doctors) are not, that in chemical-medical practice it is routine for drugs to be prescribed although the treatment is more effective than the theory.

Doctors reluctant to use natural medicines, but happy to prescribe chemical drugs, should take a long hard look into the back-up research of those drugs and ask themselves — does anybody really know how these work? The fact is that chemical drugs are regularly given product licenses although the exact mechanisms for them are not understood and, according to the American federal Office of Technology Assessment, 75% of all currently available treatments have not had sufficient scientific scrutiny. [23]

Another criticism leveled against natural therapies is that they are potentially toxic. The argument is "just because it's natural doesn't mean it's safe." Of course nature is full of dangers, as we tell our children every time they reach out to pluck unknown berries from a bush. But it is also true that nature is full of natural remedies. Natural medicines have evolved over thousands of years, time enough for people to come to know which natural products are good to eat, which are poisonous, which heal and which do not. It is this wealth of experience aromatherapy draws upon and chemical companies draw upon as they search for medications to chemically synthesize in the lab. Indeed, without certain plants, the pharmacies in cancer hospitals would have little to offer. With my hand on my heart I can

tell you that in my long experience I have rarely heard of an adverse reaction to pure essential oils used in aromatherapy treatments in Britain, other than passing skin irritation in some people. The adverse "side effects" of chemical drugs are becoming more well-known due to the efforts of the media, and there are now several good books available to the public on that subject. It is ludicrous to criticize natural therapies on the basis of their potential toxicity when so very few toxic effects have been observed or reported, not only by me but by generations of serious medical researchers and government regulatory agencies.

Meanwhile, the toxic potential of chemical drugs is well documented. In the *Journal of the American Medical Association*, (Nov 27, 1987, p. 2891), we are told that one patient in every thousand admitted to a hospital will be killed by the medicine they receive there. And according to the *Chemical Marketing Reporter* (Jan 2, 1989), as a result of the 68 million prescriptions for nonsteroidal anti-inflammatory drugs (NSAIDS) given to American sufferers of arthritis, 10,000-20,000 deaths occur each year. It is unfair to criticize essential oils for possible (unknown) side effects when chemical drugs are well-known for their adverse side effects. For example, the data sheet for Eli Lily's anti-depression drug Prozac contains not only a warning that rashes and other allergic reactions might be experienced, but a long list of "adverse effects," far too long to go into here, that includes fever, nausea, diarrhea, vomiting, insomnia, anxiety, dizziness, fatigue, seizures, pulmonary events, hair loss, sexual dysfunction, etc. Apparently, "hypomania or mania occurred in approximately one percent of fluoxetine (Prozac) treated trial patients." [24] And this, supposedly, is a safe drug.

In America, drug safety is regulated by the Food & Drug Administration but according to Representative Ted Weiss (D-NY), 102 out of 198 prescription drugs approved by them during the years 1976 and 1985 caused serious reactions that necessitated them either being relabelled or removed from the market. [25] How many of the chemical drugs currently being prescribed for the mind are destined, as time reveals their drawbacks, for the trash bin?

Natural medicines are often dismissed as being mere "placebos," chemically inactive substances that work only by the power of suggestion. The irony of this argument is that within the chemical-medical field, the placebo effect is well-known. After much worldwide research, "the placebo effect" is said to cause wellness in 30-35% of patients given nothing more than sugar pills. We are not here just talking about minor conditions. One group of doctors specializing in the treatment of angina pectoris (pain due to reduced blood flow to the heart) discovered that *pretending* to operate, by cutting the patient open and sowing them back up again, produced a cure rate equal to that produced by actual surgery (tying off the mammary artery); [26] while in a study to assess the effects of a new type of chemotherapy, doctors were surprised to find that 30% of the control group, who had placebos and no drugs, lost their hair! [27] Placebos have even been found to be as

effective as morphine in relieving pain. [28] Clearly, placebos play a part in medicine, but the placebo effect involves all branches of medicine, not just the natural ones.

Placebos cost the National Health Service at least 100 million dollars in the year 1992/3 because that's the value of the antibiotic prescriptions doctors wrote out for viral-induced colds and sore throats, which they know full well they could not possibly cure. On this subject a recent Audit Commission report stated: "Many doctors say that they often cannot afford the time to explain to patients the reasons why they do not need any medicine." [29] In other words, the antibiotics were placebos. The report also states: "Over-prescribing builds up resistance and disturbs the balance of micro-organisms in the body, permitting more severe infections to develop." [30]

When I lecture on aromatherapy, I make it quite clear that essential oils are not cure-alls. Clearly, we all have reason to be grateful to the surgeons and other medical professionals, and many people are alive today only because of the chemical drugs they take. All this, however, does not negate the fact that essential oils have their benefits too. In some cases, as in chemical medicine, essential oils may act as placebos — and why not, if that makes the patient better? But essential oils are not just placebos, and there are hundreds of scientific papers to prove that point. As a complementary therapy, used correctly, aromatherapy is a very safe method of restoring well-being and one that, if made more widely available, would bring tremendous benefits to humankind.

CHAPTER 3

THE MODERN MIND

What a crazy world! We've got people killing their neighbors on a vast scale and calling it war, children being abducted and killed, drugs being sold in the schools, workers being thrown out of their jobs, homes being repossessed, and countless pressures from all sides. I shake my head in wonder that any of us are sane. But, as our grandmothers used to say, "we've just got to carry on." The world isn't going to stop being the pressurized whirlpool it is, and unless we buy the lucky lottery ticket, we'll still have to carry on dealing with our daily problems much the way we always have. Will we ever get through?

No wonder half the population are strung out on drugs, or down at the bar, or smoking themselves into a grave! What is to be done? If you feel rotten, you can go to your doctor where, in the waiting room, you might pick up a copy of *Practical Health* and see an article entitled "The Day I Went Insane" — about tranquilizer addiction. The doctor calls you in just as you get to the bit where the lady says: "...as the years went by I began to realize that my whole character was changing. My four children were young then and I started to get aggressive, and hit them — which is something I'd never done — I'd shout and scream at them about the most minor things. I'm not an aggressive person...so I knew there was a change taking place."[1] Hoping nobody will notice, you take the magazine in with you. After you've told the doctor (in five minutes) what the problem is — your life is caving in — he pulls his prescription pad over and starts to scribble. "What's that for?" you ask. "Tranquilizers," he says. "But, eh, I was reading this..." — you show him the article. He sighs. "Oh, yes," he says, "let's hope it doesn't come to that, we'll get you off them as soon as you feel better." You ask if there are any alternatives. You're told your depression can be treated with a new family of seratonin re-uptake inhibitors, but there have been reported side effects. Like what? you ask. Like changes in personality. "Any other alternatives?" you ask. "Therapy, but the waiting list is at least six months." You say "thank you" and leave with your prescription.

Like many people, you might decide to go into psychoanalysis. Then you figure out how much it's going to cost you — $150 for each 50-minute session, four times a week, for four years equals $124,800. You decide you can't afford it, so pick up a local paper and scan the small ads — looking for help with your stressed-out life. On both sides of the Atlantic are dozens of talk-therapists of various sorts — and others who will hypnotize you so you can discover the *true* reason for your dissatisfaction with life, probably rooted in some previous incarnation, they say. Then there are the astrologers, card readers, and channellers who say they can show you the way forward. You find ads for prerecorded tapes that will subliminally teach you to have confidence, or wealth, or make you feel younger, or more assertive, less aggressive, more relaxed, or in tune with the whales. You develop a headache trying to figure out which tape to buy and which therapist to make an appointment with, then remember you've got a health magazine somewhere. You find it and flick to the ads at the back. "We can sort out your problems," they say, through rebirthing, or rolfing, bodywork, meditation, yoga,

visualization, and the list goes on and on. But which one do you choose? By now you've become so confused, you feel more depressed than you did to start with. Are you the *only* person in the world who hasn't sorted themselves out yet? You pour yourself a drink and pull out the old pack of cigarettes you stashed away when you gave up smoking two years ago.

The expression "modern-day stress" might seem like a cliché, but, boy-oh-boy, it is true. Look around you and try to think of one person you know who isn't weighed down with family responsibilities or financial obligations, or stuck in a relationship they want to get out of, or desperately looking for a relationship they want to get into, or anguished by their dysfunctional family, or sick, or worried about a sick relative, or just plain overworked. It makes you wonder — is there anyone out there who is totally, truly happy?

I remember once seeing a TV movie about people working in a factory where the interviewer went down the production line asking each person in turn what they were thinking about. About 90% said they were working out what they were going to do when they won a million dollars on the lottery — this is escapism on a massive scale. Indeed, given the amount of stress we have to deal with escapism seems to be a functional necessity. Without it, how many more of us would go mad?

I'm not going to say a word about the depleting ozone layer, or mention the scientists at the Naval Research Laboratory in Washington who have discovered a way of attaching living embryonic brain cells to computer silicon chips — the first step, apparently, in making a "bioelectronic" artificial brain.[2] We can all read the papers — and scare ourselves rigid!

What I do want to do in this section is spend a little time discussing some of the issues that immediately face the modern mind. In *The Mind-Body Connection*, we see that science is making us face up to the fact that mind and body are one. The implication is that, for physical as well as mental health, we have to address our psychological problems and deal with them. In *Drug Culture* we discuss the fact that some so-called "recreational drugs" are causing new problems, with cocaine stripping people of their character, for example, while in *Addiction*, we see that a simple cup of tea can catapult a person into a vicious cycle of tranquilizer addiction, while heavy drugs turn normal people into monsters prepared to rob and murder for a fix. *Consciousness and Control* explores the difficulty of finding, through the jungle of media interference, who we truly are, while *Spirituality* addresses the problem of religious skepticism and spiritual void. *The Untapped Mind* reminds us that there is more to heaven and earth than we understand. *Psychotherapy, Counseling* and *Other Therapies* discusses ways forward for some, while *Meditation* and *Visualization* could be a way forward for others.

I have a friend who spent time in Ethiopia working with orphans who had literally nothing — no family, no home, no possessions. If they had a pencil, they considered themselves lucky. But, they were happy, she tells me, and on returning to London after a couple of years she was shocked to see the misery in the faces of people who, materially, seemed to have it all. Somehow we have lost our capacity for happiness. Not just the happiness we feel at particularly good times — a night out with friends, and evening in with our lover, but the joyful openness and positivity we, surely, were meant to feel each new day. Life is a blessing, an adventure, a lesson with inevitable ups and downs. Okay, it's hard and rocky in places, and like sailors in a storm we have to hold on tight sometimes. But life was meant to be enjoyed and happiness is our birthright. There is much out there to help us find a way through to the light, including, as we shall later see, nature's essential oils — our little helpmates.

The Mind-Body Connection

Imagine one of the swords used in fencing, a foil, and then think of it being thrust straight through a body, but the body doesn't bleed or appear to feel pain. This was the highlight of a stage act performed at the Corsco Theater in Zurich in 1947 by a Dutch man, Mirin Dajo. A person in the audience had a heart attack and died and the show was banned, but a doctor heard about the strange exhibitionand asked Dajo to undergo scientific inquiry. At a Zurich hospital, in front of a large crowd, including doctors and journalists, Dajo's assistant again thrust the foil through his body and again there was no bleeding and the vital organs seemed undamaged. With the foil through his body, Dajo, and everyone else, trooped up the stairs to the X-ray room where it was proved that the foil was indeed going straight through his body. It was removed after a total of twenty minutes, and there were just two faint scars showing. Dajo later obligingly undertook examination by more doctors in Basel, one that thrust a foil through him. Thanks to Dajo's mind over matter, the doctor didn't have to be charged with murder.

Today, in Valencia, Spain, there is a Dr. Angel Escudero who has performed surgery on over 700 patients without using anesthetic. Instead he uses psycho-anesthesia — simply telling his patients that during surgery they will feel nothing. Observers of the procedure confirm that no hypnosis is involved. This is a different type of thought transference. The doctor says, "you will feel no pain" and the patient thinks, "I will feel no pain" — and they don't. According to Dr. Escudero, the patient having liquid saliva in their mouth is a vital adjunct of therapy. He points out that having a dry mouth is a characteristic of stress, fear, or panic. Unbelievably for more conventional doctors, Dr. Escudero uses no antibiotics yet his patients have never once developed an infection.

Dr. Escudero calls his method *noesitherapy* after *noesis*, action of thinking, and *noesiology*, the effects produced in human life by one's own thoughts. Thoughts produce changes in our arteries and in every organ, says Dr. Escudero, and he advises we think positive thoughts, not negative ones, and learn to live happier lives. Dr. Escudero takes his own advice and plays tennis regularly on the court in his lovely garden surrounding his home, which also houses the surgery and operating room. No commuting for him. In an operating room looking much like any other, Dr. Escudero is assisted by the family he loves: his son, a doctor; his daughter, a surgical nurse; and his wife, Marie-Jesus, who talks to the patient, holds their hand and generally keeps them company. The knife cuts deep into the flesh, metal rods are sometimes hammered through the limbs but the patient looks around happily, as if they were at a nice social gathering. The patient can feel heat and other normal sensation — but no pain. All this is possible, apparently, because every thought is a program in the biological computer of our brain. "Think positive" is Dr. Escudero's advice.

We've all read reports in the newspaper about people being able to do extraordinary things in extraordinary situations. The mother, for example, who lifted a car to release her son trapped beneath it, or the man who jumped a ten-foot wall to escape a rabid dog. I heard about a woman caught in a war zone who pulled apart the iron bars across a window to escape the enemy. Perhaps you or I could do the same.

In an emergency situation the brain tells the body to go on alert, and produces hormones which jolt us into action — the "flight or fight reaction." Fear also stops the instinctive sexual process. We can not only lose interest, but the penis can refuse to work and the vaginal muscles can contract sharply, preventing penetration.

On the other hand, meditation can slow the body rhythms down, and correct breathing can control blood pressure. People on biofeedback machines watch the dials and control their brain rhythms. The mind-body connection is an observable fact.

The mind-body connection is also now a proven scientific fact. One leading researcher in the field of brain chemistry, Candace Pert, says "...your mind is in every cell of your body."[3] Pert, who was formerly chief of the Brain Biochemistry Section at the American National Institute of Mental Health and is now a professor at the Center for Molecular and Behavioral Neuroscience at Rutgers University, discovered the opiate receptor and many other peptide receptors in the brain and body. For nearly two decades she has been leading the field in brain chemistry and inspiring a whole generation of scientists, who now recognize that the chemicals in the brain form a continuous circuit not only with receptors in the brain, but with receptors in the immune system, the nervous system, and the hormone system. In other words, it is impossible to physiologically separate the mind from the body.

What we are talking about here is peptides — strings of amino acids and the building blocks of proteins. The brain's own morphine, enkephalin, is a mere five amino acids long, while the peptide insulin is a couple of hundred amino acids long. There are about twenty-three different amino acids which, when put together in different arrangements, make different peptides. These peptides connect with receptors on cells, telling them whether they should divide or not divide, whether they should make a particular protein or not, and whether they should turn on one gene or another — and the thing about all this is that *emotions* and *thoughts* run this system.

In the 1980s, when Pert discovered that neuropeptide receptors were found on cells of the immune system, the scientific community went into shock and denial mode. Only after about fifteen years of further research, and after many other experimenters had replicated her work and carried out more of their own, did it slowly become accepted as fact. Pert describes neuropeptides as "biochemical units of emotion."

It no longer seems unbelievable that Jeanne Achterberg, head of research and rehabilitation at the University of Texas Health Science Center, has found that with visualization techniques people can be trained to increase the level of *particular* types of immune system cells running around in their blood. Depending on what they were asked to do, participants in the trial could increase their T-cell count or their neutrophils (a type of white blood cell).[4]

Stress is now recognized as an important co-factor in the development of cancer while, conversely, some claim to have cured cancer by reducing the degree of stress in their lives. People with cancer are told they can live longer if they keep up a fighting spirit and often take up meditation, or laughter therapy, and reorganize their lives so they can actually do what they really want. Be honest, they are told, admit your problems, air your views, say what you want, get it off your chest, decide your priorities, and act on them — all good advice for anyone.

The time has long gone since the mind and body were seen as two different things. According to Michael Talbot in *The Holographic Universe*, "deeply hypnotized persons can control allergic reactions, blood flow patterns, and near-sightedness. In addition, they can control heart rate, pain, body temperature, and even will away some kinds of birthmarks." [5] He even reports the case of a sixteen-year-old body suffering from an advanced case of Brocq's disease, a genetic condition that makes the skin thick and horny like a reptile, who was cured by hypnosis. This means that the genetic code can be mentally interfered with! [6]

Psychosomatic illnesses are defined as "physical disorders that seem to have been caused, or worsened, by psychological factors." [7] Eczema, asthma, irritable bowel syndrome, and peptic ulcers are among many conditions that are often psychosomatic in origin. The reproductive system can also be sensitive to psychological factors — think of the number of women one hears about who were infertile until they adopted a child, then suddenly become pregnant. And just as the mind can influence life, it can influence death. Stress can lead to heart disease, and the grave. Never underestimate the importance of mental health in our lives. By attending to it, we attend to our whole being — mind, body, and soul.

Drug Culture

In the modern world, drugs are a way of life. Cigarettes are sold in candy stores, alcohol is sold in the bar, cocaine is made available at "sophisticated" parties, crack is sold on the streets, marijuana is smoked in schools, amphetamines and ecstasy are part of the rave scene, while those too young to be allowed out all night may console themselves with glue and other solvents inhaled out of sight of the parents. It seems like practically everyone is looking for some addition to their lives, something to make them feel more relaxed, or "out of it," or in some sense different from their normal selves. To some extent, all this is an extension of our consumer society — we can no more help putting "extra" things into our mouths or noses than we can help buying things we don't need at the stores. The incentive comes in the form of advertising, peer pressure, or stress. Much of this is bad for us, however, and in some cases, it will kill us.

There might have been a time when "recreational drugs" were relatively harmless, but no longer. The police have found that in some instances, so-called "amphetamines" sold on the street contain as little as 2% of the drug. Today, marijuana is often cultivated using pesticides which can have a very adverse effect on health. For example, in Mexico they use paraquat which, even in small quantities, can cause irreversible lung damage; while in Jamaica, Columbia, and Belize they tend to use glyphosate. Many pot smokers have developed strange illnesses which seem to have no identifiable cause, ranging from temporary loss of sight through loss of strength or swelling in the legs and partial paralysis. Meanwhile hashish is so "cut" with shoe polish and other non-narcotic substances it can no longer be considered a "natural" drug. Cocaine is more likely to be rat poison than a derivative of the coca plant, while crack is just junk making the junkie.

So-called "recreational drugs" have other dangers. Cocaine strips people of their character so they no longer know the difference between right and wrong. Coke-heads become like soulless cadavers, a danger to themselves and everyone around them. Obviously heroin is pure evil and anyone taking it at any time needs his or her head examined.

Alcohol is by far the most widespread drug, legal and taxed, but is said to kill more people than all the other drugs combined. In America, half the accidents on the roads are caused by people under the influence, and because of them, 22,000 people die each year. In 1990 a total of 65,000 Americans died as a result of alcohol — which causes cirrhosis of the liver, heart damage, throat, mouth, and tongue cancers, gastritis, pancreatitis, brain damage, and many other things. Depression and anxiety are other effects of the drug. America consumes a third of the alcohol it did in the 1830s. Today, Korea leads the world in per capita alcohol consumption, while the Japanese have doubled their intake since the 1950s. Each country tends to have its own drinking patterns — with the Italians centering the activity around daily meals (20,000 deaths from cirrhosis

of the liver each year), while the Fins tend to binge and fall under an oncoming bus.

From all I have said, you might think I'm an old fuddy-duddy who disapproves of people enjoying themselves. Far from it, but drugs in any form are dangerous if not taken in moderation and with caution. There is a world-wide history of people wanting to escape the normal parameters of daily life, but we must somehow strive to lessen the dangers inherent in this activity and find substances which can enhance our normal hum-drum lives without killing us or making us ill.

Addiction

Although the word "addict" usually conjures up the image of a pale, skinny, hollow-eyed youth, slumped in an alley with a needle stuck in his arm, the more common addict is a nice old grandmother with a cup of tea in her hand. At least, it's now becoming clear that millions of people in America may be taking in such a quantity of caffeine — in tea, coffee, cola, and certain medicines — that they could be classified as addicts. If they don't get their fix, and even when they do, they could become ill. Estimates as to the number of cups of tea or coffee required to classify a person as a caffeine addict vary from five to twelve cups a day — twelve cups of coffee a day represents an intake of about a gram of caffeine. Someone consuming this much caffeine is liable to suffer symptoms that are indistinguishable from those produced by anxiety neurosis — including headaches, poor concentration, irritability, restlessness, insomnia, lethargy, nausea, and tremors.

You may not realize that the craving for a nice cup of coffee after a hard day's shopping is an aspect of withdrawal symptoms, or that the pick-me-up you feel after that first sip is your "fix," but caffeine is a drug and if you suddenly stop taking it you will undoubtedly feel unwell. If you suffer from any of the symptoms above, however, and want to give it a try, remember to *gradually* cut the caffeine down — and do persevere.

Because caffeine addiction is not often recognized as the root of so many troubles, a sufferer who goes to the doctor is often prescribed tranquilizers, thus exacerbating their problems. Clearly, if you suffer from the symptoms mentioned, before you convince yourself you're heading for a nervous breakdown, it might be a good idea to cut down your intake of caffeine. Switch to decaffeinated tea or coffee or fruit and herbal teas, and see what happens then — but, please, do it gradually.

Tranquilizer addiction is now, thankfully, a well-recognized problem. Although vast quantities of drugs are still handed out by doctors who don't know what alternatives there are. In Britain alone, during the year 1992-3, 540 million days' supply of benzodiazepines were dispensed. [8] Drugs classified as hypnotics and anxiolytics, prescribed for insomnia and anxiety respectively, cost the National Health Service about thirty million dollars a year.

Tranquilizer dependence is said to develop after about six weeks. Aside from the horrible effects of withdrawal, which

can be as difficult as those arising from alcohol dependency, sufferers report that, on looking back on their tranquilizer-life, they realize they had been "asleep" — so blocked-in and blocking-out, it was as if that period of time didn't exist. Whole chunks of lives are essentially lost. While on the drugs, people are more detached from life than they were when they had their neurosis, etc. They don't feel numb so much as in a dream-state — watching everything as if it were a film to which they can't consciously relate or interact with. They feel invisible.

Clearly, this is an unsatisfactory situation and if anyone reading this is caught in the trap, I suggest you get a copy of the first-ever directory of services for people who want to come off tranquilizers, which is available through the charity MIND. [9] Although I sometimes read that it takes about four weeks to come off tranquilizers, I'd say it takes very much longer than that — months, not weeks. Because the organs seem to have an addictive-type nature, the whole body becomes dependent. To suddenly stop the drug can cause the organs — like the heart or liver — to go into crisis. Whatever you do, don't get too ambitious and throw the drugs in the trash and say "that's it." Give yourself at least four months and reduce the amount of tranquilizer bit-by-bit over that time. Eventually you'll reach the point where you are shaving a few crumbs off one pill daily. *Then* take the final step.

In *The Fragrant Mind* we shall be looking at essential oil alternatives to tranquilizers, but there are other options available. Any health food shop stocks herbal relaxants which are often surprisingly effective, while homeopathic pharmacies sell homeopathic valerian and passiflora tablets. In general, valerian is calming and will stop the mind racing and is also used to treat hysteria. Homeopathy, however, is a very individualistic system of medicine and each patient coming to a homeopathic practitioner will be treated very differently. Aromatherapy, likewise, is individualistic, and therapists prescribe different combinations of essential oils for different people.

Tranquilizer addiction is itself so much of a trouble, one cannot sort out the root problems while on them because all they do is put another layer of problem on top of the underlying ones. Step-by-step though, one can reach the ideal situation — living a normal life and having natural helpmates around the house to deal with intermittent stressful situations. (See Chapter 8.)

Alcohol has been brewed by innumerable societies throughout time, with even the Bible referring to a miracle in which water was turned to wine. Poets, painters, and writers have created masterpieces with a drink in their hand, and wine buffs have invented a new language to discuss the subtleties of their chosen tipple. Alcohol is an important aspect of the social gathering — it relaxes, makes people more open and forthcoming and can't be all bad. There comes a point, however, when a threshold is crossed and instead of being "a social drinker," an innocent partaker of one of life's little pleasures, one becomes a slave to the drug — in America it's estimated that ten million

people are addicted to alcohol, while in Italy 9% of the population are thought to be alcoholics. However, it's very difficult to convince alcoholics that they have a problem, and need to change their habits.

We all know of people whose lives have been ruined by drink, of families that have been broken up by it and the promising futures which have gone down the drain. Some people become alcoholics simply because they are sociable people and the only context available in their community in which they can be sociable is the bar, and at some point their bodies become addicted. Others are driven to the bottle because they have problems which seem insurmountable and the bottle provides the only available solace. If you think you fall into the first group, then beware — you could become an alcoholic just like the millions of socialites who went that way before. The second group are, in a sense, easier to help because there are alternatives when you need help with life's seemingly endless problems; natural alternatives which don't turn you into a slave of the bottle.

Nicotine is a disgusting drug, as most addicts will admit. It makes your hair, clothes, and breath smell, makes children ill, and kills you. While fewer men now smoke than before, women continue to stick to the cigarettes and in many cases I think this is because in their busy lives of remorseless chores — encapsulated in the expression "a woman's work is never done" — the cigarette break represents a carving out of space for the woman, a little bit of space that says, "I'm having a break now, I'm going to sit here for five minutes and have a cup of coffee and a cigarette." It isn't the cigarette that's wanted so much as the five minute break!

Cigarettes are very ritualistic in that some people have to light up just before they sit down to make a phone call, or at other particular times — especially when drinking, for example. Some people convince themselves they can't *think* unless there's a cigarette in their hand, while others carry a cigarette in their hand without lighting it — like having a comfort blanket. And, of course, a cigarette often fills the big boredom void. Today there is plenty of help to get off the evil weed, including nicotine patches, hypnotism, and acupuncture — all of which work for some people. If you really want to give up, try them!

Consciousness and Control

Some people seem to float like bits of flotsam adrift on the sea of life, directed by the tide, while others seem to be fully-conscious and in control of their lives, aware of what they are doing and why they are doing it. In terms of mental health, being in control is an extremely important factor. Again and again, studies show that those who have little or no control suffer — and that is as true for rats as for people. Research has shown, for example, that patients who are allowed to control the amount of morphine given for pain relief not only achieve better pain control, they use less of the drug. Dr. Dean Ornish is rather famous in medical

history because he has shown that coronary heart disease can be *reversed* by using a combination of meditation, group therapy, walking, stress-reduction exercises, and a vegetarian diet. He says "If you believe you have some control over your life, and that you have the ability to make choices instead of being the passive recipient of medical care, or the victim of bad luck or bad genes, then you are more likely to make changes that are going to do you good in terms both of your behavior and of the direct effects of your mind on your body." [10]

But one cannot take control unless one is conscious — which the Oxford dictionary defines as "to be aware of what one is doing or intending to do." In a sense, it is quite easy not to be conscious. Schools and colleges have been criticized for not encouraging creative or original thought — the students are instead forced to learn and repeat whatever version of "wisdom" is prescribed, and not encouraged to ask the question *why*? As an adult, it is relatively easy to listen to the news but blank it out, to go to work and passively take orders, and come home and let the partner or the children take control. The world is full of people who go through life letting the forces of circumstance mold their existence. Many passive souls have woken up at age sixty and asked themselves, "what was it all about?" or bemoaned the fact that they spent so much time pleasing everyone else, they never pleased themselves.

If one goes through life not fully conscious, a mish-mash of other people's opinions and priorities, what is our state of consciousness, that is described as "the totality of the impressions, thoughts, and feelings, which make up a person's conscious being?" And whose consciousness is it — yours or your teacher's, parent's, lover's, or your daily paper? Part of mental health involves being in control — not passive, not a piece of flotsam adrift on the sea of life. Sit down for five minutes, write on the top of a piece of paper "Me," and underneath make a list of your dreams, priorities, dissatisfactions, satisfactions, etc., and try and establish where exactly you are and where you want to go in this life (as opposed to where everyone else wants you to go). Take stock, be aware, and move forward in the direction you want to go (not where the tide takes you).

The Untapped Mind

The human mind is a strange, powerful thing. Mothers walking around the supermarket are stopped in their tracks by a "feeling" that something has happened to their child. Lovers a thousand miles away from each other know when the other is in trouble — and call it "instinct." Some people can dream events before they happen — precognition. Uri Geller and many other people can, by sheer force of will, bend spoons. Others can make objects move around the room — without touching them. Archaeology uses the talents of people who can hold an ancient object and give the scientists a full history of it, and lead them to the precise site of an ancient building, far beneath the soil. Under hypnosis, people can remember past lives, complete with precise details and even in long-dead languages — which are later proven to be accurate by amazed professors who have spent their lives studying the subjects. Something is going on — but what?

Works of creation produced by people we would call geniuses are often attributed by the artists themselves to some outside force. Johann Sebastian Bach said, "I play the notes in order as they are written. It is God who makes the music." John Milton said the whole of *Paradise Lost* was dictated to him, while Robert Louis Stevenson received *Dr. Jekyll and Mr. Hyde* in a dream. Poor Samuel Taylor Coleridge was writing *Kubla Khan* in one long stream of consciousness when he was interrupted, and when he tried to go back to his writing the "inspiration" was lost — and the work was never completed. In a letter to a friend, Wolfgang Amadeus Mozart wrote that the notes of his music came from outside himself: "Whence and how they come, I know not, nor can I force them . . . nor do I hear in my imagination the parts successively but I hear them, as it were, all at once." [11] Many scientists also report that their most brilliant thoughts came to them in a flash of inspiration, as if from outside themselves. Something *is* going on — but what?

Spirituality

There is such a thing as "higher consciousness," which people experience and express in different ways. Tuning-in to whatever forces exist outside the normal world is an activity human beings have striven to do since the beginning of known time. On the Mediterranean island of Crete, 3,500 years ago, the opium poppy was employed to assist in communication with the goddess, while in Mexico for thousands of years the peyote cactus put people in touch with the spiritual realm. In India today people meditate for hours on end — to get in touch with the god within, while in churches and mosques across the world, people pray to a God high up in heaven. In a thousand ways, over thousands of years, people have reached out, and looked within, for that dimension of being we all know is there — the spiritual.

Spirituality and mind are one. To be human, to have a mind, is to be spiritual. In most places at most times the definition of the spiritual realm was pretty straight-forward — everyone around believed in the same spiritual concept and one just fell in line. Today, however, there are many spiritual options. Walking down an inner-city street you can pass a church, a Quaker meeting house, a synagogue, a mosque, a Hindu temple or a Buddhist Center. Which one are you going to walk in, if any? You might feel more drawn to a goddess-worshipping group, or a Tantric group, or any number of other groups who in their own way seek the spiritual path. On the other hand, you may not like groups, and may want to experience your spirituality in a personal, private way.

People who have a spiritual base, even if it is just a personal idea all their own, have a grounding which is emotion-ally strengthening. They feel in touch with the wider forces, and linked to other people. Obviously, this can be bad when it turns into moral superiority — "my religion is the only correct religion and the rest of you are wrong" — but it is good to feel links with other people, part of a wider family. This feeling can be experienced even when all alone — when meditating for example, or gazing at the stars on a clear night. Even alone, quietly, one can feel a connection with nature, with the natural forces, with the earth, the sky, with animals, and people. We are all connected, like a golden web, so try to connect and don't feel so alone.

Psychotherapy, Counseling, and Other Therapies

Sixty years ago in Britain some women who had children out of wedlock were incarcerated in mental institutions — the reasoning being that they must have been mad to get pregnant in such circumstances. Many women spent three and more decades behind bars for actions which today would be considered normal. Likewise, masturbation was once a certifiable offense. We have no way of knowing what judgments will be made in the future of the parameters we now apply to "sanity" and "madness," but it is quite likely that for some reason it will be considered in some respects to have been "wrong." Society tends to make rules and define "normal" behavior, or else how could we operate, but in this, many people get left out of the mainstream because they cannot conform to the rules laid down. Unusual behavior might be considered mildly eccentric, or out-and-out mad, but who makes the rules? And are *they* sane? Conformity is a straight jacket we are all forced to wear, but let us not tie the ribbons so tight we squeeze all the life out of ourselves.

There's nothing wrong with seeking help with this life. It is not an indication of failure, rather an indication that you are conscious and want to improve your emotional well-being — which is a responsible, adult, sensible thing to do. The question is, where to go for help?

Psychiatrists are doctors who have been further trained in mental illness and the emotional aspects of life and they can either take a more genetic/biochemical approach or a psychoanalytical one — seeing the source of problems as more to do with environmental factors, like family relationships, etc. Psychiatrists can prescribe drugs. *Psychoanalysts* started with Freud, and they're the ones who sit in silence as the client lies on the couch recounting their dreams and remembering their past. Key words in psychoanalysis are the Oedipus complex, the id, ego and superego, and a course of treatment can go on for years. There are many different kinds of *psychologists*, like child psychologists, industrial psychologists, clinical psychologists, etc. Carl Jung was a psychologist as much as a psychoanalyst, and took the view that inner mental forces are as much to do with intellectual

and spiritual factors, as to do with sexual ones (which is where he differed from Freud). *Psychotherapists* may only see a person a few times and give counseling — advice and psychological support — or they may see a patient for years and give classic psychoanalysis. It all depends on the particular psychotherapist and the requirements of the client.

Psychotherapy can be on a one-to-one basis, or involve couples, or the whole family. (I'd recommend family therapy for any family in which one or more members seem to be having trouble with life.) It's surprising what comes out, but it does take a lot of commitment from all sides. Couples also benefit enormously from therapy, and it's well worth trying if the relationship isn't going well.

One-to-one therapy, however, can sometimes be problematic in that the client can say whatever they want and there's nobody else there to give another perspective. This is especially likely in post-trauma stress. I recently spoke to a woman, for example, who was in therapy and who, because her records had been subpoenaed for a court case (in which she was the innocent party), was allowed to see what had been written about her. She was surprised to discover that she had been making things up. I asked her why she did it. "To please the psychoanalysist," she said, and also it was a self-protective mechanism — if she made up these stories, she wouldn't have to spend time on the things which were true but too painful to discuss. The point is, how is the analyst supposed to know the difference between truth and lies? In the records, it was obvious he had taken all she said at face value and then assessed her personality on the basis of that.

Another problem with therapy is that it is rather difficult to get referred by your doctor until you are in serious trouble — you might get an appointment with a specialist in aggression, for example, but only after you've killed someone. Places are in short supply. At least, they are if you don't want to pay. If you have not yet gone "over the hill," so to speak, and just want some general help in sorting yourself out, the doctor is unlikely to be able to help — you must find your own solution, and there is plenty of choice.

Aside from one-to-one therapy, and group therapy, there is dance therapy, art therapy, music therapy, singing therapy, anger therapy, behavioral therapy, grief counseling, rape-victim groups, sexual abuse-victim groups, and "the wounded male" groups, etc. Look around and try to identify which type of therapy might be right for you. Many people have started their own groups with people who have had similar experiences, for example there are groups for people who have had a child die of cancer, or who have a particular physical illness, etc.

It will take some homework to find the right group. The way to approach this, I think, is to say to yourself, "I'm going to make one phone call a day," and carry on until you get through the labyrinth of information to a place that seems right for you. There are several standard reference books which list organizations and they can be found in the large libraries. It might be simpler to start your own group — put an ad in the paper and see who answers.

Aromatherapy is being increasingly used in the therapy and counseling situation and specific advice on this is given later. (See Chapter 10.)

Meditation and Visualization

Meditation and visualization are both very helpful techniques and they can be learned quite easily from books, or even without them. With meditation, you're aiming to clear your mind of all thoughts. This is very difficult at first but it becomes easier with practice and even just ten minutes a day will help improve your health. You will need to focus on something. Some people use a sound — like "Om," while others think of an image — a lotus flower for example, while others concentrate on their breathing. The idea is to be very quiet, so silent you can almost hear what's going on within your body. Thoughts will come but let them float away — don't hang on to them.

Sit comfortably with your back straight. Before starting, flex your toes and then release them, then do the same with your calves, thighs, buttocks, tummy, arms, shoulders, neck, head, and face. Prerecorded tapes are available that lead you through a meditation, and they can be very helpful. Take the phone off the hook so you are not disturbed. Burning essential oils in a diffuser can certainly help the meditative process — choose one oil that you like or a combination of oils, perhaps choosing from the list of oils that help with anxiety. (See Chapter 8.)

Like meditation, visualization is an extremely ancient practice. The Hindu yogic texts known as the tantras were written between the fourth and sixth centuries A.D. and include the advice to visualize the desired lover. By making a precise image in your mind, complete with physical, mental, and spiritual attributes, and focusing on it every day, the lover could be conjured up — for real. The Tibetan Tantric texts contain sadhanas, visualization exercises, which could be used to create anything one desired. This method made perfect sense to the Tantrists, who believed everything in the world was created by thought, and continues to be modified by the collective thought of all mankind. To perfect their visualization techniques, the more serious adepts would spend years in a closed room or cave. The Sufis are another group who believe that a person's destiny can be shaped by visualization, which they call "creative prayer."

Today, in Western culture, visualization is being widely used to treat illnesses, especially cancer. In medical visualization, the idea is to imagine a "killer" destroying the diseased cells. What one imagines doing the "killing," and how you imagine the bad cells you want to get rid of, is entirely personal. The killer might be a shark progressively eating a school of little fish, or it might be a Pac-Man™ munching through the unwanted cells, or a gun blasting away bits of the tumor.

The crucial thing about visualization is to practice. I don't mean practice doing it (although you have to do that too), but practice visualizing real live objects before you start creative visualization. You can practice with anything — a flower, for example. Look at the color of the petals, and their texture, and register how many petals the flower has and look at the stamen. Whatever you choose to practice with, just have a good look at the object, close your eyes, try to see it in your mind's eye, and when you loose the image, have another look at the real thing. Keep going like this until your ability to actually see things clearly, and your ability to remember them, becomes better. Practice looking at and visualizing something interesting and pleasant, real or in two-dimensional picture form — a tree, garden, seashore, or whatever. Don't choose a cup or table or something equally boring because your interest will not be maintained.

If you decide you want to try and get rid of cancer cells inside you by imagining a shark, for example, get a picture of an actual shark and have a good look at it — look at the colors of its skin, the shape and form of its body. And if your cancer is in the colon, for example, get a book on anatomy and have a really good look at the anatomy of a colon. Also, if you are basically a pacifist, don't use violent imagery. Instead of thinking of guns blasting away at the tumor, think of it as slowly dissolving, or cracking open like an egg and pouring away, or being baked and gradually shriveled up.

As you practice visualization, burn 6-8 drops of essential oil on a burner or diffuser in the room. Use something pleasant and relaxing, something you enjoy smelling. Eventually, you'll be able to take your visualization skills out with you so you can sit on a train and, even with your eyes wide open, do your visualization exercise. If you also have a couple of drops of your usual visualization essential oils on a tissue, or on your sleeve, you can inhale them and it will help throw your mind back to your practicing and help focus your mind.

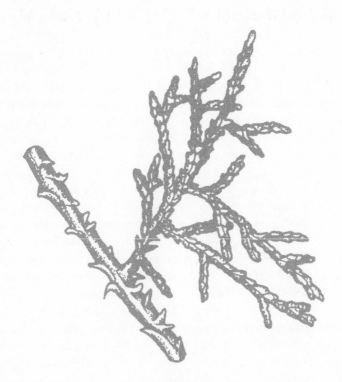

Cypress

CHAPTER 4

AROMA-PSYCHOLOGY

What's in a Word?

Before discussing what aroma-psychology means to you or me on a practical level, I just want to say a few words about the linguistics of aroma, the new language that is expanding by the day. The word *aromatherapy* refers to the clinical use of essential oils combined with physical therapy — usually in the form of massage or inhalations. Aromatherapists go through very different degrees of training — from a few weekend courses to many years of intense anatomy, physiology, chemistry, body work, massage skills, etc. Fully trained aromatherapists perform work that cannot always be done at home, and their services are sometimes indispensable. A very small minority of aromatherapists have a more medical leaning, while the majority tend toward stress-management. There are also beauticians and

cosmetologists who are using essential oils and essential oil products and call what they are doing "aromatherapy." This is the beauty and relaxation end of the aromatherapy spectrum. To some degree, anyone can be an "aromatherapist" in that much of the information required is available, and the methods do not always need outside help — one can do them at home.

Because there is so much more to essential oils than their use in a "clinical" setting or even for medicinal use within the home, several other expressions have grown up. The aromatherapist Professor William Arnold-Taylor first coined the term *aroma-tology* in 1981, and he meant by it "aromatherapy for the whole person" — body, mind, and spirit. This is a very wide term encompassing using the essential oils to re-form character and personality characteristics, and to enhance spirituality. It's a good term if you want to indicate the depths of influence essential oils can have.

The word *aroma-chology* is a trademark of the Olfactory Research Fund (formerly the Fragrance Foundation), a research institution that supports the flavors and fragrance industries. Whether referring to the use of synthetics or natural essential oils, aroma-chology is to do with influencing the mind. It encompasses the development of aromas to attract buyers into a shop and make them linger there longer, and of aromas to make keyboard operators more efficient, or customers more relaxed. The research doesn't stop here. For many years government defense departments have been exploring ways in which aroma can control crowds or influence the behavior of the enemy.

Aroma-psychology specifically refers to the use of essential oils to positively affect the mind — such as memory enhancement, learning improvement, mood uplifting, and confidence boosting. These mental stimulations have a direct impact on daily performance and practical applications are currently being utilized by a wide range of organizations.

Because the mind and body are an integrated unit, the term aroma-psychology is somewhat unsatisfactory, but it is still useful to denote the degree to which the mental or bodily functions are involved at any one time. For example, if you burn your hand and put lavender oil on it, that's a physical application although the lavender will also help with the shock and make you more relaxed. We would call that aromatherapy. On the other hand, if you're having a party and want the room to smell nice and make your guests re-

laxed, you might put some geranium, cinnamon, and melissa in a room diffuser before they arrive. The fact that these will help prevent one guest passing a nasty flu virus to another is an added bonus! This situation is aroma-psychology bordering on aromatherapy.

Man-made chemical odorants do not have this ability to perform antibacterial or antiviral activities, and although there is now a vast industry that attempts to replicate the aromas of essential oils, what they produce can in no way be compared to essential oils. It is difficult to find analogies to illustrate the difference. Perhaps one could compare essential oils to a music concert, and man-made synthetic aromas to a recording of that concert. Technicians might say the recording can improve on the real event, because in the studio they can over-dub, add echo, and "drop-in" notes or words which were less than perfect at the time of the performance. This is true, but the concert has an atmosphere, an excitement, and is a total experience in a way a recording can never be. The analogy can never really work, however, because the music in the concert will be different — *and better* — than the recording. The expression "chalk and cheese" comes to mind but essential oils are neither chalk nor cheese — they are pure, luxurious, delightful, beneficial substances, designed by God. Synthetic fragrances, on the other hand, were designed by people in laboratories and their benefits (other than to satisfy commercial interests) have yet to be proved. Indeed, synthetics are not even *meant* to be beneficial to us. They're just designed to make us choose one particular product over another, and pay more for it.

The olfactory onslaught is already upon us. Personally, I hate getting into the back of a taxi only to discover there is a horrible chemical air-freshener on the shelf behind my head. The window has to be opened and I practically hold my breath until we get where we're going. And the massive aroma bombardment that comes from most cosmetics sections in department stores is often overwhelming. But now we have a whole new dimension to aroma as the mind-altering effects of essential oils are being exploited in many so-called "aromatherapy" products, which you can find in all the major stores. What happens is that research shows a particular essential oil is relaxing, neroli for example, so the toiletry manufacturers says, "let's make a relaxing neroli bubble bath." The next thing you see is a product on the shelf purporting to be a "relaxing, aromatherapy" bubble bath, but what you don't know is that the product doesn't have a drop of neroli oil in it. Instead, it's got some combination of chemicals that *smell* like neroli.

Now, the chemists will tell you that it makes no difference. According to them, the chemical cocktails they produce in the lab and the real thing — neroli oil, say — are more or less the same thing. Some will even tell you that the chemical version is better! The logic goes like this: there are 100 components in neroli oil, say, but only 5 or 10 of these actually produce the smell, so those 5 or 10 can be tested for safety and combined to make a "neroli" product. *Real* neroli, they say, cannot be tested for safety because it's too complex. Therefore the chemical "copy" is safer than the real thing. This logic makes sense until you realize two other things. First, neroli oil, like all essential oils, is very complex — too complex to copy. No laboratory can produce a "neroli" that does what neroli does — create well-being, for example, because nobody has yet discovered what all the minuscule components of neroli actually are. We don't have names for them. The chemists say you don't *need* the 90 or 95 other components of neroli — but this really depends on whether you're trying to replicate the *smell* or the *effect*. Second, it is one thing to individually test a group of chemicals for inclusion in a product and declare them safe, but what about the product as a *whole* — how are those chemicals interacting with each other — and, more importantly, with all the natural chemicals, and cells, within our body?

Chemists are very fond of pointing out that within some essential oils there are tiny components which may be toxins, and that if they tried to reproduce them in a product, it wouldn't be allowed. Yes, maybe, but we're not making essential oils in a lab. The whole point about essential oils is that they are complex and work as a *whole*. There might be something in an essential oil that is toxic but in the context of the whole oil, in synergistic or antagonistic combination with all the other bits and pieces, it becomes nontoxic. It is this beautiful balance that gives them extraordinary potency and that cannot be replicated. James A. Duke, PhD, one of the world's foremost authorities on natural plant products makes another, important point:

> Through evolution our genes have already experienced many of the natural compounds, including toxic and medicinal compounds, often equipping us with mechanisms to deal with reasonable doses of these toxins. Our genes have no experience with tomorrow's synthetics. . . . Through maternal and/or cytoplasmic inheritance, our immune systems have also experienced many of the natural compounds, but not tomorrow's synthetics. [1]

Today, millions of people will apply essential oils to their bodies, in the form of perfume, and other millions will put them into their mouths in the form of drinks and food. Every time you chew a piece of spearmint or peppermint gum, essential oils are involved, while the soft drink industry purchases by far the largest portion of the citrus essential oils. Even ylang-ylang, usually thought of as just a perfume ingredient, is used in confectionery and baking goods. Essential oils are a vast world-wide industry. For example, the 1992 peppermint and spearmint oil production in America alone was worth $95 million and $46 million, respectively. Someone consumes all this, and as far as anyone has ever been able to say, they have suffered no toxic side effects from it. Nor, as far as I am aware, has anyone suffered toxic side effects from potatoes which, as chemists are well aware, contain toxins — especially in the peel.

Aroma-psychology and Mental States

Research into the psychological effects of aroma now attracts major funding. There are four major olfaction research institutions: The Olfactory Research Fund in New York, the Monell Chemical Senses Center in Philadelphia, the Smell and Taste Treatment and Research Foundation Ltd. in Chicago, and Warwick University's Olfaction Research Department. The Olfactory Research Fund awards grants to doctors who wish to study the psychological aspects of olfaction, and is funded by the fragrance industry, while the Monell employs fifty PhD-level scientists and carries out work on the physiology and psychology of aroma, on behalf of various funding agencies — both commercial and governmental.

In addition to these, there are innumerable commercial organizations and education facilities that now look into the psychological effects of aroma, such as International Flavors and Fragrances Ltd., the Takasago Central Research Laboratory in Tokyo, the Toho University School of Medicine, Tokyo, and Yale University. Psychology professor Robert A. Baron at the Renselaer Polytechnic Institute in Troy, New York, for example, has found that people in pleasantly scented rooms carry out their work with more confidence, more efficiency, and with greater willingness to resolve conflict. From my mailbag it is patently clear that tremendous interest in the behavior-changing potential of aroma exists among the new generation of psychology students.

As a subject, olfaction has become a hot item among a whole range of scientific researchers for several reasons. The fact that olfactory cells regenerate every 30 to 40 days makes them unique among brain and central nervous system cells, and rather exciting components of neurobiology. The olfactory receptor system also involves P-proteins, G-proteins and GABA receptors, which are interesting for various reasons, and by understanding how they work, many other physiological mysteries may be revealed. A vast body of research is also being done on the psychological effects of aroma because these have powerful commercial implications, and projects can easily attract funding.

When I read research papers involving essential oils I am more often than not surprised at the choice of oils, and the volumes at which they are used. For example, one trial exploring the sedative effects of lavender on elderly patients involved putting three drops of lavender on their pillows. Lavender is an adaptogen, meaning it has one effect in low dosage and another in a high dosage. Depending on the person on whom it is being used, one drop of lavender oil would be quite sufficient to make anyone sleep, while three could have the opposite, stimulant effect.

Another problem, of course, is that you cannot patent nature. Sorry, but Mother Nature Inc. has got the patent already. To register a patent you've got to *invent* something, and essential oils were invented a very long time ago. The people who fund research into the psychological

effects of odor want to be able to exploit the information they get. To do this, they've got to come up with a new combination of chemicals and register it for a particular purpose. Man-made aromas (like drugs) can also elicit behavioral change, a fact that pleases commercial interests who find dealing in natural products — which are prone to the vicissitudes of the weather and pests and are liable to degrade quicker — more troublesome to deal with than synthetically produced products. Consequently, the research is directed at finding which combination of man-made chemicals elicit certain responses. The end result, of course, is that you and I are increasingly going to be exposed to these chemicals as the research turns into practical applications. The important question for the future is not, "are we going to use aroma to change behavior?" That is going to happen anyway. The question is, "are we going to use man-made chemicals, or essential oils?"

Hospitals, Hospices, and Nursing Homes

Hospitals and hospices need all the cheering up they can get, and essential oils are the perfect way to do it. Aside from the fact that they deodorize the clinical and organic smells, and make the place smell fresh and charming, they can (if you use the right ones) cut down cross-infections. Fred Dale of Dale Air Products, who has twelve years experience in installing essential oil diffusion systems in hospitals, museums, and other public buildings, says that "synthetic materials, when interacting with certain other smells, won't get rid of those smells and you'll end up with a worse smell than you started with."

Essential oils, on the other hand, work very well. And they have other benefits. At the Worcester Hospital in Hereford, England, a six-month trial showed that vaporizing lavender through the air caused patients to sleep in a more natural pattern, and made them less aggressive during the day. More than that, over the six months, some patients were weaned off their tranquilizers — simply by substituting lavender in the atmosphere, which has a calming effect on the brain.

Dale has devised a "Reminiscence Pack" which he supplies to day-care centers for the elderly. Five aromas are used together with a script by care staff to elicit memories from the old folk. As you may know, elderly people tend to have bad short-term memory but very good long-term memory, and if that long-term memory can be evoked through aroma, their minds can be kept active recollecting their school days, youth, and happier times. It is apparently very effective and much appreciated by all concerned. Meanwhile, an American diffuser system company, AromaSys of Minneapolis, are also working with nursing homes for the elderly to explore ways of reducing "wandering." Here too, aromas are being used to create a nostalgic stimulus to kindle more dynamic mental states.

AromaSys have installed six hundred aroma-diffusion systems in the United States, including one at the St. Croix Valley Memorial Hospital in Wisconsin. In this fully registered general hospital, essential oils are diffused throughout the lobby, at a nurse's station and in the emergency waiting room. Here, family members wait to hear news of their sick relatives and it is obviously an extremely stressful place, made more bearable by the anxiety-relieving essential oils that are diffused in the atmosphere. The hospital also has two "floaters," mobile systems, that can be taken to any areas where they are particularly required, including the chemical dependency unit where people with drinking or drug problems are seen. Various aromas are used in different areas, at different times, depending on the requirements. The hospital administrator, Steve Urosevich, says his aim is to make the patient's hospital stay "more humanizing, more personal, and demystifying." [2]

In 1992 Dr. William Redd and Dr. Sharon Manne at the Memorial Sloan-Kettering Cancer Center in New York conducted tests to see whether aroma could reduce the anxiety of patients undergoing magnetic resonance imaging procedures. They compared stress levels between 42 patients who breathed normal air with 38 who breathed air containing molecules of heliotropin — a sweet, vanilla-like fragrance naturally occurring in pepper oil. Sixty-three percent of those exposed to the aroma experienced reduced anxiety levels.

Stress reduction is a major concern of the London Lighthouse — a specialist facility for those with HIV-related problems. For many years now they have been offering complementary therapies in addition to the usual medical treatments.

Aromatherapy treatments have an extremely high uptake rate, but because of financial restrictions, demand outstrips supply. The main benefits are perceived to be general relaxation and stress and anxiety relief, which in turn positively affect the immune system. Wendy Peters of the medical and complementary health services department says that aromatherapy treatments seem to prevent the onset of the disease, although this can only be an anecdotal observation as each client will be undergoing several different treatments at the same time. I find it very touching that many clients, or their family and friends, ask that essential oils are diffused in the atmosphere during the death process itself.

At the St. John's and St. Elizabeth's Hospital in London, all eleven midwives have become trained aromatherapists. They have no doubt as to the benefits of essential oils. They offer them to women during the antenatal stage, during the birth itself, and in after-care — for both mother and child. They use essential oils for physical ailments such as nausea, swollen legs, muscular pains, mastitis, infections, etc. (See *The Complete Book of Essential Oil & Aromatherapy*). But anxiety, stress, and tension may also accompany pregnancy and birth, particularly for women who have had previous bad experiences, and blood-pressure levels must also be controlled.

There is a growing interest in aromatherapy on the part of nurses, who were inspired by the good work done by members of the International Federation of Aromatherapists, as part of the "Aromatherapy in Care" project. These practitioners worked with children, cancer and Aids patients, among others. The Royal College of Nursing, in recognition of the interest, has produced its own literature on the subject, and many small-scale studies are being carried out all over the country. At the Royal Sussex County Hospital in Brighton, for example, a trial involving thirty-six patients in the intensive care and coronary care units were put into three groups that would receive either aromatherapy massage, massage without oils, and nothing — i.e., the control group. (Massage was done to the feet.) Over a five-week period various measurements were taken. Systolic blood pressure measurements showed a reduction in the control group of 16% over the five weeks, while the aromatherapy group decreased by 50% (massage alone was 40%); decrease in respiratory rate was 16% in the control group, and 75% in the aromatherapy group (41% massage alone); while reduction in heart rate was 41% for the control, and 91% for the aromatherapy group (58% massage alone).

Hopefully, as ignorance and prejudice break down, more trials will be instigated. Experience has shown that no harm comes of aromatherapy, and that patients very much appreciate its benefits. As "patient care" becomes a buzz-word in the restructured National Health Service, we should see more attention being given to aromatherapy.

Offices

The Japanese have a long tradition of using aroma, and they have much respect for it. Perhaps then, it is not so surprising that it should be the Japanese who have most easily accepted the logic of using aroma as a management tool. In 1985 research into the mind-altering affects of essential oils was started in Japan by Dr. Shizuo Torii who, by measuring brain waves, showed that some aromas can have a stimulating effect and some can have a relaxing effect. Things have progressed somewhat since then, and to my knowledge there are now fifty aroma diffusion systems in place in both commercial and municipal offices.

Japan's third largest construction company, the Shimizu Corporation, has specialist engineers who incorporate aroma systems into the new "intelligent" buildings which use aroma to improve efficiency and relieve stress. In one bank designed by the company, lavender or rosemary are diffused into the customer areas, while lemon or eucalyptus are used to keep workers alert at their computers. Commercial diffuser systems are capable of pumping different aromas into the atmosphere at different times of the day, to relax or stimulate as required. The fragrance company Takasago have shown that key-board punching errors fell by 20% when lavender was diffused in the atmosphere, by 33% with jasmine and 54% with lemon. By changing the aromas around periodically, smell sensitivity (tolerance) — and efficiency — can be maintained.

Another Japanese construction company that has taken aroma to heart is the Kajima Corporation, which now also sells aroma diffusion systems. In their state-of-the-art "intelligent" head office in Akasaka, Tokyo, sensors monitor atmospheric conditions like temperature and humidity and the building's computers blend appropriate fragrances, which are diffused into different areas of the building, taking the time of day and the male-female ratio of any one department into consideration. While a lavender and rose combination creates a calming, stress-relieving, and blood-pressure reducing effect for general purposes, the after-lunch drowsiness is combated, they say, with lemon and jasmine, which have a refreshing and reviving effect. Many combinations of aroma are possible, and Kajima are using lemon in the morning, floral and wood aromas during the day to maintain a relaxed atmosphere, with a final flourish of lemon at the end of the day to give workers the boost they need to fight their way home through the traffic. And after a good night's sleep they can be woken by Seiko's Hattori clock, which releases the aroma of pine and eucalyptus just before the alarm goes off — to both create the impression of waking in a lovely natural environment, and invigorate the worker so they can get going again.

The logic of using aroma to keep workers happy, relaxed, and efficient has not been lost on certain American companies either. In Ohio, the 10,000-square-foot offices of hair care distributors Frederick's Inc. have been fitted with an adjustable aroma-diffusion system. Their chairman, Frederick Holzberger says, "I have seen an absolute major attitude change." [3]

Retail Outlets

Retail Planning Associates of Seattle, USA, are one of the new breed of companies who specialize in creating fragrances for retail outlets. Their president, J'Amy Owens, says that aroma is "...one of the best ways to influence the customer that's legal.... It's the 'come into my parlor' approach, one more piece of netting in the web."[4] A unique, personalized store aroma, which can be used in the air conditioning system, can cost anything up to $20,000 to create.

Aroma diffusion does not have to be an expensive business, however. Anyone can create their own, unique, personal range of preferred aromas when they have a few bottles of essential oils to work with. There is a very effective diffuser available, which doesn't use electricity or candle-heat and, because it's portable, can be used in your office as well as your home.[5] Even when using essential oils on a commercial scale, the cost is not excessive. The Radisson Mart Plaza Hotel in Maimi, for example, fragrances its 7,000 square-foot lobby for $21 a day.

According to Alan R. Hirsch, neurologic director of the Smell and Taste Treatment and Research Foundation in Chicago, "Odorants are potentially more efficacious than any other modality in increasing sale ability of consumer products. This is true regardless of whether the odor is actually related to or synergistic with the product." In other words, you can put a false aroma of popcorn into the environment, a cinema foyer for example, and increase your sales of actual popcorn, or you can use a floral aroma to make the customer buy something that has nothing to do with flowers — a pair of tennis shoes, for example.

In 1990 Dr. Hirsch recruited thirty one people at a shopping Center and asked them to look at trainer shoes in two rooms. The Nike shoes used in the trial were identical, but one of the rooms was perfumed with a light mixed floral aroma. Twenty-six or 84% of the people indicated that they were more likely to buy the shoes in the scented room, and on average, they said they'd pay $10.33 more for them. Although the test attempted to make the aroma detectable to the participants, many couldn't smell it although they too preferred the product in the perfumed room. This means the "buy-me" reflex is operating at a subliminal level too. All this is very tantalizing to sales managers, especially as the technology now exists to release a variety of odorants into a closed atmosphere in standardized but adjustable concentrations.

In another trial, in a gambling casino in Las Vegas, Hirsch discovered that if a particular aroma was put into the atmosphere around a group of slot-machines, the amount of money put into the machines by gamblers increased by an average of 45.11%. As part of the trial, Hirsch had also used a second aroma around another group of machines and taken a non-perfumed area as his control. Neither of these areas saw any increase in their takings, so obviously there was something in "aroma #1" causing the increased sales effect. Finding exactly what makes people spend their money so freely is what the new aroma research is all about, and what more and more businesses will find themselves having to pay for, as aroma-competition heats up.

Although Japan does not at present use aroma to an extensive degree in retailing, Toyota does use floral aromas to attract women into its showrooms. Meanwhile, an unnamed American car manufacturer is supporting research to find a scent which makes its salesmen appear "more honest and trustworthy to customers." [6]

Of course, making a sale is only half the problem — then you've got to collect the money. Aroma can help here too. Imagine if there was an aroma you could spray on your invoices to induce the customer to pay up. There is. It's called *Aeolus* 7 and smells like sweat. Apparently, it is a much faster way to get payment than sending a lawyer's letter and, of course, *very* much cheaper.

Schools and Colleges

The first hard proof that aroma can be used to improve memory (and thus learning and passing exams) came from psychologist Frank Schaub at Yale University. He gave seventy-two undergraduates a list of forty adjectives and asked them to write down their opposites. They were not told that the next day they would be required to remember them. At various stages of the experiment students were given the aroma of chocolate, and some were not. On average, those not given the

aroma remembered 17% of the answers and those given it, 21%. These results were replicated later using the aroma of mothballs. The crucial factor, apparently, is that the same scent is used in each session — remembering and recalling. Aromatherapists believe essential oils can improve on 21%, but then we don't use mothballs!

More recently, Dr. Hirsch and his team in Chicago found that students in the senior calculus class at Lincoln High School, Portland, Oregon, could be made to increase their speed of learning by using a chemical-mixed floral aroma in the room. The students had to do a test three times, wearing a mask, either with or without the odorant. When the same test had been done on adults, they improved their score from 14% to 31%, while the high school students improved their scores from 14% to 54%. Dr. Hirsch has proposed several mechanisms that may explain why aroma should have a positive impact on learning as the exact reason is not yet clear. What is most clear is that there is still much work to be done. If these findings can be replicated, however, the implications for education are staggering.

It is not too hard to imagine a future in which our children are exposed to aroma in the classroom — but what aromas are they to be — natural or chemical? Already, our children (and we ourselves) are exposed to pollutants in the water; to pesticide, herbicide, and fungicide residues in vegetables; and metals and hormones, etc. in meat; as well as to air pollution, chemical air-fresheners, cleaners, toiletries, etc. There has to come a point at which we say "too much." And the classroom has to be it. On the other hand, it is true that aroma can enhance memory, and there is a way to do it — using essential oils. Although one is adding something to the room, it is something that can be found in nature — which is, after all, where children throughout the eons have sat and learned their lessons. With essential oils, we're putting back some of the benefits of the natural environment, things you would experience in the country — trees like pine, eucalyptus, or cypress, fruits like bergamot or grapefruit, herbs like basil or rosemary, flowers like geranium or rose.

The Future

In the case of aroma-psychology we are standing on the threshold of a new era and there is no reason not to take the natural route. From a world-wide supply and demand point of view, one might say that if all the products that now use fragrances were to switch to naturals, there wouldn't be enough space on the planet to grow them. The answer to this may be in biotechnology, which the perfumery and cosmetics house, Estee Lauder, are looking into as a way of producing rose and jasmine oil — which are notoriously expensive. The method their research and development department are exploring involves isolating the oil-producing cells in the flower petals and culturing them in a soup of nutrients. If this method works, it may be a good thing in that it will provide a source of "rose" and "jasmine" that can be used in perfumery. These would not be substances, however, that I or my colleagues would use for traditional aromatherapy. Whatever science may tell us, we believe that *real* essential oils can only be produced by chlorophyll-bearing plants which absorb the sun's rays and synthesize organic compounds. We prefer bio-dynamics over bio-technology. For fragrancing alone, however, the new biotechnology may provide a solution to supply problems.

From the future of the planet point of view, plants are already being explored as a means of helping the ozone layer. Much international interest is being taken in *Vernonia galamensis*, from the Compositae family (which includes chamomile and helicrysum) because its oil can be used in paint manufacture and reduce the pollutants in the atmosphere. Because of its low viscosity, *Vernonia* can be used as a solvent which, uniquely, actually becomes part of the dry paint surface and does not evaporate to pollute the air. In America and Germany, according to a report in *Herbalgram*, "research is underway in university and industry laboratories on its use for lubricants and lubricant additives, adhesives, and epoxy resins and in the synthesis of dilbasic acids currently obtained from petroleum and used in the manufacture of industrial nylons."[7] As a cash-crop for the third world *Vernonia* has the distinct advantage of being able to grow in as little as eight inches of annual rainfall and is distasteful to animals. As a benefit for the whole world, consider the fact that in the Los Angeles basin alone twenty-two tons of volatile organic compound emissions from paints and varnishes rise to create smog *each day*.[8] Any reduction in that has to be a blessing.

Citrus essential oils, meanwhile, are a good alternative for petrochemicals used in paints, household cleaners, and solvents used to clean computer chips. This is good news for the 20% of people who suffer headaches caused by the common solvent, trichloroethylene.[9]

The human mind was not designed to inhale the plethora of man-made chemicals and we are only just beginning to understand what effects they are having on us. In the year 2020, children may not know what it feels like to walk, exhilarated, through a pine forest, and they may associate the aroma of pine with synthetic cleaning fluids. Already olfactory researchers are having difficulty finding people who make natural associations with aroma. For example, because of its widespread use in confectionery, synthetic strawberry flavor is more often identified as "real" than the real (i.e. natural) thing. Natural aromatic connections are in danger of being lost!

Part 2

Emotional Healing and Aromatherapy

*"Miracles occur naturally as expressions of love.
The real miracle is the love that inspires them.
In this sense everything
that comes from love is a miracle."*

– A COURSE IN MIRACLES

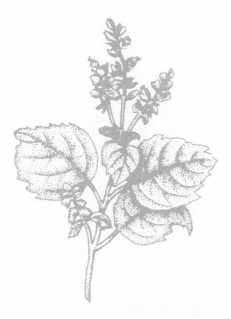

CHAPTER 5

HOW TO USE ESSENTIAL OILS FOR THE FRAGRANT MIND

There's always been something for people to get depressed about. When there weren't any supermarkets filled with foreign goods, the crops were all-important. If they failed, or the pests came, life became hell. People starved. And you might hear rumors about a strange army moving toward your area, on horses, carrying weapons, intent to pillage and rape. You might spend half your life anxious about what might happen to your children — now and in the future. People have been under stress for as long as we can imagine and, among the balms, unguents, ointments, and salves of ancient times, you can be sure there were plant essences being used specifically to ease the burdens of the mind. Even the frankincense given to Jesus was (and is) a mind alterant — in fact, it uplifts the spirit and helps dispel earthly problems. By the time Dioscorides came along in 60 A.D., he could name 1,500 medicinal plants, many of which were in aromatic oil form. This was the materia medica our ancestors grew up with, which we have developed to the point where we can see the rich diversity of help nature can provide, including that for the mind.

Over the years many different systems of medicine have developed. These are not necessarily in conflict, as a wise person somewhere once said — you can take many routes to get to the same place. In India, the traditional method of medicine is Ayurvedic, and in that the personality and character of the patient are taken as part of the diagnostic procedure. The type of person would (and still does) determine the particular plant prescribed. This diagnosis by character is today routine in homeopathy and herbalism, while personality, in all its forms, is a routine subject of discussion for perfumers. Personality and character, in relation to essential oils, is the subject of Part Three of this book.

Part Two deals with all those things for which aromatherapy is best known — stress, tension, etc. They are included within the A-Z of emotional problems — which goes from Abuse, Additions, Aggression, through Trauma, Withdrawal, and Worthlessness. In between the down's, there are ups — Confidence, Contentment, and Joy. It is these potentials that have contributed so much to the growth of aromatherapy in recent years. Essential oils are positive additions to one's life, including one's mental life. And the great thing is, you don't have to be sick or even troubled to use them. They are there to enhance, to strengthen, and to delight.

Complexity and Flexibility

Essential oils are like people — complex. One person called Rosemary might be a fabulous ballet dancer, and a computer buff, a mother, a cook, a driver, a chess player, a tennis player, and a poet. Likewise, the essential oil, rosemary, can do many different things. Just because you might have read somewhere that rosemary oil is used for rheumatism, for example, don't assume that is its only use. It's also good for depression and fatigue. Essential oils are flexible and adaptable — like people.

In a clinical setting, an aromatherapist will individualize the formula of essential oils she or he uses on a client. No two people are alike, and even if they were, circumstances or situations can be different. In a book it is obviously impossible to individualize, but the format of this book allows us to get around this problem to a certain degree. Alongside the standard clinical formulations I give for each situation, you will find a list of essential oils that you can choose from to design your own formula, tailor made for you. Look at the individual oils listed for a particular problem, Emotional Violence say, and cross-reference them with what else is said about them throughout the book. Smell the actual oil next time you go into a store. If you like it, buy it. You can personalize a formula for yourself that might change with time and circumstances. There are many possibilities because essential oils are so flexible; there are lots of formulas to try.

One of the great things about aromatherapy is how you get a synergistic effect when you blend two or more oils together. Bergamot is a great confidence booster, but blend it with geranium which is an emotional balancer, and you have a winner. Single essential oils can be vibrant and dynamic on their own but put in a blend, they become more than the sum of their component parts — with a unique character of their own, and with an extra energizing and harmonizing potential. With approximately 300 essential oils in common use, you can see how many permutations there are to try. Two of this and one of that, two of that and one of this, or two of each — all these are different formulas. It would take a mathematical genius to work out all the possible permutations, even given certain restrictions.

Synergy and Creative Blending

When you put two essential oils together you create an entirely new compound. The number of permutations — using blends of two, three, or more — are incalculable. Throughout this book you will find formulas that contain several essential oils but, because these formulas are meant to be taken as a *whole,* and because particular essential oils cannot be taken out of context of the entire formula, do not assume that if a particular oil is included in a formula for stress, say, then that oil can be used on its own for the same purpose. Sometimes this is indeed true, but not always. Please therefore use either the formula given in particular sections, *or* a single oil listed for that purpose (which may also be in a formula), *or* a combination of oils from that list, made up to suit your choice.

Adaptogens

Many herbs, roots, and essential oils are adaptogens — natural balancers. Lemon works on the nervous system, active as a sedative or tonic, as required. Lavender is another adaptogen — small quantities are usually relaxing, while high concentrations can be stimulating. With essential oils, balance is all, and when balanced, the body and mind can perform to their best. Bear all this in mind when you see a particular oil appearing on two lists of opposing conditions — the *quantities* of these oils can be all-important, as is the

quality or nature of an individual person at any given time.

Chemotypes

The same species of plant, grown in different growing conditions, produces a different essential oil with unique properties. Altitude, water quality, soil fertility, the magnetic pull of the earth, methods of growing, and weather are all factors that have an effect on the way the plant develops, and thereby influence the properties a particular batch from a particular country produces. Think of it like wine. People transport vines with them as they emigrate, and produce a wine that is related to, but not exactly the same, as that produced in the valley from which the vine came. The word *chemotypes* describes these branches of the same family, which can do somewhat different jobs, and gives another indication of the broadness of the possibilities inherent in essential oil use.

Purity and Quality

It used to be the case that you could be pretty sure where a particular species of plant was grown and the essential oil came from — lavender used to come from either England or France, for example. Lavender still comes from England and France, but it also now comes from China, from where it is sometimes shipped to France — and re-exported as "French." It used to be the case that French lavender was grown under clear skies, fresh and clean. Now you can see lavender growing in fields adjacent to motorways, under skies thick with the smoke rising from chemical plants. It now makes a great deal of difference where, *exactly*, in France the lavender comes from — the high Alps are preferred partly because the air is cleaner there. For an aromatherapist it is also important to know whether a helichrysum, for example, is grown in Corsica or the former Yugoslavia, because the two essential oils have different therapeutic qualities.

It used to be the case that some essential oils were sold at auction. Today, wholesalers tend to have a more direct access to the source — the field in which the crop is grown, and the farmer — often through a middleman. This gives purchasers more control, which is necessary, because there are more factors to consider. Aside from the question of which country, and *exactly* where in that country, the oils come from, aromatherapists who use essential oils for clinical use want to know which, if any, chemical pesticide, fungicide or herbicide is used on the crop. Bear in mind here that we are talking about tiny quantities of biocide residues. These things also exist — in very much larger quantities — in the foods we eat every day. Plagued as they are by insects, insect eggs, snails, rodents, weeds, and fungi, farmers are tempted to use chemicals (known as "biocides"), and it is the job of the middle-man or direct buyer to make sure they're not. Just how much biocide residue is left in any particular essential oil depends on the integrity of the line of supply. For serious aromatherapists, this is the thing they look for when choosing essential oils. The various aromatherapy oil trade organizations recognize the public's desire for purity and as the acceptance of biocides grows less, growers are responding by trying to cut down on them, or omit them altogether.

Essential oils are tested by gas chromatography, mass-spectroscopy, thin layer chromatography and high performance liquid chromatography, which are methods used for separating essential oils (and other things) into their components parts and analyzing them. The gas chromatograph (GC) is basically a hollow column which is lined inside with a chemical resin. A tiny amount of essential oil is diluted with a solvent and injected into one end of the column and then a gas — hydrogen or helium — is forced through the column, under constant pressure, forcing the components of the essential oil to stick to the sides. The most sophisticated machines have columns that are 0.25 mm in diameter and 100 meters long. A detector at the other end identifies each component as it releases from the resin and comes to the other end of the column, the most volatile being evaporated first. Then the column is heated, releasing more components, which are likewise registered, one after the other. As they arrive at the detector, the components are burned, which causes electrical activity, which is recorded as a series of peaks on a piece of paper. The unique pattern of the peaks, showing the relative positions of the components, creates a "fingerprint" of the oil.

There are however, several problems with this, and other, methods of analysis.

As we have already noted elsewhere, each machine responds somewhat differently, and records differently, so fingerprints cannot be accurately compared one machine to another. This means that a library of characteristic fingerprint patterns has to be built up, for each machine, so there are accurate fingerprints for the tested material to be compared against. What tends to happen however, is that the fingerprint is compared to one of the set of "standard" fingerprints used as a reference by the industry, so the idiosyncrasies of each machine are not always taken into account. Also, interpreting the fingerprint is done by humans, who can have different opinions on the matter. Nevertheless, the GC can help identify adulteration of essential oils to a certain extent. For example, a common adulterant is linalol, an alcohol found in many essential oils. Linalol produced artificially contains traces of other compounds — dihydrolinalol, for example — while natural linalol does not, so if any dihydrolinalol shows up on the fingerprint, it shows the oil has been adulterated. However, it is also possible to add a naturally produced linalol, extracted from another plant, and this form of adulteration cannot be detected by this method. Once the essential oil components have been separated by the GC, there are other machines that can further help identify them, including mass spectrometers and infrared spectrometers. Essential oils contain hundreds of components and not all of them have been identified by science yet. Because of this, certain peaks on the various printouts that come from the various machines cannot be named. (It means that the complete essential oil cannot be exactly reproduced in a lab.)

If one were to apply all the known technology to an essential oil to be analyzed, although one couldn't get a *complete* picture, a fair enough picture would emerge of its age and chemical composition. This process, however, would be very expensive. What often happens instead is that a substance is tested for the main constituents that are supposed to be in it. "Eucalyptus essential oil" will be tested to see whether it has the correct proportions of eucalyptol and 1,8-cineol, for example. This doesn't tell us much about the tested material, which might even be an entirely man-made chemical composition.

The term "essential oil" can, in law, be applied to a liquid that has nothing whatsoever to do with nature. Also, bottles can be labeled "essential oil," but bear no relation to what description is given on the bottle — "tuberose absolute" could, in fact, be a mixture of other absolutes and essential oils cleverly blended to smell like tuberose. It is also possible to buy bottles labeled "aromatherapy essential oils" that have a few drops of essential oils blended in with carrier, vegetable, oils. In some cases these mislead people into thinking they are buying undiluted essential oils.

Most essential oils are distilled from the plant material, which is placed in a still and exposed to steam, forced through from below, which makes the volatile aromatic molecules detach from the plant. These rise with the steam and after condensation, turn into liquid form. At this point, the essential oil is separated from the water — as it is lighter than water — and is siphoned off the top. Citrus essential oils are produced by another method known as *expression* which involves highly sensitive machines extracting the essential oil from the rind, without using heat. In this process, whatever biocides were used on the fruits are inevitably included with the essential oils. All these aspects of cultivation and extraction have to be considered by wholesale purchasers of essential oils, who more and more are coming to the conclusion that it is better to lease your own fields, so control over growing methods can be maintained, and the biocides eliminated. Ultimately, they all know the end-user would prefer to use organically grown essential oils, and by collectively pressing this point, we, the consumers, can pressure suppliers to aim for the highest purity.

Professor George Dodd at the Olfaction Research Department at Warwick University has developed an electronic nose capable of picking up and identifying small components of aroma. Perhaps in the future this will be a tool in essential oil analysis but until then, despite all the latest technological developments in essential oil analysis, the human nose is still the most sensitive aroma-detector going, and it is sometimes still used, instead of a machine, at the receiving end of the GC column. The best way to assess an essential oil is to smell it, but, like the CG machines, each of us has to build up our own library of aromas. Obviously this takes time, but the powers of discrimination should soon build up providing you have access to pure, fresh essential oils. At the end of this book you will find the address of the Aromatherapy Trade Council who will be able to help you identify reputable suppliers.

The Art of Smelling

The professional "noses" employed by perfumers and essential oil houses go through many years of training before they are able to identify which components are in a particular product, but apparently any healthy human nose can be trained to distinguish between 10,000 different aromas. It does take experience and practice to develop a nose capable of distinguishing between essential oils, and determining the country of origin and quality of them, but one also needs to know something about the art of smelling.

Take an open bottle of essential oil, or a perfumer's smelling strip (simply a thin strip of blotting paper on which a smear of essential oil has been put) in your hand and swing it around in a circle about six inches under your nose. This creates a vortex in which the aroma molecules become "excited" and more easily detectable. Then move the bottle or strip, under your right nostril and sniff, then under your left and sniff, and then under both and sniff. When you sniff, inhale the aroma so you can feel it at the very top of your nose, then take it (visually) to the crown of your head, and through the whole body. To do this, you must have a fully conscious intent about what you're doing. Really concentrate to experience the aroma. If you do it correctly, you can feel the aroma in the back of the mouth, and feel its effect on the brain. After trying four oils, take a rest from concentrated sniffing — olfactory overload will reduce the ability to perceive accurately. The smelling strips can be used afterwards as book markers or put in drawers to fragrance clothes.

How Much?

Less is sometimes best. It is not the case that by doubling a quantity of essential oils being used, you double the effect. Also, if you are looking at a choice of formulas in a particular section and you see that the first formula has 30 drops, say, and the second has 28, and the third 26, do not assume that the one with 30 drops is the stronger. Each oil has its own potency, so fewer drops of certain oils may be required in particular formulas. Also, when essential oils are mixed with each other, an energetic potency is achieved, through the synergistic effect. If you just stick to the proportions used in any one formula, you'll be fine.

Unless you are a qualified practitioner, do not use essential oils neat (undiluted), massaged on the skin. There are a few medicinal circumstances when essential oils are used neat — lavender on a burn, for example — but this is a particular situation. There is *no need* to use essential oils neat on the skin for emotional problems, no matter how desperate

you may be feeling. Don't worry — the problem can be sorted out — just be patient and don't panic.

How Long?

There are no hard and fast rules about how long a particular formula or essential oil should be used for a particular purpose. It all depends on the person, the problem, and the root cause of that problem. For the purposes outlined in this book, try a formula or oil for a couple of days and if it doesn't work, simply switch to another.

Which Method?

There are many methods of using essential oils, as you can see from the following chart on page. When you visit an aromatherapy clinic you are most likely to be massaged — using a system *particular* to aromatherapy. A more general massage can be done at home and this is a very effective method because, as we have seen earlier, the essential oils get directly through the skin and into the body, and the aroma molecules can also be inhaled at the same time. It is thought that essential oils get into the body when they're used in baths, although in lesser quantity, through the process known as osmosis. Water molecules are too large to penetrate the skin but the molecules of essential oils are tiny and easily pass through. One also gets the benefits of the aroma molecules as they rise with the steam and are inhaled. But simply sniffing the oil directly from the bottle, from a tissue or handkerchief is also very effective. The subtle way to use essential oils is in the room methods — diffusers, candles, room sprays, water bowls, humidifiers, and heat-sources. Which method you use depends upon your degree of requirement and also the particular circumstances you happen to be in. If you're at the office, for example, it is obviously impractical to have a bath, so you can use a diffuser or simply inhale from a tissue or bottle. The diversity of methods-of-use match perfectly the diversity of situations we find ourselves in over the course of the day. Experiment.

Spoons, Bottles, and Droppers

Throughout this book I advise you to make formulas or use individual oils diluted in base oils that can be measured by spoonfuls. Spoons do vary in size so buy a set of accurate measuring spoons from a chemist, cooking store or hardware store. Generally, modern cutlery measures as follows: 1 teaspoon = 5 mls (.2 oz); 1 dessertspoon = 10 mls (.34 oz); 1 tablespoon = 15 mls (.5 oz).

You will need clean, brown glass bottles to mix your massage oils in. You can wash thoroughly and then sterilize bottles you happen to have in the house, or obtain them from any pharmacy. The volume of the bottle is usually imprinted on the base — the figures "20," "30," or "50" refer to milliliters. In this book I usually refer to formulas mixed in 30 milliliters (1 oz) of base oil, and for these you only need a bottle with 30 ml or 1 oz

capacity because the essential oil addition will not increase the volume substantially and this size of bottle is perfectly sufficient. Bottles are made so that the intended capacity, written on the base, will reach to the shoulder of the bottle, not to the neck.

If you are purchasing them, try to get round bottles because these are much easier to roll between the hands — an important component in the blending process. The bottles must be stored in a cool, dark, dry place. Keep any bottle with essential oil in it, or any essential oils, well away from homeopathic preparations because the essential oils may alter the homeopathic preparations if kept too close to them. This is the case whether the essential oils are well sealed or not. (Also, do not buy homeopathic preparations that have been kept near essential oils, or near strong smelling perfumes, soaps or other toiletries. Classical homeopathic preparations are very subtle, and are said to be adversely effected by any strong aroma).

Most essential oil bottles have a dropper in the lid. In the rim of the dropper-top there is a little hole. This should always be uppermost because it allows air in, and the drops of essential oil to come out in nice, equal drops. If you don't do this, the essential oil may not come out of the bottle or the drops will fall out in a long stream, ruin your calculations, and you'll have to start again! Some essential oils are sold without a dropper-top and this is against the guidelines of the Aromatherapy Trade Council because if children find the bottle they may drink from it. Also, of course, it makes it difficult to measure drops. However, pharmacies do sell droppers on their own, and can be used in this case. But, you'll have to have many droppers — one for each essential oil. Do not use one dropper for all your essential oils because small residues may still be left in the dropper and these will get mixed in the next time you use it.

Base or Carrier Oils for Massage

Aromatherapists use a wide range of base oils including sweet almond, apricot kernel, grapeseed, macadamia, and hazelnut oils. We also use wheat germ, avocado, carrot extract oil, borage, and evening primrose oil for certain medical conditions, and rose-hip oil for regenerative purposes. There are many other carrier oils available, from the mundane, like corn oil, to the exotic, like Monoi oil from Tahiti. And there are many other oils that have been around for some time, like cherry seed oil, kukui nut oil, kiwi seed oil, coprah oil, camellia oil, passion flower oil, and orchid oil, whose benefits are being rediscovered by aromatherapy.

Because the various benefits of these carrier oils do not directly relate to the workings of the brain (although almond oil is used in India to heighten intellectual ability), I do not intend to go into any detail on them here. A few pages of *The Complete Book of Essential Oils & Aromatherapy* have been devoted to this subject, and the interested reader may want to refer to them.

When choosing a base oil, almond is the easiest to obtain, although you could also try sunflower, safflower, or grapeseed oil. Buy the one that looks the most pure — that is to say, any one labeled "organic" — that is grown without biocides (without pesticides etc.), and/or "cold pressed" or "virgin." If you can find an oil labeled with all three, that would be perfect.

Methods of Use and Dosages

One of the great things about essential oils is that there are so many ways to use them. If you don't have a diffuser for dispersing the aroma around the room, simply put a few drops on a cotton ball and tuck it behind a hot radiator, which will heat up the aroma molecules and release them into the atmosphere. And if you don't have a radiator, you can put a few drops into a bowl of hot water, which again heats the aroma molecules and releases them into the room. If you don't have a bath, they can be used in the shower, and if you don't have time to see an aromatherapist, you can massage yourself.

The quantities recommended for use in the room methods may seem rather small, and if you prepare them and wait to experience the effect, they may seem hardly perceptible. In fact, the aroma is there but the olfactory tricks we play on ourselves make it seem that it isn't. Think of how the smell of cigarette smoke can seem completely overpowering when you walk into a smoky bar or party, and yet after a few minutes it is not so noticeable.

Likewise, with essential oils, we get used to them quickly. When you come to prepare a room method, therefore, do what has to be done and then leave the room, closing the door behind you. When you return a few minutes later you will get a much clearer idea of their true impact on the atmosphere, and you'll be better able to judge whether you have used too little or too much.

The following chart outlines the various methods, and gives the dosages you should use. Following this is another chart that gives the quantities of essential oil that should be used in various quantities of carrier oil for massage.

CHART 5:1 METHODS OF USE AND DOSAGES

Amount to Use	Method
	BATH
As directed or a maximum of 8 drops	Run the bath and then add the essential oil. Close the door so the vapor doesn't escape. Soak for at least ten minutes, relaxing and inhaling deeply through the nose. The essential oil can be diluted in a small amount of vegetable oil before being added to the bath. **Unless otherwise indicated, certain *oils* should *not* be used in baths. They are basil, cinnamon, clove, peppermint, and thyme.**
	SHOWER
As directed or a maximum of 2 drops	Wash as usual. Then put the essential oil onto a wet washcloth or sponge and rub it over yourself briskly, still standing under the hot water, inhaling deeply through the nose.
	JACUZZI
3 drops per person	Same as for bath.
	SAUNA
2 drops per 600 ml water (appx 1 pint)	Only use eucalyptus, tea tree or pine as these three enter the body with inhalation and leave by perspiration. They are excellent cleansers and detoxifiers. Mix the oil with the water beforehand and put on heat source as usual.
	TISSUE OR HANDKERCHIEF
1 drop	Just inhale when required.
	INHALED AS A VAPOR
2-3 drops	Pour hot water into a bowl and add the essential oil. Place your head over the bowl, about 10 inches away, and cover with a towel so the sides are completely closed. Eyes must be shut. Breathe deeply through the nose for about one minute.

CHART 5:1 METHODS OF USE AND DOSAGES

Amount to Use	Method

MASSAGE OIL

As directed or a maximum of 1 drop to each ml base (vegetable) oil.

See chart at end of section for complete guide of volumes to use.

Add the essential oil to the base oil: use sweet almond, hazelnut, peach kernel, grapeseed, soy, peanut, sunflower, safflower, etc. Mix in a clean, brown glass bottle — available from any pharmacist (the volume it contains should be imprinted on the base.) If using more than one essential oil, blend those in the bottle before adding the base oil. Blend essential oils into base oil by turning the bottle upside down a few times and rolling briskly between the hands. To ascertain how much to use for a body-massage, pour oil into cupped hand. The amount held there without pouring over the sides of the hand or into the finger creases is adequate. As hand size is relative to body size the amount used will vary. Generally, one dessertspoon should be sufficient. *If you have allergies* to soaps, perfumes, or cosmetics, do a skin test 24 hours before using massage oil.

WATER BOWL

1-9 drops

Room method. Pour hot water into a small bowl, add essential oil. Make sure windows and doors are closed. Allow 5-10 minutes for aroma to permeate atmosphere; replenish if required, but the aroma should not be overpowering.

DIFFUSERS

1-6 drops

Diffusers are especially designed for use with essential oils. They have a bowl section which is heated by candle flame or electricity. This bowl should be made of nonporous material so it can be wiped clean after use, ready to take a different aroma if required. Usually diffusers are made of pottery. Always put water in the bowl before adding the essential oil. Diffusers heat and release aroma molecules into the atmosphere. There is now a model which does not use a heat source — of particular interest to those with children or pets. See suppliers for details.

CANDLES

1-2 drops

Light a candle and wait for the wax to melt a little. Add the essential oil to the melted wax. Essential oils are flammable so take great care not to get them on the wick, or too near the flame.

RADIATORS

1-9 drops

Put the essential oil onto a cotton ball and lodge it either on the radiator or by the pipe — in contact with heat.

HUMIDIFIERS

1-9 drops

Add the essential oil to the water.

CHART 5:1 METHODS OF USE AND DOSAGES

Amount to Use	Method
	ROOM SPRAYS
4 or more drops per half-pint (280 ml) water	Use a new plant-sprayer. Put warm (not boiling) water in, add the essential oil and shake. Spray high in the air, and also on curtains, cloth-covered furniture and carpets. Do not spray over polished wooden furniture or velvet — as you would avoid putting water on these or other vulnerable items.
	LIGHT BULBS
4-6 drops	You can buy specially designed rings — usually made of metal or pottery — which can sit on top of a lightbulb in a table-standing lamp. They have a hollow section which can take the essential oil. Always put the ring on the lightbulb when it is turned off and cool. Take care not to spill the essential oil onto the attachment because essential oils are flammable (as well as wet).
	LOG FIRES
1 drop per log	Use pine, cypress, sandalwood, or cedarwood essential oils. Put 1 drop on each log half an hour before using, although the essential oil will still be effective if the log is used many weeks later. Three drops of essential oil per log fire is sufficient.
	SILK & PAPER FLOWERS
1 drop per flower	Simply put the essential oil onto the flowers and place in a vase. Some essential oils are colorless and have the texture of water, others have a slight color and are more viscous, so depending on which oil you use, and the color(s) of the flowers, place the essential oil on a petal, stamen, or stem.
	PILLOWS
1-3 drops per pillow or pillows	Some essential oils will leave a mark on pillows (and other cloth material) so, depending on the essential oil you use, place it directly onto the corner of a pillowcase or onto a cotton ball, which can be placed in the corner between the pillow and pillowcase. Alternatively, the cotton ball can be tucked under the pillow.
	CLOTHING
1-2 drops	Again, some essential oils are colorless and have the texture of water, others have a slight color and are more viscous. Bear this in mind when choosing the oil to use by this method. The essential oil needs to be placed where its aroma can be appreciated. If it is put on the cuff, it can be smelt easily when required. If it is put on a collar, the aroma will rise to the nose over the course of the day (or evening).

CHART 5:1 METHODS OF USE AND DOSAGES

Amount to Use	Method
*	**PERFUME** Essential oils can be used as a perfume. For the purposes outlined in this book, they can be diluted either in jojoba oil or vodka (alcohol). Use one third volume essential oil to two thirds *either* jojoba or vodka. If it's in vodka, it can be further diluted in 50% water. The bottle can also simply be opened and sniffed from when required.
*	**JEWELRY** With the rise in interest in aromatherapy, more manufacturers are producing neck pendants and even earrings in the shape of a little bottle — designed to hold perfume or essential oils. The bottle can be opened at any time and sniffed.
10-15 drops per 50 mls or 1.7 oz	**LOTIONS AND CREAMS** Essential oils can be added to prepackaged lotions and creams or you can make up your own (see *The Complete Book of Essential Oils and Aromatherapy*). If adding to a prepackaged product, it must be perfume free. Buy the simplest, purest product you can find. Pots: add the essential oil and stir. Bottles: empty the contents into a bowl, add the essential oil, mix and replace in the bottle.

ESSENTIAL OIL FORMULAS USED IN CHAPTERS 7 AND 8

All the blends used in this book are in the amounts one would expect to use for initial clinical aromatherapy bodywork (i.e., 5% dilution). However, there are those who may wish to use smaller amounts of essential oil. This can be done simply and effectively by halving the number of drops in the formulas while keeping to the correct proportions, and using the same amount of base oil specified in the blends. By using lower amounts of essential oils it is often the case that one must use the blend more often and for a longer period of time.

CHART 5:2 BLENDING ESSENTIAL OILS WITH BASE
OR CARRIER OILS — QUANTITIES TO USE

Number of drops of essential oils to use: Blend the number of essential oils on the left into the volume of base oil on the right.

Essential Oils   **Vegetable Oil**

MIN to MAX drops	Per ml.	teaspoons	dessertspoons	tablespoons
1/2 - 1	1	1	-	-
1 - 5	5	1	1	1
2 - 10	10	2	1	1
3 - 15	15	3	1	1
4 - 20	20	4	2	1
5 - 25	25	5	2	1
6 - 30	30	6	3	2

These are the minimum and maximum quantities that should be used, unless otherwise stated in formulas or blends mentioned elsewhere.

When buying essential oils it is useful to know how many drops there are in a bottle. These can only be approximations because droppers do vary slightly. Here is a guide:

1ml (0.035 oz) essential oil = 20 drops   2ml (0.07 oz) essential oil = 40 drops
5ml (0.175 oz) essential oil = 100 drops   10ml (0.35 oz) essential oil = 200 drops

Many of the expensive essential oils and absolutes are sold in 2.5 ml to 5 ml bottles. Most essential oils are sold in 10 ml quantity.

PREGNANT OR LACTATING WOMEN

should always use the minimum quantity of essential oil stated here, and reduce the number of essential oils used in formulas or blends by half. Please also see page 402 for the list of oils you should not use at all during pregnancy or while lactating.

PEOPLE ON MEDICATION

For all methods, use up to half the maximum recommended dosages. If you are using them as medicines, inform your doctor. If using homeo-pathic medicines, inform your homeopath. It is thought that essential oil use may negate the effect of homeopathy.

TRANQUILIZER ADDICTION

During addiction all essential oil dosages should be half the maximum general dosage.

SUBSTANCE ADDICTION

During addiction all essential oil dosages should be half the maximum general dosage.

ALCOHOLISM

When using alcohol to excess all essential oil dosages should be half the maximum general dosage.

CHRONIC OR LONG-TERM CONDITIONS

Use formulations at half the minimum to maximum strengths.

Blending and Mixing

The very fact that you can smell the aroma of essential oils being used as a massage oil proves the point that they evaporate. Indeed, *most* of the essential oils being used will evaporate before they have a chance to penetrate the skin. For this reason it is wasteful to mix essential oils in an open bowl. (The essential oils start to oxidize on contact with air so it is also wasteful to leave the bottle of essential oil open while treating yourself or others.) These factors have been taken into consideration in the formulas and volumes suggested in this book for home use and if you follow the guidelines above sufficient quantities will be absorbed.

HOW TO MAKE A DILUTED OIL USING MORE THAN ONE ESSENTIAL OIL.

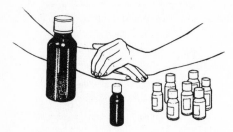

1. **Collect the things you will be using: essential oils, empty bottle, and base (vegetable carrier) oil.**

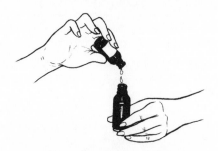

2. **Drop the various essential oils into the empty bottle. Put the top back on and roll the bottle between your hands to thoroughly blend the essential oil molecules together.**

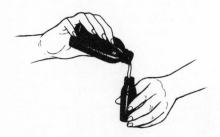

3. **Then add the base oil to just above the level of the bottle's "shoulder."**

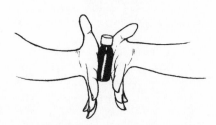

4. **Put the top on the bottle and roll between the hands vigorously to thoroughly mix the essential oil and base oil together.**

HOW TO MAKE A SYNERGISTIC BLEND CONCENTRATE OF ESSENTIAL

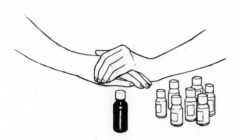

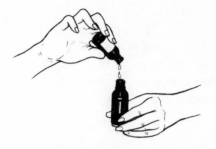

1. Collect the things you will be using: essential oils and small, empty brown bottle.

2. Put the required number of essential oils into the empty bottle, starting with the more viscous essential oils first.

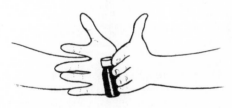

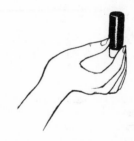

3. Put the top on the bottle and roll well between your hands to thoroughly blend the essential oil molecules together.

4. Turn bottle upside down.

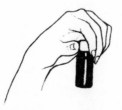

5. Turn bottle right way up.

USING ONE ESSENTIAL OIL IN A MASSAGE OIL.

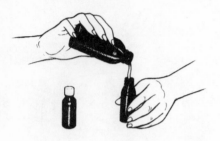

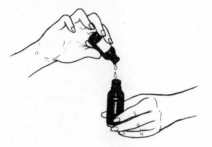

1. Pour the base oil into your empty brown bottle so it reaches to the "shoulder."

2. Add the essential oil.

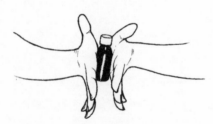

3. Put the top on the bottle and roll between the hands vigorously to thoroughly mix the essential oil and base oil together.

CHAPTER 6

HOW TO GET THROUGH LIFE IN ONE PIECE

Someone somewhere once said, "Life's a bitch and then you die!" I'm not sure it's quite that bad, but it does have its moments. I think we can all agree that if you can get through it in one piece with your sanity intact, you're doing okay. In this chapter, I discuss a few areas of particular stress in which essential oils can help: education, offices, industry, farming, plane and car travel, the police, and prison services.

Schools and Colleges

Essential oils can play several roles in helping us get through the education process — happily, confidently, efficiently, and healthily. To a large extent, of course, just how well we perform within the education system depends on factors we can't control. If we come from a family of ten

children and live in a small overcrowded apartment, it's going to be more difficult to find the peace and quiet needed to study, and our parents will have less time to apportion to each of us when it comes to helping with homework. Essential oils can't do much about that. What they can do in a general sense is help us maintain good health so we don't have to take time off. If we catch the "flu" and miss school for three weeks, that can be a setback that is difficult to recover from. Physical health, however, is not the subject of this book and I have covered quite a bit that could be said on that subject in another publication, *The Complete Book of Essential Oils & Aromatherapy*. But the other factors — happiness, confidence, and efficiency — are certainly things that essential oils can also help with.

Again, in a general sense, the mood we are in when we arrive at school or college goes a long way to determining how we approach the material being supplied to us, and how we absorb it. In the next chapter there are many formulas and suggested essential oils that will help you to overcome the negativity that prevents us from performing to our maximum potential. Included among these, for example, is enhanced confidence, which can help if you're on the receiving end of bullying, as it can help when you're sitting in a classroom of thirty people who are listening to every word you say, and every mistake you make.

Of course the main objective of education is to fill your head with as many facts as possible, in a way that you'll be able to remember them later — in an exam, or in the work situation. This is very much a matter of memory, an area in which essential oils are well known to be very helpful. It also depends on the teachers being in a frame of mind best suited for the communication of ideas. Essential oils used in the staff room can help here too. Then, there is the larger environment, the buildings themselves, in which everyone has to operate for a large portion of the week. As we shall see, essential oils can have a beneficial effect on this in various ways, not least in the control of infections. If one person comes into the building with the "flu" a week before exam time, with the domino effect, by the time the big day arrives half the school or college — both student and staff — could be out of action. Even during other times in the term, lost time still has to be made up — only putting more pressure on everyone concerned.

Memory Enhancement, Mental Clarity, and Efficiency

As we saw in Chapter Two in *The Sense of Smell*, when an aroma molecule hits the olfaction receptors on the cilia of the olfactory bulbs, they are actually connecting with a part of the brain. The olfactory bulbs are embedded in the "limbic system," a part of the brain that deals with, among other things, memory. Usually we experience this connection *passively*, when an aroma reminds us of something that happened in the past. In aromatherapy we use this connection in an *active* way, by stimulating the memory to recall information we previously studied.

Basically, what happens is this: while you study, and your mind is absorbing information, you use a particular essential oil nearby — in a diffuser or on a tissue or hankie that you can occasionally sniff. The information then becomes associated with this particular aroma. When the exam comes along, you use that same aroma nearby — this time not in a diffuser, but again, on a tissue or handkerchief. You can discreetly sniff the aroma, an action that transports you back to the time when you were studying, and this helps your memory recall the information. There are several rules to follow in this process:

1. Try to use a fragrance you have never used before because an aroma used previously may have associations that probably have nothing to do with the subject being absorbed. Or make a

unique formula especially for each subject.

2. If possible use one fragrance (or formula) per subject, and then not too much.

3. Only inhale the aroma when you need to remember the studied information — in a test or exam for example, and not at other times. If you use it all the time, your memory will get confused. Be very precise about this.

4. Be discreet. There are no rules, as far as I know, forbidding the use of essential oils during exams, but it could be construed as an unfair advantage.

5. Do not rely solely on this method. The aroma-memory connection is meant to be an additional aid, not a replacement for hard work. Don't just scan your text books expecting everything to magically sink in. Sorry, it's not that easy. You'll have to put the time in and read your material thoroughly, and check with your teachers that you have understood it.

The memory has a horrible habit of slipping away. You can listen to a general knowledge quiz on TV, merrily shouting out the answers but, if you were actually in the studio, in front of TV cameras and glaring lights, aware that millions of people were watching, that same information you know, slips away. You go blank! Essential oils won't make you remember things you simply don't know, but they'll help you bridge the gap between knowledge and recall. This advantage can be the difference between pass and fail. As I have said, you can use any essential oil to do this but good choices, for example, would be Basil, Bergamot, Lemon, or Rosemary — or a blend of two or more of these. Basil gives the mind tremendous clarity while Bergamot is terrific for giving confidence. Rosemary is renowned for memory and Lemon is great for concentration.

Years ago I heard a young man being interviewed over the radio. He'd just passed fifteen "O" levels in that school year — the highest number passed in Britain by one student. The interviewer asked him how he'd done it. Apparently, he'd put a tall pile of books and papers relating to all his homework on his right, on the desk, and took the first book off the pile, opened it, and worked at it until he got to the point where he couldn't continue. Without wasting time worrying about his inability to finish, he moved that book to the left of him. He then took the next book/papers and carried on with them until he got stuck, immediately putting them to the left, and so on. So he worked through the pile on the right, actually finishing a couple of homework projects, leaving him with the pile on the left. He moved the whole lot to the right, and continued the process again. By the time he'd gone through this process a few times, he was left with a couple of subjects he was truly stuck on and the next day he referred to the teachers for help. The point was, when he came to look at the sticky subjects, either on the second look, the third or fourth or fifth, his mind could approach them slightly differently — the "lateral thinking" effect I suppose it would be called — and on these subsequent looks he could grasp the point, solve the problem, or whatever. When you're completely overburdened (as I have been myself on occasion) his advice comes in very handy. Try it.

The Staff Room

Trying to keep thirty and more children under control and actively engaged in useful activity is a very hard task, and I take my hat off to all those who do it. Using essential oils in the staff room should be directed at reducing the "frazzled" element in the day by creating a little peaceful haven where teachers can relax and re-charge their batteries. With the agreement of all those concerned, I suggest using the relaxing and calming essential oils in a diffuser. The relevant oils are listed in the main chart at the back of this book.

Also, because the staff room is an enclosed space, it is the perfect environment for the transmission of germs, especially those that cause coughs, colds, and flu. Essential oils used in a diffuser can prevent infection spreading, if they are of the antibacterial and/or antiviral type. I would suggest using eucalyptus, rosemary, thyme, clove, cinnamon, or, especially in times of major flu epidemic, a special mixture called "Dermatect" (see *Suppliers* on page 405).

The School Buildings and Halls of Residence

In Japan large offices are using essential oils diffused throughout the building to enhance efficiency and create a relaxing environment. Different aromas are used at different times of the day to create different moods (see *Aroma-Psychology*, page 51) and there's no reason why this principle shouldn't be applied to education facilities. For a stimulating effect, especially after lunch when everyone is feeling a bit deflated and needs a little boost, I suggest using one of the citrus essential oils — lemon or grapefruit, lemon eucalyptus (E citriodora), or a light floral. These would not be irritating, and most children like them. The aroma should not be overpowering, but barely perceptible.

Leaving home for the first time to go to university or college can be stressful, if liberating. Everything is new — the place, the people, the home, and the work. The temptations to go out every night and socialize are powerful, and while there is no harm in it, that's only so long as it doesn't blind you from the object of the exercise — study. Central to study is the ability to concentrate — to focus your mind — and essential oils are useful in this. What you can do is use one oil or a special blend of oils in your room at the halls of residence or in your digs, as an environmental cue that "this is my study time." Set the scene: arrange your desk, make your coffee, and try to forget what happened at the bar last night, what dramas and gossip are still cluttering up your brain. Then light your diffuser, or arrange whatever room method you're going to use, add the essential oils, and say to yourself, "now I'm going to concentrate on this" — and do it! Having an aroma around can focus your mind on the task at hand — pull you in, as it were.

Offices

Today offices are more stressed out than they ever were, with the threat of redundancy hanging over everyone and new technology buzzing away all day. As we all know, work-related stress is a major problem for this country, as for others, and the number of days lost through it costs every company a small fortune. Some of the more forward-thinking companies employ in-house aromatherapists who give treatments to stressed-out executives and other personnel. When an executive is earning $100,000 a year, you can see the financial logic of doing what you can to make sure he or she is actually sitting behind their desk every day, and not lying in bed suffering from stress-related disorders. However, there is no joy in anyone being ill, and no advantage in it as companies more and more keep a tight check on the number of days taken off for illness. Being ill these days can easily loose you your job. It makes sense then, all around, to employ the benefits of essential oils in the workplace.

The crucial thing to bear in mind about essential oils is that people have different reactions to aromas. Because of the memory connection, someone might have a negative association with one particular aroma, for a multitude of reasons. You have no way of knowing which aromas may cause a bad reaction, and to whom. For this reason, if you share an office, you must get the agreement of all concerned before putting a diffuser on your desk, which will, of course, let the aroma into an area extending beyond the confines of your desk. Bring several aromas into the office for everyone to sniff before actually using them in the shared space. As there are so many essential oils to choose from, it should be easy to find something that suits everyone and still does something positive for you. If you have your own office, obviously you can use whichever oil you like.

Which particular oils you use rather depends on the situation. If there's a bad flu making the rounds then use something that is antiviral and protective. If you are under constant pressure, use something relaxing, and if you've got a rush job, use something stimulating. As we have already seen in the chapter entitled *Aroma-Psychology*, essential oils have been shown to reduce keyboard errors significantly. You will find information as to which oils to use Chapter 8, *The A-Z of Emotional Problems,* and also in the large chart at the end of the book, but you may consider grapefruit or eucalyptus lemon (*E citriodora*) to combat lethargy, and basil, cardamom, or bergamot to help concentration. Stale air is another problem in offices, and I'd suggest to combat this: lemon, lavender, rosemary, grapefruit, eucalyptus lemon, or cypress.

If you work in sales, you should really be aware of the recent work into the affect of aroma on clients, as discussed in *Retail Outlets* in the chapter *Aroma-Psychology*. As researcher Dr. Hirsch says, "odorants are potentially more efficacious than any other modality in increasing sales ability of consumer products." The thing about aroma is that it's subtle — it can work on the subconscious — and people can be favorably impressed without even knowing why. This dynamic can be used in all sorts of ways. Essential oils can be diffused through the atmosphere when you show clients your latest products and they can be used to infuse brochures and other paperwork with an aromatic impact. Light florals have been shown to be particularly effective.

Industry

All the problems and solutions discussed above are relevant for industry in general, and as time goes on, with everyone looking for things to give them the market edge, aroma is being used more and more. The process known as "micro-encapsulation," best known for the "scratch and sniff" perfume samples we find in our magazines, is shortly going to arrive on supermarket shelves. Your bleach container will be micro-encapsulated with the aroma of the bleach inside, and released when you pick up the product from the shelf and squeeze that area with your hand. In five years time we'll probably be able to walk into huge supermarkets and find the toiletries department or the coffee shelf simply by following our noses — there's going to be a major aromatic experience in-store!

Aromatherapy works in a different way. It's not about informing you of the aroma inside a bottle before you open the

top. It's about convincing the customer, subliminally, that your product is best, and your product doesn't have to have any aroma whatsoever — although, as Dr. Hirsch showed in Chicago, if it does, it's more likely to sell, and at a higher price.

Companies spend a fortune sending out catalogs and promotional literature — and much of it ends up in the trash, so anything you can do to make sales literature more appealing has got to be a help. It's been shown in various trials that people will linger longer when a pleasant aroma is in the atmosphere. So, if there's a pleasant aroma on your paperwork it stands a better chance of lingering on your potential customer's desk. Essential oils can do better than this, however. Certain essential oils instill confidence. Now think of the possibilities. The client gets your brochure and for some reason unbeknownst to them, feels compelled to keep it out on the desk; and for some reason (unbeknownst to them) they feel confident when they pick it up. "Let's use this company," they say, "I have a good feeling about it . . ." and you're half-way there.

To make brochures and other paperwork aromatic, simply drop some essential oil on the cardboard box in which they're packed, then wrap the box in a black plastic garbage bag for at least 24 hours. Keep it closed, of course. The aroma will permeate the box and, eventually, the papers inside. Although the aroma may seem hardly perceptible, especially when it's gone through the postal system, remember that aroma works subliminally — it doesn't *have* to be perceptible. As an experiment, aromatize one box of catalogs and keep another unaromatized box for a control. It's no good using a floral essential oil if your firm doesn't want to project a feminine image so choose something that reflects confidence and prosperity. In this case, I'd suggest using cardamom, petitgrain, coriander, lemon, or bergamot. When you send both boxes of brochures out, keep a record of which potential customers each type of brochure was sent to, and see which brochure — aromatic or not — produces the most inquiries. What have you got to loose? I'll tell you — sales!

In the future I'm sure we're going to see aroma used in many more subtle ways. Already, fragrance houses produce "corporate aromas" for clients who use it in their customer waiting rooms and on their paperwork. If, let's say, there is an element of lemon in that corporate aroma, each time a customer smells lemon (in other contexts) they will be reminded of the company. Now that's clever. If you can get your potential customers to think about you when they're cooking dinner, out at a restaurant, walking through a market, or washing their hands with a lemon-scented bar of soap, you are really in their mind — where you want to be.

Smart corporations have already grasped the fact that aroma can be diffused into their offices to make their workers relax when they come in at 9 a.m. after struggling through the rush-hour, or perk up after lunch. Errors on keyboards are reduced with aroma, customers are relaxed, sales staff made more confident, and illness is reduced by pumping antimicrobial essential oils into the air conditioning system. All this is happening now throughout the world. Factory floors may seem difficult to aromatize in this way because the floor areas are usually so large, and the ceilings so high. There are commercial diffuser systems, however, that can get around these problems so workers on factory floors can also reap the benefits of essential oils. Some factory jobs are very tedious and if you drift off to sleep after lunch while on an assembly line, you could loose your hand, as well as your job. Accidents at work are often caused by a moment's loss of concentration and anything that can be done to reduce them has got to be a good thing.

Farming

The growing interest in aromatherapy is creating a greater demand for essential oils, but meanwhile farmers in Europe are being paid subsidies by the European Community (EC) to let their fields lie idle. It doesn't make sense. British growing conditions are ideal for certain species of plants that essential oils are extracted from, including chamomile roman, lavender, clary-sage, sage, rosemary, peppermint, spearmint, rose, melissa, marjoram, and thyme. We also need base oils, which are distilled from borage and evening primrose, just for example. Some of these plants grow so fast one would hardly have to do much to propagate them — such as melissa and borage — while others are easily propagated from cuttings, such as lavender and rosemary. The seeds of some species, such as chamomile roman, are harvested simply by putting bags over their heads at the right time of year.

The growing demand now is for oils distilled from organically grown plants, and if farmers turned their attention to this method of farming, I'm sure they could easily find a market. Indeed, it would help all of us if farmers approached essential oil distributors directly and asked if they'd like to lease their fields for this use, with the farmers doing the work required. It would cut out the middlemen and reduce prices, give the essential oil company a guaranteed source of supply and the farmers a guaranteed buyer. As I have discussed in *The Complete Book of Essential Oils & Aromatherapy*, the system of inter-cropping known as companion gardening can easily be applied to essential oil production and it does away with the need for biocides — pesticides, herbicides and fungicides — that damage the environment. It can't be very pleasant being a farmer when you're obliged to use these products because the food seed companies (which are now owned by chemical companies) engineer food plants so they *require* certain chemicals, (which are supplied, of course, by the chemical companies).

Essential oil production is a very environmentally friendly occupation. Not only is there no need to use biocides, the unrequired and dried part of the plant can be used to fuel the fire in the still. The ashes can go back onto the land, as fertilizer. Stills in Egypt are cleaned using dried basil, followed by lots of water, and that basil is also grown on the land — again, no need to buy expensive, environmentally unfriendly, chemical cleaning solutions. In many parts of the world farmers club together and buy a still as a cooperative. They share it, so the initial financial outlay is not too great. All in all, essential oil production is a very viable alternative to the production of foodstuffs when the market doesn't require it. Plus, the farmers would be producing something that does everyone so much good.

Planes and Car Travel

If you travel in *Virgin Airways* "Upper Class" you can stop off at the "Club House" at Heathrow airport and get an aromatherapy treatment. On selected flights they also provide "Upper Class" passengers with in-flight beauty therapists who can give an aromatherapy neck and scalp massage, as well as a manicure. They're also looking into the possibility of providing essential oil-impregnated pillows, which, on request, can be given to those who'd like to sleep, helped along by the relaxing properties of the chosen essential oils. Next time you detect a delicious aroma coming from the Upper Class section, you'll know how the other half live! Passengers in "First Class" or "Club Class" on *British Airways* flights, meanwhile, are given, along with other goodies, miniature aromatherapy products — rehydration face and hand gel and rosewater face spray. Aromatherapy has clearly taken off.

Flying is a very stressful experience for some people — so much so that they simply won't do it. This is a major nuisance if you dream of going to visit relatives in Australia. Airlines fully appreciate this and would, if it were practical, diffuse relaxing essential oils into the atmosphere. They are certainly aware of their potential, but the problem is that each person has a unique reaction to aromas and there is no way of anticipating which aroma might bring back unpleasant memories for one or more passengers. On an individual basis, however, the stress and anxiety related to air travel can be alleviated by having a relaxing essential oil bath or shower before leaving for the airport, and take with you a tissue or handkerchief that can be taken from your pocket and inhaled when required. I would suggest you use one of the following oils singly or in a combination of your choice: marjoram, lavender, clary-sage, bergamot, ormenis flower (chamomile maroc), chamomile roman, nutmeg, or the more expensive linden blossom. Although by all means use any essential oil or combination that you have previously found relaxing. I find the combination of clary-sage, marjoram, and lavender particularly effective. Bear in mind though that you are in an enclosed space with other people so don't wave your hankie around the place. Just keep it in your pocket and take it out and hold it to your nose as and when required.

When traveling by car, as a driver or passenger, you definitely don't want to use essential oils that are going to make you feel relaxed — and make the driver fall asleep at the wheel. Avoid lavender essential oils and other relaxing oils that could slow down reactions. Yet, driving is a stressful experience, especially in traffic jams and there are essential oils that can help deal with this while, at the same time, keeping you alert. The only essential oils that should be used in cars are peppermint, lemon, lime, grapefruit, cypress, bergamot, juniper, rosemary, petitgrain, eucalyptus lemon (*E citriodora*), and eucalyptus peppermint (*E piperata*).

The Police and Prisons

Nobody goes into police stations or prisons for fun. Police stations are places you go to when you've been robbed, raped, or mugged, and if you go to a prison it's because you or somebody you know has (allegedly) been naughty. To say they are stressful environments would be an understatement, perhaps especially for the people who have to work in them day after day. In Essex, England the police are regular clients of aromatherapists, who try to relieve the stress associated with being on alert all day and having to deal with some very nasty characters. Indeed, the police forces need to have special counselors to help police officers come to terms with some of the unpleasant experiences they go through in their job, which in point of fact, put them in life-threatening situations on a regular basis. When you're a police officer, the unexpected is to be expected and if you don't keep your wits about you, you could easily end up dead. On top of that, you have an enormous amount of paperwork to deal with. Stressful? Yes!

I know of at least one police counselor who has trained as an aromatherapist, and gives officers massages as they recount the dramas of their day. I hope in the future there will be more trained aromatherapists within the police service. I also know of successful businessmen who have regular aromatherapy treatments to alleviate their different kind of stress — like doing deals that could make them a million or lose them a million. Keeping your nerve can take several forms!

Precisely because police stations are stressful environments, they would be ideal candidates for the benefits of essential oils. Lavender would be inappropriate in police personnel areas because officers need to be alert, but lemon or grapefruit would take the edge off things when a whole pile of paperwork is looming after a hard night on the beat. The waiting room, on the other hand, where distressed victims of crime wait to be seen would be far more pleasant environments if anxiety relieving essential oils were gently diffused in the atmosphere. You could try lavender, bergamot, geranium or clary sage. These same oils could be used in interview rooms where victims are required to recount their unpleasant experiences, sometimes for hours on end. This gruesome procedure, on top of the crime itself, is a tortuous nightmare, often carried out when the victim is extremely tired, both physically and emotionally, and I know if it were me, I'd find the essential oils a tremendous help.

There was, unfortunately, a time not so long ago when rape victims were made to feel the guilty party — by the police as well as by the courts and society at large. Today police authorities make an effort to make the victim feel more relaxed, even to the extent of creating less institutional environments in which the victim will be seen by the doctor, be interviewed, and counseled. Because the day a woman is raped will probably be the most traumatic and terrifying day of her life, it is extremely important to take a sensitive approach to the use of essential oils. The woman *must* be given a choice in the matter. For one thing, by using a particular essential oil, no matter how relaxing she may find it at the time, it may in the future be associated with this horrific event. Some women may prefer to go through the interview and counseling procedure without essential oils being diffused in the atmosphere for the simple reason that they don't want the aroma to be negatively associated. Yet, essential oils can help alleviate stress, give courage and, moreover, give a gentle air of femininity and humanity to what is an otherwise crude and inhuman experience. Therefore, if essential oils are to be used in a rape counseling environment, they must be placed openly where the woman can see them, she must be given a choice of oils and, above all, the choice of whether she wants them used at all. When I acted as a victim supporter on one occasion we used essential oils that helped the victim be open and expressive about the experience. She found this invaluable, especially in the long term.

As for the criminals, there are no essential oils which will make them spill the beans, although research is currently being carried out into aromas that can break down resistance. The police cells, however, are another matter. The enclosed space is enough to drive anyone to distraction and, even though belts and shoelaces are taken away, people do hang themselves or somehow kill themselves. Others just scream and shout all night or throw themselves against the wall — all of which helps no one. An essential oil like lavender, gently diffused in this environment would help to keep everyone calm and quiet.

Essential oils used in prisons to keep prisoners calm and less violent seems a better option than giving them drugs. What essential oils do is give a positive attitude. They don't just numb, they bring out the best in people. Anyone who is in prison needs all the positivity they can get, to get through the experience and consider their future role in life. Prisons today are overcrowded not only with lawbreakers but with people who have been released from mental institutions and, basically, have nowhere to go. Any prison doctor will tell you they are their most serious problem. Now, consider what it's like to be locked up with a whole load of people who are basically off the rails — it's enough to drive you crazy yourself. Aside from relocating those who really shouldn't be there, those who are in charge of our prisons should seriously consider using essential oils to diffuse this situation. They could start with prisons for women because the prisoners, being female, will have less resistance to essential oils — which may be perceived by some men as "feminine."

———

CHAPTER 7

EMOTIONAL HEALING

"A journey of a thousand miles must begin with a single step."

– LAO TSE
Chinese Proverb

Introduction

The brain drives everything: Every word is projected from it, every mood emanates from it, and every feeling passes through the brain at some point. But the brain and body are one, they work together all the time, part of the same system. The brain says "get up" and the legs swing out of bed. But, also, as discussed in Chapter 3, *The Modern Mind*, there are receptors throughout the body that are directly connected with chemicals we also find in the brain. It is no longer possible to discuss neurology, immunology, and endo-

crinology as three different fields because they are all related, like bits of a telephone system. You can't have one without the other. Psychoneuroimmunologists are now telling us that, scientifically, body and brain are one and the same.

What happens in the brain decides whether you're going to be happy or sad; it decides whether life is worth living or not. But we are very passive about the brain, we don't pay much attention to our emotions until something goes wrong. We don't take our brain to the emotional gym for a workout, like we exercise our body to feel fit and stay well. But, with a strong mind, we can do anything, even cure disease in our own body. With a weak mind, we can't do a thing. Some people do, of course, control their brain, or at least attend to its well-being: meditation, yoga, and tai chi are just three practices that are carried out by millions of people each day around the world. And no doubt it has a beneficial effect on the emotions of them all. Other people go to counseling or therapy of some sort, and clearly this is extremely helpful to many people. Essential oils have a different approach, which is clearly complementary to the others: to help a person obtain emotional equilibrium — allowing happiness and joy, our birthright, to come out. Essential oils are facilitators, balancers and, at the risk of sounding poetic, drops of pure positivity. They can put the sparkle back into life.

Essential oils are a chest of goodies you can dip into at any time. Got a tough interview ahead? Just put a drop of bergamot on a tissue and take a deep sniff before you go in. Feeling really vulnerable but got to get through the day as usual? Sniff some Rose Otto — it will help. Just want to feel bright and on top of it today? Have a grapefruit shower. The variety of essential oils are there to dip into, for a variety of different emotions and feelings, a rich treasury courtesy of mother nature.

The first part of this chapter explains how essential oils can help us keep in tip-top emotional condition, under the headings *Alertness, Assertiveness, Concentration, Confidence, Contentment, Creativity, Focus, Happiness, Joy, Memory Enhancement*, etc. Then comes a much larger section, concerned with the negative emotions that exist in this world, *The A-Z of Emotional Problems*. Under "A," for example, you'll find *Abuse, Addictions, Aggression, Amnesia, Anger, Anxiety*, and *Apathy*. There are so many entries under this negative emotion section because there are so many problems out there in the world, and at home. And, as we need all the help we can get, in Chapter 9, *Taking Control,* I briefly discuss *Autogenic Training, Breathing, Massage, Meditation, Relaxation*, and *Visualization*.

In an ideal world, happiness would be the norm. We'd all go around smiling. As it is, we sit on the train each morning with our heads hung low, like everyone else. There is so much to worry about. Rapists stalk the street; jobs can disappear; people get ill; and war is ubiquitous. And here comes the mailman with another bill in his hand. How is one supposed to find happiness in all this? Ironically, it is those who have been through a near-death experience who usually have the answer to this question, and we read their stories in magazines and newspapers every day. For example, there's the man who had a heart attack and realized he was wasting time taking an antagonistic approach to people close to him. He realized he loved them, and that they were more important than his job. From that moment he lived life to the fullest; before he walked around saying, "How is one supposed to find the happiness in all this?" Now he knew, you look to your loved ones, and treat them right. That is happiness.

Love is the most important formula we have for solving problems — it dissolves them away like mist in the sun. Love is an energy that radiates from every person, young and old, and lifts the darkness. It is instinctive, the blossoming flower within, the opener of hearts, the bringer of joy. The vibration of love is the greatest gift we can bring to this life, if we contribute a good share of that, our life has purpose. Ideally, none of us would be emotionally damaged in our youth, and our hearts would be open to love — love of our neighbor as well as our family and friends. But it is not an ideal world and many of us arrive in it damaged in some way. Essential oils can help a person recognize and repair this damage, allowing the love to recover and strengthen the soul.

The problem with love, of course, is that it opens us up to emotional pain. To love is to hurt. Children are hurt by the parents they love and children hurt parents in return. Lovers hurt each other, with a careless word or more. We are all vulnerable to pain and sometimes we hurt. That is unfortunate, but our pain is not unique, it is a part of the human heritage, something we know and, to a certain extent, something essential oils can help deal with. They can assist us as we repair the damage and get back on our feet. Being alive is to feel — to feel sad watching a sad movie, or feel a rush of adrenaline with fear. These are the feelings of life, they are to be expected now and again. But to be overcome with a negative feeling a lot of the time is not good.

We seem to have gotten in a mind-set that says, "being miserable is normal, life is so hard, if only I had this or that I'd be happy." Happiness is like the butterfly we never quite catch. But being happy is normal — it's normal to babies and children, and normal to many poor people and rich people, around the world. What is it exactly that stops us, too, from being happy? I don't think it is the number and severity of life's knocks that make the difference. From my experience of people, it's the attitude they take toward life. Those who realize that life is short and precious see the good things in life — of which there are many. Each day people set off to do volunteer work for people less fortunate than themselves, in terms of money, physical health, or whatever. Each day people pull out their check books and send money to charity. We all do each other "favors" all the time. If we can see this as the norm — people being kind, people showing love, life going on, then the bad episodes can be put in perspective — small windows in the long wall of happy normality.

It does sometimes seem indulgent to think about oneself and do something for oneself, and it might seem altogether easier to use essential oils, for example, to help make a friend feel better. Ourselves, we forget. But we deserve attention too. The fact is, we are born alone and shall die alone, and must take care of ourselves in between. Only we can find the purpose of our lives; only we can make sense of it. We have the right to deal with problems in our own way. If that involves sitting on a sofa for three weeks, hugging a cushion and crying, so be it. If that involves three weeks of cleaning the house from top to bottom, so be it. Just be yourself, and you will be beautiful. Indulge yourself, be good to yourself — it is not a crime. You could say it's your *responsibility* to make yourself happy, because when you're happy, those around you are too.

It helps to have a philosophy of life, and some people have religion. But anyone can have a reverence for the beauty of nature — the design of a flower, the call of the birds, the wind in the trees, or the moving shadows of clouds on a hill. How magnificent it all is, there, a constant reminder of the beauty in life. And nature is full of surprises, and lessons too. I remember one day driving in Europe — a long and tiring haul toward a destination and meeting I didn't want to reach — fed up, when I saw a huge, perfect rainbow ending right there, in the grass between the road and a wooded area. I pulled the car over and leapt out, looking up at the huge miracle reaching across the sky above me. It was so close and real I could jump into it, I thought, and I did. But the rainbow moved away, again and again, and then I realized that rewards are not the goal — if one seeks the ultimate, it will elude you. The reward is life itself, in its richness, in its sadness, and joy. Humbled, but happier, I continued my journey and did what I had to do.

All experience is good because that is the truth, the reality of our life. We must embrace it and make it work for us, transmute the bad experiences into lessons for the future, wisdom for our soul, compassion for others, and understanding for the world. Good experiences are the sugar on the porridge, the bit that makes life sweet. But it is all real, and there is purpose in it all, even if we cannot see it now.

If we could expect nothing more than to be happy, we would be happy. But we expect too much. Some of the happiest people I know have nothing, or have lived and worked among people who have nothing. Every small thing then becomes a gift, not an expectation. Let us stop and thank our lucky stars for what we do have, for the people we love (and tell them), for our humble home, our memories. We can't expect to go through the hurdle race of life without getting a few knocks — that's what it's about. All we can do is appreciate the people around us, be kind to them and ourselves, and hang on tight during the rough patches. Essential oils appreciate the drama of life — they have been there, so to speak, they are part of it. We're all in this together, and essential oils are there to help.

It is our birthright to be spontaneous, joyful, confident, loving, trusting and free — free in mind and spirit, free to soar, create, and laugh. And it is our human responsibility to be compassionate, sympathetic, and aware. Deep inside us, there is a spiritual connection that we can find if we just stand still long enough, and quietly absorb. That spiritual connection is the reference point we should take as "normality," that quiet, reassuring wholeness, more soothing than mother's breast. If this could be our normality, rather than "depressed," "anxious," or "stressed," how much happier our lives would be. It is not a question of how many knocks one has, because those who have had more than anyone are often the first to say that the knocks are not what's important — the good is what we should focus on.

The mind comes with certain gifts — like intuition. Our intuition says of someone, "not aura friendly" — so we keep away, to protect ourselves. Our mind gives us individuality, to approach things our own unique way. That is good. By contrast, co-dependency, relying on others for gratification, a form of vicarious living, is a bit of a cop-out, like hitching a lift through life on the back of somebody else's truck. Patience is a gift we often ignore and even feel contempt for, calling it passivity. But impatience causes frustration and anger. Patience is the better quality, along with positivity, hope, enthusiasm, and the capacity for enjoyment. These are the gifts within us that essential oils seek to bring out, philosophically, deeply, naturally. And, by seeking a solution to our problems, we show our awareness — that we are alive and kicking, confident and optimistic.

Positive Mind, Mood, and Emotion

Alertness

Twenty thousand years ago, being alert was the difference between life and death. You couldn't wander around the countryside ignoring the sound of a twig cracking behind the bush (an animal about to charge) or the sight of a plant crushed on the ground ahead (potential dinner nearby). Well you could, but you might not have lasted very long or had much to eat. Being alert is a survival mechanism, now as ever. Women walk down the street late at night acutely aware of the footsteps behind them, and alert to shadows in the alley up ahead. Drivers are alert to the vehicles in front and behind, and mothers are alert to their children's movements in the playground. We are all alert, to greater or lesser degrees, because our life or someone else's life might depend on it. Also, our future and job might depend on it. Managers make sure they're alert in meetings while students must be alert to what the teacher says if they want to stay in the course. Certain jobs require more alertness than others. If a pilot, air-traffic controller, or train driver is not alert, just for a minute, a major disaster can result.

Being alert is more than vigilance and attention, like soldiers on guard. It's about mental responsiveness, being alive in the head. Alertness extends beyond our physical surroundings, it's about being alive to the people around us too. Can we hear the twig breaking and can we sense what people are feeling? Alertness is not just about staying alive, it's about *being* alive — on the ball, in the game, sensitive.

The following two blends can each be

ESSENTIAL OILS THAT HELP TO BRING ABOUT ALERTNESS	
Basil	Black Pepper
Cardamom	Coriander
Cinnamon	Juniper
Petitgrain	Thyme
Eucalyptus	Peppermint
Rosemary	Pine
Grapefruit	Bergamot
Lime	

diluted into 30 mls (1 oz) base oil and made into stimulating massage oils, or made up into a synergistic blend using these proportions and used 5 drops in a bath, or 1-3 drops in inhalations, or 8 drops in one of the room methods:

ALERTNESS BLEND 1	
Juniper	14 drops
Pine	8 drops
Rosemary	8 drops
ALERTNESS BLEND 2	
Grapefruit	10 drops
Lime	10 drops
Black Pepper	5 drops
Peppermint	5 drops

The following blend is for use in difussers only. Again, it is stimulating, and helps make one alert:

DIFFUSER BLEND — ALERTNESS	
Eucalyptus Citriodora	15 drops
Peppermint	5 drops
Basil	5 drops

Assertiveness

I once overheard someone in a hospital say, "The trouble with being ill is I'm not my usual assertive self. I can't seem to get the staff to tell me anything and I'm put off all the time." This happens to sick people a lot, in and out of the hospital, because they're so busy fighting the illness there's nothing left over to fight for their rights. Assertiveness is all about not being afraid to ask for what you want, or feel is rightfully yours. It's about doing what you feel instinctively should be done, whatever anyone else says; and it's about defending your right to be who you are, not what someone else wants you to be. Assertiveness is about defending our integrity and, at times, maintaining our sense of who we actually are.

Assertive people get what they want. They stand their ground when they've been given shoddy service, they get recompensed by the manager they insist on seeing, they're not frightened to ask the man or woman of their dreams out for a date, and may find true love. In women assertiveness is often mistaken for aggression, but these are two entirely different things.

Essential oils are wonderful in the way they work to bring out assertiveness, and I really don't know how they do it — but they do! Over the years I've seen countless people coming to their first aromatherapy treatment all meek and mild, but blossoming into frank and open, assertive people after several sessions. One particularly unforgettable case was an older lady who'd been under the thumb of her family for years, who wouldn't say "boo" to a goose but who, after a few months of aromatherapy, found herself walking into a friend's house, straight over to the fruit bowl, from which she picked up a peach and promptly bit into it. At this point she "woke up" and realized what a

ESSENTIAL OILS FOR ASSERTION

Sweet Fennel	Basil
Jasmine	Cedarwood
Cypress	Ginger
Frankincense	Patchouli
Ylang Ylang	Black Pepper
Bergamot	Coriander
Carnation	Tuberose
Pimento Berry	Lime
Cardamom	Cistus
Litsea Cubeba	
Ormenis Flower	

in people. Choose individual oils from the list, or combinations from the list to suit your choice, or try one of the blends below. They can be used in a bath, massage oil, diffusers, or other room methods, in the steam inhalation method, or inhaled from a tissue. The change will not happen over night, and will take about two weeks of regular use. You may not recognize the change yourself until someone says to you, "Oh, I liked the way you handled that, what's come over you?"

Basil should not be used in baths. For the assertion blends, use these quantities each blended with 30 mls (1 oz) base oil for a massage oil, or make a synergistic blend using these proportions. See Chart 5.1 for quantities to use and methods.

cheeky thing she'd done, unimaginable a few months ago — and the lady and her friend had a good laugh over it.

All the above oils have been used successfully to bring out the assertiveness

ASSERTION BLEND 1

Cistus	2 drops
Litsea Cubeba	10 drops
Jasmine	6 drops

ASSERTION BLEND 2

Patchouli	10 drops
Frankincense	10 drops
Bergamot	10 drops

ASSERTION BLEND 3

Cedarwood	15 drops
Cypress	5 drops
Lime	10 drops

Concentration

There's a lot to be said for concentration. It certainly helps to get jobs done more efficiently, and it's more fun doing them too. There's nothing worse than a stream of interruptions when writing, for example, and I'm sure a mechanic banging away under a car hood needs to be able to concentrate just as much. Lives may depend on it. But people have different requirements for concentration — some can do it with a radio in the background, and teenagers seem *only* to be able to do it with the volume turned up high! It is difficult to concentrate when children are running around demanding things, but I've seen women concentrating on complicated lace work at the same time as giving instructions to half a dozen kids.

Others have immense difficulty finding the quiet to concentrate. One writer friend was plagued by roadwork outside her window and then a guinea fowl settled in a large tree in the garden and started squawking from five o'clock in the morning. Concentration was difficult to achieve. And the phone rings. And the doorbell goes. And so many distractions — programs we *must* watch on TV and phone calls we *must* make. Finding the time to concentrate is difficult and jobs are often rushed. What we've learned to do is concentrate on several things at once. I knew a woman, for example, a mother of four who wrote TV screenplays who could hold a conversation, accurately scan the credits on the TV screen after a show, read the paper, tell you stories from it, and paint her nails, all at the same time.

Whatever it is you do, it helps to be able to concentrate — to cut outside interference and direct your mental energy to the subject in question. The job is done better, and gives a greater sense of satisfaction. It's also much easier to organize life when you can concentrate on a job long enough to get it done, and it gives you confidence to positively change other aspects of life. Concentration helps toward clarity of thought, which is a marvelous thing.

Essential oils have been well documented for their ability to enhance the powers of concentration. They can be inhaled from a tissue, gently diffused throughout the room, perhaps during work or meditation. They can also be used in the bath, which is a good time to con-

ESSENTIAL OILS FOR CONCENTRATION	
Lemon	Basil
Lemongrass	Litsea Cubeba
Cardamom	Bergamot
Orange	Cedarwood
Rosemary	Eucalyptus
Peppermint	

centrate on oneself. To help overall concentration, use the essential oils in a massage oil. There are many approaches to take. Also, aside from the oils listed below, people find certain other essential oils help their concentration, jasmine and rose for example are great for getting the mind to concentrate on romance. (See *Aromantics*.) For concentrating on efficiency, better choices would be lemon, basil, litsea cubeba, or frankincense.

The following can be used in all the usual ways except basil and peppermint should not be used in baths. See Chart 5.1 for quantities to use and methods.

CONCENTRATION BLEND 1	
Lemon	20 drops
Basil	6 drops
Rosemary	2 drops

CONCENTRATION BLEND 2	
Litsea Cubeba	10 drops
Cardamon	10 drops
Lemon	10 drops

ESSENTIAL OILS FOR SPIRITUAL CONCENTRATION	
Frankincense	Neroli
Rose Otto	Narcissus
Chamomile Roman	Hyacinth

Confidence

Self-confidence makes us sure of our-selves, unafraid to walk tall, go anywhere or do anything, feeling free. Confidence means you don't let opportunities pass you by, and generally make the best of what life has to offer. Confidence is attrac-tive, and we all know it when we see a confident person walk into the room. They have an air about them that says "take me or leave me as I am." Being con-fident gets us the job, and makes us bold enough to buy that fabulous dress the less confident woman wouldn't dare be seen

in. In some sense, to have confidence is to allow us to enjoy life to the fullest.

Essential oils can't do it all for you, but they can certainly boost confidence, a fact established by countless people who have had aromatherapy treatments over the years. From the list choose an essen-tial oil that you feel akin to when you breathe it in deeply through the nose. You will feel something emotionally, and if that feeling is negative, don't use that par-ticular oil because it won't work. The oil you choose should make you feel good, and you should like it. Essential oils work on confidence by relieving the fear, stress, and nervous tension that often prevents us from doing things.

In the blends below, add the quanti-ties in each to 30 mls (1 oz) base oil, to make a massage oil, or use these propor-tions to make a synergistic blend of oils, which can be used in baths, inhaled direct

ESSENTIAL OILS FOR CONFIDENCE	
Cedarwood	Cypress
Coriander	Cardamom
Sweet Fennel	Ginger
Bergamot	Grapefruit
Jasmine	Pine
Rosemary	Orange
Linden Blossom	

CONFIDENCE BLEND 1	
Orange	10 drops
Cedarwood	5 drops
Ginger	5 drops
Jasmine	6 drops

CONFIDENCE BLEND 2	
Grapefruit	10 drops
Orange	10 drops
Bergamot	5 drops

CONFIDENCE BLEND 3	
Cedarwood	10 drops
Cypress	12 drops
Pine	8 drops

CONFIDENCE BLEND 4

Rosemary	20 drops
Fennel	10 drops

CONFIDENCE BLEND 5

Cardomom	5 drops
Ginger	15 drops
Coriander	10 drops

CONFIDENCE BLEND 6

In 30 mls (1 oz) base oil use 15 drops of *either* Jasmine or Linden Blossom

from a tissue, or diffused in the room. See Chart 5.1 for quantities to use.

Contentment

When people are asked what they want out of life one of the things high up on the list is "contentment." For some reason, contentment conjures up images of animals — the cat that got the cream lounging in front of the open fire, a big dog sitting at your knee. We might feel content after a good meal, especially if we prepared it. Contentment isn't being complacent, it's about being satisfied with your life, or with a job well done — whether finishing the ironing, tidying up the tool shed, or mowing the lawn.

Few people go through an entire day feeling content, and some might say that would be boring anyway because a whole range of other feelings would be missed out. But there has to be some kind of balance. Consider the extreme — the discontented soul, dissatisfied with everything and everybody, who dismisses contentment as an impossibility. Some people don't want to believe they can be content, and may have unreal ideals or expectations. To them I say, look at your life and name one small area you could say you feel content with, love of music say, and build on that, extend your contentments one by one.

Don't expect essential oils to do your inner work for you, but they can help by reducing the tenseness that discontented people feel, and any other stress or unhappiness. The person may then be able to see clearly enough to find at least a small piece of contentment. Use the oils in all the usual ways.

The quantities in the individual blends below could be diluted with 30 mls (1 oz) of vegetable oil to make a massage oil, or make a synergistic blend using these proportions. See Chart 5.1 for quantities to use and methods.

ESSENTIAL OILS FOR CONTENTMENT

Rose Otto	**Cypress**
Lavender	**Neroli**
Bergamot	**Orange**
Sandalwood	**Patchouli**
Ylang Ylang	**Clove**
Chamomile Roman	**Benzoin**

CONTENTMENT BLEND 1

Bergamot	10 drops
Clove	5 drops
Sandalwood	10 drops
Ylang Ylang	5 drops

CONTENTMENT BLEND 2

Chamomile Roman	5 drops
Orange	10 drops
Lavender	10 drops
Cypress	5 drops

Creativity

Apart from nature, the delights of this world are due to the creative spark in the human spirit. The things that make life a joy are music, paintings, books, and for some, designer dresses, and a good dinner. Imagine a world with no creative people — no TV or movies, no computers, no cars, no planes, no newspapers, no radio. Hang on, it's starting to sound good. But no beautiful buildings and gardens? It all sounds a bit bland.

Creativity is like shaking hands with tomorrow. It's the interface between the known and the unknown, and about the art of the possible. To be creative, the imagination has to soar. It can be painfully satisfying but takes confidence and belief in oneself, especially when treading into an area where nobody has gone before. Creativity is a joy and delight, both to the creative person, and to the one who enjoys the fruits of that creativity. Art saves lives.

It is the thing people turn to when under most pressure — a piece of music, a book, a picture; these things hold us tight in a sometimes difficult world.

We are all creative, to some degree or another. Look around you, isn't there something you've created — a piece of sewing, a model, a picture, a photograph, a garden? But some people seem better able to access those parts of the brain that facilitate the flow of ideas. They have gone beyond focus and concentration, and tapped into that gem, intuition. Baudelaire, the French writer, loved his essential oils, and it's reported that Leonardo da Vinci liked to have "perfumes" around, particularly neroli. William Shakespeare's father was a glover, a profession that used liberal amounts of perfumes, which, at that time of course, were essential oils. Perhaps they were a contributing factor in Shakespeare's prodigious and brilliant output — they certainly didn't hurt! Today, rock musicians write songs using essential oils and I even know a

ESSENTIAL OILS FOR CREATIVITY

Bergamot	Lemon
Frankincense	Geranium
Neroli	Rose Otto
Rose Maroc	Jasmine
Bay	Clove
Carnation	Mimosa
Litsea Cubeba	Sandalwood
Cypress	Juniper

vicar who writes his sermons with the help of their fragrance. They are just as uplifting as they ever were.

When it comes to choosing a single oil or oils to blend, pick aromas that appeal to you, that feel right. Choosing essential oils is almost as individual as creativity is. However, the oils listed below have been found useful by people I know and other colleagues. The essential oils for creativity can be used in all the usual ways (except clove should not be used in baths). See Chart 5.1 for quantities to use and methods.

ESSENTIAL OILS FOR FOCUS	
Thyme Linalol	Lemon
Fennel	Bergamot
Basil	Cedarwood
Cypress	Juniper
Lemongrass	Ginger
Cinnamon	Clove
Ylang Ylang	Nutmeg
Litsea Cubeba	Rosemary
Linden Blossom	

Focus

Being able to focus on the task ahead is often the difference between doing well and just scraping through, and gives a great sense of satisfaction. To focus is being able to direct all your attention and energy to one place, focused on the job at hand. Meditation teaches people to focus — both when doing meditation and, as a "side" benefit — throughout their daily lives. Focus is a great attribute and we owe many of our inventions and creations to people's ability to do it.

In this noisy world it is difficult to find a quiet place to focus the mind: neighbors play loud music, children slam doors, kittens climb up large house plants. And, given all that, there is only one word to think about — "selfish." *You* need to be selfish, so take the phone off the hook, ignore the doorbell, send everyone away and meditate, or at least sit still for five minutes and focus the mind on what you are doing, and why. Identify the side-tracks and decide to ignore them.

The following essential oils are renowned for helping people focus. Use them in all the usual methods, following the dosages recommended in Chart 5.1. It's not going to help to use aromas that already have a memory-connection because those memories will flood in, and not allow focus on the job or thought at hand. So it may be better to choose essential oils that have no previous connotations.

Use the quantities in the blends below, each blended with 30 mls (1 oz) base oil for a massage oil, or make a synergistic

FOCUS BLEND 1	
Thyme Linalol	10 drops
Lemon	6 drops
Rosemary	10 drops
Basil	4 drops

FOCUS BLEND 2	
Fennel	5 drops
Cypress	5 drops
Juniper	10 drops
Litsea Cubeba	10 drops

blend using these proportions. See Chart 5.1 for quantities to use and the list of oils that should not be used in baths.

Happiness

Happiness is that magic state we all aspire to, and if we achieve it, we've clinched life, gotten it right. The happy person exudes a radiance and seems to have found a philosophical position that banishes misery from the soul. Their aura is a delight. But happy people can sometimes attract unhappy people, energy vampires of whom one should beware.

Happiness is a very personal thing — what makes one person happy would not necessarily make another one happy.

SOME ESSENTIAL OILS FOR HAPPINESS	
Orange	Rose Otto
Rose Maroc	Jasmine
Coriander	Ginger
Clove	Cinnamon
Benzoin	Carnation
Pimento Berry	Geranium

However it comes, though, happiness is glorious. In a sense, it is nothing more than the ability to accept who we are and how we are living, instead of striving to be someone we could never be. Accepting our limitations is one door to happiness; having self-worth is another.

Essential oils will not put a person in a happy state if they have been miserable all their lives, but they will certainly help in a subtle way to bring out happiness. Traditionally, of course, aromas have been used for celebrations and other happy occasions. When it comes to choosing a single oil or oils to blend, pick aromas that appeal to you, that feel right. You might want to refer to other sections of the book.

On the list below, clove and cinnamon should not be used in baths, although if you used 4 drops of one of the blends below, their inclusion is actually tiny — much less than half a drop, and okay to use when included in such blends. See Chart 5.1 for quantities to use and methods.

HAPPINESS BLEND 1	
Orange	19 drops
Rose Maroc	5 drops
Jasmine	5 drops
Clove	1 drop

HAPPINESS BLEND 2	
Pimento Berry	5 drops
Geranium	10 drops
Cinnamon	5 drops
Ginger	10 drops

Joy

Joy is pure, unadulterated delight. It is the feeling a small child has when they see the packages Santa left under the tree. It is the feeling a son gets when his father hands over the keys to the car. Joy can be felt in a football stadium when the home team makes a goal. Joy is when you open the envelope containing the exam results, and find that you have passed; it's the feeling someone gets when they finally get a date with the love of their lives. Joy is boarding a plane to a dream destination; and for those traveling the spiritual path, the ecstatic joy of becoming one with the universe. And with joy, comes peace. Joy is healing too. It makes every cell in the body feel good — a tremendous pleasure, a gift!

Use the essential oils in all the usual ways, and create your own formula for joy!

ESSENTIAL OILS FOR JOY	
Sandalwood	Lemon
Bergamot	Orange
Rose Otto	Neroli
Ylang Ylang	Frankincense
Pettigrain	Mimosa
Linden Blossom	
Chamomile Roman	

Memory Enhancement

This section is not intended for people who have memory loss or forgetfulness, amnesia and so on, but for people who wish to improve upon what they already have — perhaps at certain times, like before starting a new job or college, or just in general. No magical memory tricks will appear. To do that you'll have to read a book on mnemonics and other aids to memory, and do some practice, but essential oils will have cumulative benefits, perhaps not noticed at first. Things will become easier to recall, and the details of situations and events will be remembered in more detail. Creative people, in particular, appreciate being able to recall the details of a landscape or the design of a flower.

Essential oils can be diffused, inhaled, used in a bath, or as massage oil. A world-famous artist told me that he uses essential oils to prepare himself before looking, and also during the creative process. A businessman told me he diffused them on his desk when writing a report, so he would remember all the little details he wanted to put in. Using essential oils regularly seems to give access to areas of our memory that might otherwise be overloaded with the plethora of daily events, or ignored by a conscious mind that has its own ideas about what is important. Aromas are the direct route of access into the brain, stimulating brain cells to respond. Aroma probably works well to retrieve memorized information because it stimulates the hippocampus, which seems to be responsible for storing information, both about experiences (*episodic memories*) and facts (*semantic memories*), in the brain. Aroma evokes memories — it presses a button and flash, the memory is there. How it does this, we do not know. The following essential oils have been found by essential oil users and therapists to be particularly useful in enhancing memory.

<table>
<tr><td colspan="2">ESSENTIAL OILS FOR MEMORY ENHANCEMENT</td></tr>
<tr><td>Ginger</td><td>Basil</td></tr>
<tr><td>Lemon</td><td>Grapefruit</td></tr>
<tr><td>Thyme Linalol</td><td>Rosemary</td></tr>
<tr><td>Cardamom</td><td>Black Pepper</td></tr>
<tr><td>Pimento Berry</td><td>Coriander</td></tr>
</table>

The essential oils can be diffused, inhaled, used in the bath (except basil and thyme unless as a small part of one drop, taken from a blend), or in a massage oil.

MEMORY ENHANCEMENT BLEND 1

Ginger	7 drops
Lemon	8 drops
Cardamom	10 drops
Pimento Berry	5 drop

MEMORY ENHANCEMENT BLEND 2

Rosemary	10 drops
Basil	5 drops
Thyme Linalol	7 drops
Grapefruit	8 drops

Use the oils singly or in blends. The quantities in the blends below should each be blended with 30 mls (1 oz) base oil if making a massage oil, or mixed in these proportions if making a synergistic blend. For quantities to use, see Chart 5.1.

Peace

Ah, peace, how magnificent it is! Peace is a state of grace, a spiritual restfulness that reaches to every cell in a body. It can come anytime, even standing in a crowded commuter train. Peace may be the view from the top of the mountain, the reward for a job well done. It might be the peace of knowing we have tried our best to mend a rift or put right a wrong. But how many of us have "tied up the loose ends" of our life, or as regression expert Dr. Roger Woolger says, "finished our unfinished business?" Until we do this, will there ever be peace in our hearts?

Having inner peace doesn't mean you don't get angry at injustices, or never shout, and it doesn't mean being passive either. But it is about having an all-embracing stillness inside — in the muscles and nerves, in our minds and spirits — the still vibration of the universe. It may be fleeting, but peace will be unforgettable. It may come when fully absorbed reading a book, or during meditation. Peace is there within us, like a quiet pool beneath the rocks, there for us to draw on when we take the time to find it. And we can find it if we listen with every cell in our body, not just the ears, and feel with every atom of our being, not just our hands.

The following essential oils create a peaceful environment that encourages peace within. Use them in a massage oil or diffuser, inhaled, or in the bath method. Aroma is so individual and subtle, what might be a peaceful oil for one person will not be so for another, so these can only be guidelines. Smell the aroma of them and see what they do for you, or perhaps use another unlisted oil.

ESSENTIAL OILS FOR PEACE	
Neroli	Juniper
Frankincense	Rose Otto
Melissa	Spikenard
Yarrow	Jasmine
Angelica Seed	Carnation
Chamomile Roman	

Performance

Cars "perform" well, we say, by which we mean they achieve toward the upper limit of their mechanical ability. Humans "perform" too, but we don't know what our upper limits of performance are, and there are few "mechanical" limitations to us. Who knows what we could do if we were trained, and if we tried. Perhaps we could become astronauts flying to the moon.

Professional performers give im-

mense pleasure to others, whether they act or dance on stage, or play in an orchestra or rock band, and they try to excel each time. It is onwards and upwards for them. But we all strive to perform better, whether we're performing for others, or performing for ourselves. Being able to perform well gives us confidence and self-esteem, and enables us to focus and channel our creative nature into an ever better performance of skill and control.

Essential oils will not make a person perform to an ability they do not possess, but by giving confidence, they allow a person to perform to their maximum potential, if they apply themselves. Professional performers use essential oils to overcome stage fright, to give confidence and assurance, and make them feel good.

Use the quantities in the following blends, each blended in 30 mls (1 oz) base oil for a massage oil or make a synergistic blend using these proportions. For quantities to use and methods see Chart 5.1.

ESSENTIAL OILS FOR BETTER PERFORMANCE	
Lemon	Bergamot
Lavender	Grapefruit
Helichrysum	Rose Otto
Rose Maroc	Jasmine
Geranium	Bay
Frankincense	Cypress
Ormenis Flower	
Eucalyptus Citriodora	

PERFORMANCE BLEND 1	
Helichrysum	8 drops
Geranium	12 drops
Bergamot	10 drops

PERFORMANCE BLEND 2	
Frankincense	4 drops
Cypress	8 drops
Lemon	10 drops
Ormenis Flower	8 drops

Positivity

Thought is perhaps the most powerful tool we have. Some say you can think up your future — determine whether it will be full of happiness and cash, or miserable and lonely, and workshops are held on this subject every day of the year. We are the architects of our own future, we are told, so think positive. Anticipate a positive outcome to get one, and take control. The classic test of a positive or negative personality is to show the person a half full bottle of wine and ask how much is in it. If they say, "it's half empty," they're negative, and if they say, "half-full," they're positive. This simple test does make an important point — our view of reality is altered by our attitude, whether positive or negative. We know this from our own experience, and from watching other people. The trick is to *get* a positive attitude, but how is it to be done?

Dr. Seymour Epstein, of the Psychology Department of the University of Massachusetts, is one of the new breed of positivity gurus, and one of his pieces of advice is to "dispute" a destructive thought every time it occurs. To help you do this he suggests you wear a rubber band on your wrist, then each time a negative thought comes up you shout "stop" and snap the elastic at the same time. This kind of programming could be thought pointless because we're human and going to react in an emotional way to whatever happens. This is the "you can't stop negativity, it's human" theory. I might once have agreed with that but over the years I have seen people deliberately adopt a positive attitude and, sure enough, change for the better. I can think of a couple, for example, who determined ten years ago never to argue, and they haven't, despite all the usual ups and downs that could give a couple an excuse. But not only do they not argue, they don't gripe, complain, criticize, or make bitchy comments toward each other. They tell me their relationship gets easier and more respectful all the time and is more blissful by the day.

Another piece of advice from Dr. Epstein is to accept your failures without judging yourself too harshly, which "only feeds your mind's habit of thinking destructively." [1] As another guru said many years ago, "Today is the first day of the rest of your life," so don't labor over past misfortunes. Take the lessons from them and move on. All is not lost.

Interestingly, eccentricity could put ten years on your life. At least, research carried out by psychologist Dr. David Weeks of the Royal Edinburgh Hospital has shown that unconventional people live longer than their staid counterparts — by between five and ten years longer. "Unconventional" is defined as having a strong sense of purpose, robust sense of humor, and curiosity (which doesn't say much for "conventional"). Staying involved and stimulated is important for a long life, we are told.

One of the qualities that distinguishes "winners" from "losers," apparently, is that winners know when to extricate themselves from situations that are leading them nowhere, while losers, on the other hand, tenaciously hang on to a project even when it is worthless. But persistence is not always a virtue, and like gamblers we have to know when to quit, and let things go. This can be difficult if there are few other options to turn to, which reminds me of a piece of advice given by a very positive American lawyer — "Put all your pots on the stove." What she means by this is explore all the avenues and let the projects roll, put them on the stove, and see which ones come to fruition and which fizzle out. Because that's the point — not all projects will work out well, so don't rely on one pot.

Positive people construct strategies to improve their chances of success — they are pro-active. Rather than leaving things to chance, they put the odds in their favor by careful planning and learning to deal with different situations. Positive people don't daydream that one day it's all going to get better; they set themselves realistic goals and go for them, step by small step, and they don't blame themselves for every little mishap. Mishaps are to be expected. They are part of the drama, so expect them but just don't expect them to rule your life.

Life is about good and bad and the trick is to find a balance in which there is more good than bad. That is all one can do. According to the Oxford dictionary, "optimism" is "applied to any view which supposes that good must ultimately prevail over evil in the universe." Pessimists tend to see the worst aspects of everything, which we can all do — the bottle is half empty syndrome. But how can we think that good must prevail over evil when the world is such a rotten place? We can read, hear, and see that on the news. But forget the news for five minutes and phone those long-lost dear friends, and make good contacts again. There is positivity out there, but one has to reach out for it.

Because I work with essential oils every day, and see them dispel negativity, I find it easy to say good will prevail over bad. Positivity is part of my day. But the essential oils are there for anyone to use. They're like little packages of positivity, a helping aid in the move toward optimism. They gently nudge a person with positivity, and you find yourself saying, "oh, maybe things aren't so bad" or "oh, maybe I can get out of this." You'll have to help yourself too. Because it's easier to deal with small problems, cut a large problem into several smaller ones. Think of your successes, not your failures. Know what you want and why you want it then write it down, and draw up a plan of how you're going to get it. Don't wait until tomorrow — if you do just one small thing toward your goal every day, you will get there.

I don't know of an essential oil that *doesn't* add positivity, but the following have been chosen for their traditional use in this area. Like other things in life, essential oils work better with positivity. Use them with positive thought, intent and purpose. In the diffuser method they create a positive atmosphere, at work or at home. They can also be used in massage oils and inhaled from a tissue.

Basil should not be used in baths. The quantities in the following blends can each be diluted with 30 mls (1 oz) base oil for a massage oil, or make a synergistic blend using these proportions. For quantities to use see Chart 5.1.

POSITIVE BLEND 1	
Geranium	10 drops
Pimento Berry	8 drops
Bay	8 drops
Frankincense	4 drops

POSITIVE BLEND 2	
Cedarwood	10 drops
Pine	5 drops
Cypress	5 drops
Petitgrain	10 drops

ESSENTIAL OILS FOR POSITIVITY

Basil	Lemon
Grapefruit	Cedarwood
Pine	Vetiver
Patchouli	Juniper
Cypress	Cardamom
Petitgrain	Geranium
Frankincense	Rosemary
Pimento Berry	Bay

Restfulness

We all need to rest, not only to sleep but to balance and ease our minds. Restfulness is a joy, as we allow our minds to drift and the equilibrium to return. But some minds never rest — they are constantly filling with new ideas, projects, things to

do, ever searching, learning, probing, ever on the move. There's nothing wrong with having an active mind, providing it's smart enough to know the benefits of rest. As a wise person once said, to be a perfect human being one needs the stillness of a sage and the action of a king. Balance is all, and restfulness is part of the equation. Any of the following oils will work equally well on their own or in mixes.

The quantities in the following blends can each be diluted with 30 mls (1 oz) of base oil to make a massage oil, or make a synergistic blend of oils using

ESSENTIAL OILS FOR RESTFULNESS

Lavender	Geranium
Rose Maroc	Clary Sage
Linden Blossom	Neroli
Marjoram	Petitgrain
Rosewood	Sandalwood
Mimosa	

these proportions and use in all room methods, inhalation methods, and in the bath. See Chart 5.1 for quantities to use.

RESTFUL BLEND 1

Neroli	10 drops
Petitgrain	20 drops

RESTFUL BLEND 2

Geranium	20 drops
Lavender	5 drops
Clary Sage	5 drops

ESSENTIAL OILS FOR SELF-AWARENESS

Clary Sage	Ylang Ylang
Cypress	Geranium
Pine	Sandalwood
Ormenis Flower	Bay
Pimento Berry	Jasmine
Clove	Mandarin
Coriander	Angelica Seed
Sage	Cistus
Myrtle	

Self-awareness

Being able to connect with who we really are is a useful tool in the striving for fulfillment. Not only does self-awareness bring us closer to our spiritual selves, it helps identify our hopes, fears, and joys. If we have an awareness of how we feel and react, a strong sense of who we really are, it contributes to emotional well-being. There are many routes to self-awareness, including Gestalt therapy, which is based on the idea that a person reflects his or her true personality through the things they do or need to do, and tries to make the person aware of their thoughts, feelings, and actions. The aim is to view the life clearly, uncluttered by outside thoughts, and try to understand what it is that is wanted from it. People are encouraged to feel free to be who they are, and to feel content with themselves. The message is *appreciate yourself*.

We don't all need to go into therapy. A great deal of self-awareness can be had from simply observing ourselves, and asking other people how they see us. By understanding the effect we have on other people, we can gain insight into our motives and hidden agendas. What the essential oils can do is help bring out parts of ourselves we may not have recognized, or been aware of, before.

Self-esteem

There's nothing wrong with having a favorable appreciation or opinion of oneself. If you can't appreciate yourself, who else can? But I am constantly amazed at the number of people who put themselves down with comments like "I could never do that" or "I'm not smart enough for that." In fact, they are perfectly capable of meeting the challenge, or at least having a jolly good go, but have low self-esteem so do nothing.

Simply, self-esteem is recognizing your potential and worth, taking pride in what you do, and trusting your judgment in most things. When you have self-esteem you are secure in yourself, despite the weak points, because you recognize your strong points and appreciate them. okay, you're not perfect, but who is? You're as good as the next person. So Mr. Jones next door grows bigger cabbages — so what? Your potatoes are bigger than his! We cannot go around making value judgments about other people compared to ourselves, it is a totally useless exercise. Everyone is different; that is the beauty of it, and we all have our good points, which should give us self-esteem.

Essential oils won't miraculously turn you overnight from someone with low self-esteem into someone brimming over with high expectations of themselves, but they will subtly and gently help you deal with any corner of your life you feel unhappy with, and so build up your self-esteem and your estimate of what you can do in this world. Use an oil or oils with no previous

SELF-ESTEEM BLEND 1	
Ylang Ylang	10 drops
Bergamot	4 drops
Vetiver	2 drops
Sandalwood	12 drops

SELF-ESTEEM BLEND 2	
Hyacinth	8 drops
Bergamot	4 drops
Rose Maroc	8 drops

memory-connection that could have negative associations.

The quantities in the following blends can each be diluted with 30 mls (1 oz) of base oil to make a massage oil, or make a synergistic blend of oils using these proportions and use the synergistic blend in baths, room methods, and the inhalation method. For quantities to use see Chart 5.1.

(The second blend here uses a particularly powerful combination of oils and only 20 drops are needed in 30 mls (1 oz).)

Self-image

If we can see ourselves as a positive, happy, vibrant, radiant person, other people will be more likely to see us in the same way. Of course, having a good self-image isn't very easy if you've been battered down by life's events, but it is possible to raise oneself out of this hole by thinking positively. In the early 1970s practically everyone wore a yellow badge with a smiling face on it, and

ESSENTIAL OILS FOR SELF-ESTEEM

Hyacinth	Sandalwood
Vetiver	Ylang Ylang
Rose Maroc	Jasmine
Carnation	Bergamot
Geranium	Cedarwood
Ormenis Flower	

the word "smile" underneath. This icon of an era worked — people wore it and smiled. Smiling makes you happy, just as being happy makes you smile. If we can visualize ourselves as positive, smiling people, and project that image into the outside world, perhaps that is exactly what we shall become.

Essential oils can help in raising self-image by seeking out the hidden reserves we have within us, and bringing them forward. They find our best qualities and fortify them, which improves our self-image. This is an intensely personal area and so only use those oils you feel drawn to. Certain aromas could already have a negative memory-connection — associated, for example, with someone who put you down. Obviously don't use them. The following oils can be used either singly, or in blends.

The quantities in the following blends can each be diluted with 30 mls (1 oz) of base oil to make a massage oil, or make a synergistic blend of oils using these proportions to use in baths, diffused in the atmosphere, and in the inhalation methods. For quantities to use see Chart 5.1.

ESSENTIAL OILS FOR SELF-IMAGE

Orange	Lavender
Melissa	Neroli
Ylang Ylang	Rose Maroc
Jasmine	Sandalwood
Cypress	Juniper
Cedarwood	Pine
Black Pepper	Frankincense
Mandarin	Nutmeg
Myrtle	Bay
Chamomile Roman	

SELF-IMAGE BLEND 1

Rose Maroc	10 drops
Orange	5 drops
Mandarin	10 drops
Ylang Ylang	5 drops

SELF-IMAGE BLEND 2

Sandalwood	5 drops
Black Pepper	10 drops
Frankincense	5 drops
Jasmine	10 drops

CHAPTER 8

THE A-Z OF EMOTIONAL PROBLEMS

Abuse

Emotional and Physical

The word "abuse" is expected to explain a whole range of experiences suffered by an individual — from regular violent beatings from a so-called "partner," or daily sexual violation as a child, to verbal attacks or put downs that are within the boundary of so-called "normal" behavior. For example, countless parents all over the country say of their child, "they're a monster" or say "come here you little monster" — half-joking, half meaning it. If, as an adult, someone called you a monster, you'd be pretty upset, but children are expected to take this abuse as some kind of punishment for crying, demanding food at inconvenient times, producing dirty diapers, or taking the parent's freedom away. But if a child is called "a mon-

ster" just four times a day, by the time they reach five years of age, they've been called a monster 7,300 times. The danger of this is, the child may come to believe that they are, in fact, a monster. When one includes this kind of verbal abuse in with the discussion of "abuse," and adds in the nastiness siblings can inflict upon each other, one could come to the conclusion that there are few people in our society who have not been through some kind of abuse or other.

Of course, some forms of abuse are more damaging than others but it is most often inflicted upon us by someone we love: babies get called a "monster" by the mommy they love, little girls are abused by the fathers they love, and lovers are abused by each other — both physically and verbally. It is this, the mixing of hate and love, that is so damaging in the long term because later, in other relationships, it can become difficult to extricate the hate from the love and future love becomes a love-hate relationship, somehow never entirely satisfactory.

As the word "abuse" covers so many experiences, which may affect us all to some degree or other, it is impossible to say what emotional damage results from it. These may include the inability to accept love, or feel love, the inability to share, lack of self-confidence, low self-esteem, insecurity, shame, an inferiority complex, depression, fear, and guilt. It may express itself as a general feeling of anxiety — inexplicable perhaps, and general, a sort of permanent discomfort with life. If any of these feelings are left unexpressed, they can eat away at the very fabric of a soul or personality, like woodworm silently eating away a timber-framed house, which one day may fall.

Thankfully, abuse is now a widely discussed subject, partly thanks to the frankness of certain famous people, and it's no longer thought to be the victim's fault. Although it may be easy to understand *intellectually* that abuse was not our fault, coming to understand that *emotionally* is another thing altogether — and much more difficult. Help is often required, and although there are now counseling services available for people who have experienced sexual abuse as a child, and domestic violence, it is very difficult to find a context in which to discuss the less dramatic types of abuse, the type that is part of "normal" behavior. Doctors aren't as a rule very sympathetic when a person goes to them and says, "Doctor, I feel permanently anxious because my big sister used to verbally

abuse me, remorselessly, until I left home at eighteen, and now I just feel permanently anxious and unconfident." He or she is unlikely to consider the case important enough to refer the person to a free counseling service, and may just tell them to "buck up." What they need to do, however, is discuss the problem, get to the root of it, look at it, examine it and, having done that, throw it away like so much garbage.

Sexual abuse is altogether more difficult because it is so appalling, often "blanked out" altogether — until something triggers the memory, perhaps decades after the events. One dreadful aspect of sexual abuse is that the abuser often makes the abusee think that they are responsible or somehow compliant in the acts. It is not only physical invasion but mental manipulation too. Figures show that it is very widespread — horrifyingly so. In *Women: A World Report*, the authors looked at statistics from Britain, America, Australia, Israel, Egypt, and India and extended them world-wide, coming to the conclusion that they could imply that "as many as 100 million young girls may be being raped by adult men — usually someone they know — often day after day, week after week, year in, year out." [1] These men aren't obvious demons, they're men we see walking down the street, men we work with, men we see driving cars or on the bus. They *look* and, disconcertingly for the girls concerned, behave normally most of the time. One woman I know, who we shall call Linda, was regularly abused by her father on the evening her mother went to a night class. Like most abusers he made her feel as if it were her fault, that she had somehow invited it or deserved it. She couldn't tell her mother, then or even to the present day, because she knew, and knows, it would destroy her, and still feels she should somehow get through the experience without putting her mother through the anguish, and that is her choice. I recently went to Linda's wedding and marveled at the way she got through the whole event without once looking at her father, embracing him or in any way recognizing him. If he was standing on her right, she talked to someone on her left. If he stood on her left, she talked to someone on her right. It was a masterstroke of polite avoidance. But, I wonder, hasn't her mother noticed that Linda never actually looks at her father or speaks to him? It is not only the abusee that "blanks" it out. Like many abusers, Linda's father is a respectable, professional man, and one would never guess from looking at him that he was capable of such ghastly deeds.

Another abusee I know, who we shall call Jill, grew up on a farm with three brothers, a mother, and a violent father. He would beat Jill's brothers at the slightest excuse — so badly they would often have to miss school for a whole week to allow their physical marks to heal. Like many mothers and wives, Jill's mother was so passive (and terrified), she just let the whole business pass. As Jill entered adolescence she discovered that she could prevent her father from beating her brothers by interrupting him and becoming like a young Lolita, stroking his face, kissing him, saying, "Please daddy, stop." This calmed him down long enough to stop the beating. However, being a nasty, manipulative man, he also saw that Jill's "solution" could be exploited and as time went on he wanted more than a kiss on the cheek and a hug. By the time she turned fourteen, only full intercourse would "calm" the man down and, predictably, Jill's father would find more and more excuses to thrash the boys, knowing that Jill would "placate" him.

It's easy enough to say children or young girls or boys should "tell," but very difficult for them to actually do it. I know of a recent case involving two eleven-year-old boys who were regularly "felt up" by a classmate's father who came along to "help" when that class went swimming. The boys kept it all a secret for about six months, and then one told his mother. All hell broke loose, the man was taken to court but, because it was their word against his (and he was a highly respectable member of the community) he got off the charge. In his summing up, the judge noted that the boys hadn't mentioned the first (alleged) incident and apparently thought the boys were having pre-adolescent fantasies, and advised the jury accordingly. The whole experience has left the boys devastated, distrustful of both men and authority.

I know of so many cases of sexual abuse it is quite easy for me to believe the horrifying statistics, and difficult to find the space here to recall them all. But one thing that recurs through all these experiences is the fact that the abusee, for many reasons, doesn't tell, or makes the one person they tell *promise* not to tell. *Not telling* and abuse seem to go hand in hand.

It is then, precisely telling that's required before the events can be "processed" by the mind, allowing the abusee to continue with their life without this experience gnawing away at them. This is where essential oils can help. We know that aroma molecules do reach and activate the limbic system, which is the home of memories and emotions, thereby facilitating the release of the pent up experiences, while at the same time certain essential oils are calming, seemingly, as research shows, because they expedite the production of beta-waves in the brain.

Someone who has been abused needs to discuss it and work it through. It is irrelevant how long ago it all was. Not everyone needs to go to counseling or to a special therapist. Linda, mentioned above, kept her experience a secret until she was thirty years old, then went through a crisis period during which she discussed it with a few close friends, and came out of it all a much more confident and assertive person. She no longer apologized for everything she did, and felt she deserved the little space she took up in the world (which was a profound change for her). After much thought, she decided group counseling was not for her. But the point is, she had to discuss it with *someone* to get it off her chest, and it didn't much matter who that someone was, or who those somebodies were, so long as they were genuinely supportive.

Of course, it is upsetting to recall the abuse, and it often involves coming to the realization that the abuser is a horrible person, even if he is your father. However, it has to be done. The alternative may be to live with a whole range of feelings that slowly destroy the abusee — and nobody deserves that to happen. Abuse generates feelings of betrayal, suspicion, mistrust, self-doubt, dread, terror, panic, resentment, violation, guilt, and many other things that could possibly be dissipated with sympathetic help.

Some essential oils are better suited to use in cases of abuse and have been empirically shown to help the wounded child or adult. Also, refer to other sections in this book — those dealing with emotional hurt, anxiety, depression, lack of self-confidence, etc. — and see which essential oils seem most relevant to each particular experience. Also see the large chart at the end of this book.

ESSENTIAL OILS THAT HELP OVERCOME EMOTIONAL ABUSE

Ormenis Flower	Melissa
Rose Otto	Neroli
Mandarin	Benzoin
Chamomile Roman	

ESSENTIAL OILS THAT HELP THE HURT INNER CHILD

Geranium	Lavender
Neroli	Melissa
Mandarin	Benzoin
Rose Otto	

e — Using a Blend

As each case of abuse is so individual, create a formulation using essential oils particular to your needs. For example, if you experience a lot of panic, see that section and include an oil or oils from that list. Make up a synergistic blend of essential oils in a bottle. From that, you can use the oils in various methods, in the quantities given below. For example, you might put into your synergistic blend bottle some mandarin or chamomile roman for gentleness, some rose or neroli to deal with the sadness, and some geranium to deal with the insecurity. Here are a couple of suggested blends you might like to try, remembering that these quantities indicate proportions to be used when making a synergistic blend, and not the maximum number of drops.

SYNERGISTIC BLEND 1

Chamomile	
Roman	2 drops
Mandarin	4 drops
Neroli	6 drops

SYNERGISTIC BLEND 2

Rose Otto	4 drops
Geranium	2 drops
Mandarin	4 drops

Once you have made your synergistic blend of oils you can use it in several ways. Use 5 drops to a teaspoon of base oil for a massage. This doesn't sound like much, but it will go further than you think, and it can be effective if massaged into the solar plexus area (middle, where the ribcage separates), upper chest and across the shoulders. Alternatively, use 3 drops of synergistic blend in a bath. Also use the synergistic blend in any of the room methods. Using the essential oils in this way will help you express yourself during counseling, or help you generally as you try to deal with the problem by facing it and expressing your feelings about it. Use the essential oils daily and change the formula as you progress.

Addictions

When the body cannot react normally without a particular substance, it's said to be "dependent," and the body will go through "withdrawal symptoms" if that substance is not provided. This is addiction, and it can be caused by many substances — heroin, cocaine, diazepam and other tranquilizers, amphetamines, alcohol, the nicotine in cigarettes, and the caffeine in tea and coffee. Addiction involves physical processes and is not simply a psychological demand — like a baby crying because their comfort blanket is not in their hands. It is even possible to become addicted to chocolate. Don't blame yourself, it's the chemicals in the chocolate.

Whether the addictive substance comes in the form of little pills from the doctor or in the form of tea bags from the supermarket, it is a drug. By taking it into the body on a regular basis, the cells in a body adjust themselves to it, so they then *expect* it. When the head decides to "give up," the body may not be ready, so, whatever the drug, unless the person is prepared to go through rather unpleasant "withdrawal symptoms," they'll have to reduce their intake of the drug slowly, allowing the cells to gradually adjust back to their old selves. With some drugs, the cells adjust and keep adjusting so that as time goes on they require more and more of the drug to achieve the same effect. Heroin is a classic example of this, but so is alcohol. One becomes inexorably drawn into addiction, deeper and deeper, day by day.

This section is arranged as Drug Addiction, Alcohol Addiction, and Nicotine Addiction, and please refer to the section which applies to you. Keep in mind, most addictive substances are poisons and they need to be cleared out of the system. Fruit juices, water, fresh foods, and vitamins are all useful aids in the process of withdrawal. Change to a wholefood diet; avoid junk foods, refined food products and soda drinks (which can themselves be addictive if they contain caffeine). Eat plenty of fresh green vegetables, salads and fruits, and drink sparkling water combined with fruit juices, as this lifts low blood sugar levels. It's important to eat three meals a day, especially breakfast: have cereal or an egg on toast with fruit juice, something light but nutritious. Also consider going to an acupuncturist, who may be able to help.

Use the following oils in diffusers, in massage oils, inhaled in the water-bowl method or, in any other way that is found helpful, following the dosage guidelines in Chart 5.1.

ESSENTIAL OILS TO USE IN THE FIGHT AGAINST ADDICTION	
Vetiver	Narcissus
Helichrysum	Basil
Rose Otto	Frankincense
Spikenard	Benzoin

HYPNOTICS THAT CAN BE USEFUL IN THE FIGHT AGAINST ADDICTION	
Narcissus	Jonquil
Rose Maroc	Hyacinth
Carnation	Jasmine
Hops	Valerian
Tonka Bean	Vanilla
Tuberose	Spikenard

OTHER ESSENTIAL OILS THAT MAY BE OF USE TO COMBAT ADDICTION	
Marjoram	Bergamot
Juniper	Patchouli
Bay	Clary Sage
Nutmeg	Cistus
Chamomile Roman	

Drug Addiction

When tranquilizers first came on the market, nobody knew they were addictive, not even the companies that made them — who are currently embroiled in expensive legal battles with people who were prescribed the drugs by their doctors. Now we all know what trouble they can be. As the dangers of tranquilizers were becoming known, people were reassured that antidepressants were not addictive, but now of course we know that they are. Patients are told that the panic, anxiety, and depression they may feel when they stop taking antidepressants is a symptom of *withdrawal*, and not a sign of relapse, and to reduce the dose gradually over a four week period, at least. It's got to be worth a try. In an article in the magazine *She*, one woman gave a very moving account of antidepressant dependency. Her memory was like porridge, she said, she couldn't remember what happened yesterday. And decisions took days. She experienced mental confusion — "like being hopelessly drunk," her thinking "fogged and slow," her limbs "leaden," and her joints "aching." Plus her life was full of dread — as in dreadful.

When you're addicted to drugs, your whole life revolves around them. Are they in your handbag when you go out? Where is the next fix coming from? Likewise, withdrawal takes over the life. How am I going to get through the next five minutes? The addict needs support. There are several useful addresses at the end of this book, of organizations that advise on support groups people can join.

There are two ways to get addicted to drugs. Tranquilizers are often prescribed for far too long. Instead of seeing the person through a rough patch of anxiety or depression, the pills are continued because the problem itself isn't being sorted out, and even when time has passed and dissolved it anyway, the tranquilizer addiction remains — probably causing more problems than the original problem. Of course tranquilizers, sleeping pills and antidepressants have their place in the pharmacopoeia, but to take them over long periods when they are no longer required is to use them incorrectly. Another way to get into drugs is to be drawn to them, like an animal to water, because of some very hurtful dynamic in the early family life, or a traumatic experience. Drugs provide comfort. If this is the case there is only one answer — counseling, in some form or other.

People often become addicted to drugs because they were mistreated as children — not in dramatic ways necessarily, but in ways that hurt. Simone, for example, was brought up by her grandmother because her mother was sixteen and single when she had Simone, and couldn't cope. The father was nowhere to be seen, and the grandmother resented Simone for having "ruined" her daughter's life. Not surprisingly, Simone grew up feeling unloved and later turned to drugs — including heroin.

David's parent's were similarly unloving, but in a different way. His father was a sparkling, successful professional man — charming, liked, amusing, rich, and much adored by the mother. David and his siblings were always second in line — "Stop that now, your father's talking," or working, or whatever it was. Not that David had much time to interrupt his perfect father, because like many other middle class boys of his generation, he was packed off to boarding school at the age of seven. Because father was the center of the domestic universe, mother dismissed David like a little inconsequential boy, even when he was thirty years old. He too turned to drugs. Many problems like this are still unresolved in the minds of junkie-type personalities, and it's not really their fault. I know David's family and to look at them you'd say, "Oh what a perfect family," so it's difficult for David to openly blame them for his indulgent behavior, or at least it may seem so to him. But his situation is real and unresolved, something trained counselors would recognize, and have sympathy with. That's what they're there for.

As for the physical effects of withdrawal, these must be overseen by a medical practitioner because it can be dangerous to do it on your own. Plan to cut down over a long period, cutting down the number of pills taken each day, cutting them in half, then into quarters, then scraping small bits off, gradually — and very slowly — reducing the amount of drug that is taken in each day. Withdrawal from drugs such as the opiates morphine and heroin, or amphetamine; synthetic diet pills; and barbiturates, tranquilizers, and sleeping pills, causes the body to go into crisis. It's tough for all those little junkie cells. They're not used to it and they have to readjust. People think of drugs as "head" things. They're not. Benzodiazepam receptors (and benzodiazepines are the most commonly prescribed drugs for anxiety and stress) are

found all over the body, not just in the head, and more drug receptors are being found every day — in the least expected places. The whole body is into drugs, not just the head, and consequently the whole body is going to react with a whole range of symptoms that might include sweating, palpitations, shaking, nausea, breathing difficulties, tremors, rashes, aches and pains, diarrhea, or constipation. The brain, meanwhile, could be suffering with headaches, distorted vision, anxiety, confusion, panic attacks, insomnia, paranoia, and hallucinations. No wonder addicts trying to get off drugs wonder if it's worth the trouble. But it is — well worth it.

During the withdrawal process essential oils can help in two ways — by contributing to a sense of well-being, and by treating the physical problems that go along with it. The essential oils listed below can be used to supplement and support any other treatment. Use the oils in warm baths, inhaled as a vapor, and diffused in the room. If possible, arrange

---

ESSENTIAL OILS FOR USE DURING WITHDRAWAL FROM DRUGS

Vetiver	Helichrysum
Spikenard	Valerian
Ormenis Flower	Nutmeg
Juniper	Bergamot
Basil	Clary Sage
Geranium	Hyacinth
Narcissus	Tuberose

to see an aromatherapist, at least once a week to begin with, and then monthly. This may not be possible for financial reasons, but you can massage the oils in yourself. (See page 200, Massage).

There are many essential oils to choose from. As well as those listed above, refer to particular sections throughout this book, or try one of the synergistic blends below. Use these quantities each blended with 30 mls (1 oz) of vegetable oil to make a massage oil, or make up a synergistic blend using these proportions and use 8-10 drops in a bath, or use in the inhalation or diffuser methods. See Chart 5.1 for quantities to use.

DURING DRUG WITHDRAWAL BLEND 1	
Vetiver	10 drops
Basil	5 drops
Bergamot	5 drops
Clary sage	10 drops

DURING DRUG WITHDRAWAL BLEND 2	
Nutmeg	10 drops
Ormenis Flower	5 drops
Spikenard	4 drops
Bergamot	5 drops
Juniper	6 drops

The above blends can be altered as time goes on, when a lighter emotional blend may be needed. The essential oil of helichrysum has been used on its own very successfully in some cases of withdrawal, as have the floral absolutes — which are very expensive but as a very small amount is required, not as expensive as they first appear.

When withdrawing from drugs, as well as using the essential oils suggested in the lists and blends in this section, take 100 grams of vitamin B-complex twice a day, and 500 grams of vitamin C-complex twice a day, or a multi-vitamin and mineral supplement. Homeopathic remedies may help as well, such as capsicum, ignatia, or nux vomica (x6). Also, consider going along to the meetings of "Narcotics Anonymous," or contacting the organizations Tranx or MIND, who can give advice about coming off drugs and put people in touch with local support groups.

Alcohol Addiction

There seems to be something in human nature that drives people to brew alcoholic drinks, which we make from just about every grain, berry, and fruit going. Even grandmas brew up elder flower champagne and plum wine in their back kitchens. Drinking is a part of life and we flock to the bar for a drink, are encouraged to buy wine with our meal in restaurants, and cannot avoid it at parties. It's not all bad, of course, and alcohol can help us to relax and communicate, it keeps us warm in winter and, according to some doctors, drinking two glasses of red wine a day is actually good for the heart and digestive system, something the French and Italians have been saying for years.

Drinking is so much a part of life that "to go out" is synonymous with "let's have a drink." But for some people, a social drink becomes a problem drink, from which there is no going back. Once an alcoholic, they say, always an alcoholic — it's as if the body can let you give it up for ten years and then, a couple of drinks lapse, and you're in its grip again. That's why they say drink is evil.

People get driven to drink by the manifold pressures that face the average human soul — financial problems, marital break-up, depression, unemployment, boredom, frustration, lack of confidence, insecurity and so on and so on. The drink is in the cupboard, it's there in that friendly bar, and so it draws us to it, solace in a bottle. Some people, we are told, have a genetic predisposition to alcoholism — it's wired in the genes. As many people who are married to alcoholics know, from trying over and over again to get their loved ones to stop, alcohol is a deep, dark abyss from which it is difficult to escape.

In Los Angeles today, the *Alcoholics Anonymous (AA)* meetings are full of movie stars, and all over the world other less-famous types of people stand up in AA meetings and bravely admit they too are hooked. AA is a wonderful organization but families need support too, and *Al-Anon* is there to do that. Doctors can prescribe a drug such as Antabuse that will make the person feel sick if they have a drink, but it usually takes more than this to get to the root of the problems.

As with drug addiction, essential oils have been shown to be very helpful, espe-

ESSENTIAL OILS FOR USE IN WITHDRAWAL FROM ALCOHOL	
Helichrysum	Juniper
Lemon	Bergamot
Marjoram	Clary Sage
Eucalyptus Citriodora	

cially during the first stages of withdrawal. You might like to try the following oils, used singly or in blends.

Or try either of the following blends, which are both synergistic blends. Either add one of the blends to 30 mls (1 oz) of base oil for a massage oil, or mix the essential oils in these proportions for a synergistic blend to be diffused in the atmosphere, or add 8 drops to the bath. See Chart 5.1.

DURING ALCOHOL WITHDRAWAL BLEND 1	
Helichrysum	10 drops
Lemon	10 drops
Juniper	10 drops

DURING ALCOHOL WITHDRAWAL BLEND 2	
Marjoram	10 drops
Bergamot	10 drops
Clary Sage	10 drops

After a while, different oils should be substituted to deal with the withdrawal symptoms — try chamomile roman for a calming effect and geranium to ease anxiety. But look at the other sections through this book and find what is specific for each person, during the various stages. This is one of the great advantages with essential oils — aside from detoxifying, and making one feel positive, they can run with you — providing specific help every step of the way.

Nicotine Addiction

Cigarettes are so dangerous, manufacturers are obliged to print, "Cigarettes can kill you" and other such warnings on the packet and advertisements. This doesn't stop people from buying them. Indeed, people buy nicotine sticks by the zillion, despite the fact that there isn't a good word to be said about them, even by the people who smoke them. Cigarettes cause all kinds of cancer, heart disease, strokes, and respiratory tract disorders, including bronchitis and emphysema — sufferers of which often have to carry their own life-saving supply of oxygen around with them. Cigarettes make the skin gray or yellow and the breath, hair, and clothes stink. Plus, aside from killing yourself, you may be killing somebody else, who passively inhales your smoke — and increasingly, court cases are being fought and won on this point. It's a myth that smoking reduces stress — that's official. Clinical psychologists have shown that smoking at the same time as experiencing stress just compounds the bad effects on the

heart. You can't even console yourself with the thought that at least tobacco is a crop that provides a living for someone somewhere, because tobacco is an invidious crop that sucks all nutrients from the earth and leaves it useless, and farmers say it requires much more tedious manual work than almost any other crop and the work must go on right throughout the year. Other crops would be more useful, in more ways than one.

Nicotine is highly addictive, and rumor has it that manufacturers are putting more and more chemicals into the tobacco and rolling paper each passing year. Old Granddad smoking his pure roll-ups for eighty years might have survived, but I don't know that smokers will live that long in the future. Giving up isn't easy, however, and help is required. Essential oils can provide relief for some of the specific symptoms of withdrawal such as grumpy moods, depression, anger, nervousness, and sheer panic — and please look to those sections to see what is required with each passing day, if not hour. Also try vitamin therapy to build up your strength and replenish some of the supplies smoking inevitably drains. Vitamins B_1, B_6, B_{12}, and vitamin C are especially important now. Or get a daily multi-vitamin with B-complex and mineral supplement, and take it with a minimum of 200 grams of vitamin C each day.

Aggression

Aggression is part of our survival system and shouldn't be entirely wiped out because aggressive tendencies can actually help protect us from what the world throws at us today. Nevertheless, it's perfectly clear that some people are too aggressive. You can see it in certain children, in men who get in a fight, and people who seem to thrash it out with the wall when they hang wall-paper. Supposedly, aggression is due to the hormone testosterone, of which men have more than women. We expect men to be more aggressive than women, to the point where if a man and woman were behaving in exactly the same way, he would be called assertive, and she would be called aggressive. Aggression is hostile action or behavior — rough, hard, and unpleasant. It may only become a problem when it is already well and truly established as part of the personality. Little Billy is "a bit of a rebel," then he grows up into a thug.

In some cases, we know which components in essential oils bring down the level of aggression, in some we don't. But they are proven to do so in animals as well as in people. Thankfully, essential oils quite easily reduce aggression in most cases. Relaxation exercises are also most helpful, particularly the tension-releasing ones, which make one very aware of the mind-body connection. It is very effective under these circumstances to use essential oils in a diffuser at the same time as doing breathing exercises. Also, take a regular warm bath using one of the essential oils listed below (or a blend of oils) and then take that same oil (or blend) out with you on a tissue or handkerchief and whenever you feel the aggression coming on, just

ESSENTIAL OILS FOR GENERAL AGGRESSION	
Geranium	Frankincense
Sandalwood	Grapefruit
Cedarwood	Vetiver

OTHER ESSENTIAL OILS THAT HAVE A SOOTHING EFFECT	
Neroli	Lavender
Clary Sage	Spikenard
Benzoin	Marjoram
Litsea Cubeba	Coriander
Valerian	
Chamomile Roman	

Plus the more expensive absolutes of Rose Maroc, Tuberose, Mimosa, Carnation

pull it out and inhale. Think of the nice, relaxing bath you had last night.

Aggression can also turn inward, and there may be feelings of aggression towards oneself. Try the soothing essential oils for this — lavender and litsea cubeba are also useful for this situation. Alternatively, try one of the following blends — adding these quantities to 30 mls (1 oz) base oil for a massage oil, or making up a synergistic blend using these proportions and using 8 drops in a bath, or in a room diffuser method, or 3 drops inhaled directly from a tissue.

In the case of aggression toward other

AGGRESSION TOWARD SELF
BLEND 1

Clary Sage	10 drops
Vetiver	8 drops
Grapefruit	12 drops

AGGRESSION TOWARD SELF
BLEND 2

Frankincense	15 drops
Geranium	5 drops
Sandalwood	5 drops

AGGRESSION TOWARD OTHER
PEOPLE BLEND 1

Cedar Wood	5 drops
Grapefruit	15 drops
Frankincense	5 drops
Geranium	10 drops

AGGRESSION TOWARD OTHER
PEOPLE BLEND 2

Chamomile Roman	10 drops
Litsea Cubeba	6 drops
Clary Sage	2 drops
Sandalwood	12 drops

people, use suggestions made elsewhere in this section, or one of the blends below. Use these quantities added in 30 mls (1 oz) base oil for a massage oil, or make a synergistic blend using these proportions and then add 8 drops to a bath, or in a diffuser, or 3 drops on a tissue or hankie to be inhaled when required.

Children can be aggressive too, and it's a bad habit to acquire. Those under five years of age should only be exposed to chamomile roman and lavender, while those over fifteen years of age can follow the adult lists and blends. Children in between — over five and under fifteen — can use the ones below.

CHILDHOOD AGGRESSION
AGES 5 - 15 BLEND

Chamomile Roman	5 drops
Lavender	5 drops
Frankincense	2 drops
Geranium	3 drops

Blend these quantities with 30 mls (1 oz) base oil to make a massage oil or make a synergistic blend using these proportions and use 4 drops in a bath.

Amnesia

It's bad enough to wake up after a wild night out and not remember where you went, or who with, but try to imagine what it's like to wake up in a hospital after a car crash and not remember a thing about last night, the night before that, and all the days and nights of your life. Even your mother is a stranger. It is truly terrifying.

Forty percent of people involved in road accidents suffer brain damage and some degree of amnesia. Most of these victims are under twenty-five years of age. Amnesia can also come about as a result of various illnesses, such as meningitis or encephalitis; alcoholics can have it as a result of their thiamine deficiency; drug addiction can cause it; as can epilepsy, stroke, and brain tumors. Amnesia can also come about for no apparent, physical cause, but because of emotional trauma. Perhaps something so painful happened in the past, that period of one's life is simply wiped out as a self-protection mechanism. Shock or hysteria can also cause amnesia.

There's retrograde amnesia — forgetting things that happened before the incident that caused the amnesia, and anterograde amnesia — forgetting things that happen after the incident. People who have retrograde amnesia also often cannot remember things that happen after the incident very well. Amnesiacs have dreadful problems to deal with, frustrating, exasperating, and debilitating. Essential oils obviously cannot help all these problems but where they may be able to help some people is in alleviating some of the confusion that results from the condition. Also, if the amnesia was caused by shock or fear, essential oils can work on them, and thus may perhaps beneficially affect the amnesia. It's certainly worth a try.

The two following blends can be added to 30 mls (1 oz) base oil and made into massage oils, or they can be made into a synergistic blend and used in diffusers or other methods. See Chart 5.1 for quantities to use.

AMNESIC CONFUSION BLEND 1	
Cardamom	10 drops
Bergamot	10 drops
Ginger	5 drops
Petitgrain	5 drops

AMNESIC CONFUSION BLEND 2	
Helichrysum	10 drops
Petitgrain	5 drops
Geranium	2 drops
Grapefruit	10 drops

ESSENTIAL OILS TO HELP SHOCK-INDUCED AMNESIA

Mandarin	Ylang Ylang
Rose Maroc	Rose Otto
Neroli	Melissa
Peppermint	Lavender

Also see the essential oils listed under the Trauma section.

ESSENTIAL OILS THAT HELP THE CONFUSION OF AMNESIA

Cardamom	Tuberose
Ginger	Black Pepper
Bergamot	Geranium
Petitgrain	Helichrysum
Grapefruit	Basil

Both these following blends can be made into a massage oil by adding each to 30 mls (1 oz) base oil. They can also both be made into a synergistic blend and used

TRAUMA SHOCK BLEND

Peppermint	10 drops
Lavender	20 drops

EMOTIONAL SHOCK BLEND

Rose Otto	5 drops
Neroli	5 drops
Mandarin	15 drops

FEAR-INDUCED AMNESIA BLEND 1

Chamomile		
Roman		15 drops
Cypress		10 drops
Vetiver		5 drops

FEAR-INDUCED AMNESIA BLEND 2

Sandalwood	15 drops
Lemon	5 drops
Orange	10 drops

in a diffuser or sniffed from a tissue or the bottle. The Emotional Shock blend can also be used in a bath — use 8 drops. The Trauma Shock blend, however, should not be used in a bath.

ESSENTIAL OILS TO HELP FEAR-INDUCED AMNESIA

Sandalwood	Cypress
Vetiver	Lemon
Bergamot	Neroli
Geranium	
Chamomile Roman	
Cedarwood Orange	

Also see the essential oils listed under the Fear section.

The following two blends can be added to 30 mls (1 oz) base oil (each) for a massage oil; they can both also be made into a synergistic blend and used in the usual methods including diffusers and baths — 8 drops per bath.

Anger

Many people working in the medical and therapy fields have commented that unexpressed anger can result in many chronic symptoms including chronic tiredness, apathy, the inability to concentrate, back ache, intestinal problems, rashes, skin disorders, and many other more serious physical problems, including heart disease. At the same time, too much anger can cause a rise in blood pressure and the possibility of a stroke. Just as it can kill you, anger can make you loose control and kill someone else. The French recognize that anger is a built-in safety valve to our program for psychological well-being and have tolerance for crimes of passion, but not every country is so broad-minded and anger can send you straight to the electric chair if you don't watch out.

Clearly, the trick with anger is to keep it in balance — have enough to express what is really felt, but not enough to get someone into trouble. We know we shouldn't bottle it up, but when a job is at stake it might seem more sensible to bite our tongue and pretend nothing happened. Inevitably, in our nice civilized world, much anger remains unexpressed, festering away in our body and soul.

The colors of anger are red, black, and white — as in "to see red" and have a red face, have a black scowl of fury, or white, clenched knuckles and a face white with rage. People can go very still and quiet — seething with anger, while others shake, tremble, or feel weak. Some people express their anger at a moment's provocation, others bottle it up and explode like a volcano hours, days, or weeks later, while others still tuck it away and pretend they don't have it. Everyone reacts in a different way. And there are people who seem to be angry for no reason at all, or no reason they have yet understood. And there are people who are angry with others; and those who are angry with themselves.

The essential oils have been arranged in this section under three categories: essential oils to calm down anger; essential oils to help cope with anger; and essential oils to help express anger. We start with the oils that can help calm an angry person down, long enough for them to look at the heart of the matter and hopefully try to find help.

There are many ways of coping with anger, from relaxation techniques, yoga, holding your breath, doing deep breathing exercises, counting to ten, and punching a cushion instead of a face. I know a man who used to jump in his fast car when he had an angry argument with his wife and drive like a maniac until he cooled down. He and quite a few other people were lucky they didn't end up dead. Essential oils are a much safer bet. Choose from the following list.

ESSENTIAL OILS TO CALM DOWN FEELINGS OF ANGER	
Tuberose	Vetiver
Lavender	Bergamot
Rose Maroc	Rose Otto
Petitgrain	Patchouli
Chamomile Roman	
Chamomile German	
Linden Blossom	

ESSENTIAL OILS TO HELP COPE WITH ANGER	
Vetiver	Ylang Ylang
Rose Maroc	Valerian
Black Pepper	Spikenard
Myrtle	Benzoin
Chamomile Roman	
Linden Blossom	

The following quantities of oils can each be blended with 30 mls (1 oz) of base oil for a massage, or made into a synergistic blend and used in other methods. For quantities to use see Chart 5.1.

Anxiety

COPING WITH ANGER BLEND1

Spikenard	10 drops
Bergamot	10 drops
Chamomile Roman	10 drops

COPING WITH ANGER BLEND 2

Rose Maroc	10 drops
Linden Blossom	10 drops
Chamomile Roman	2 drops

ESSENTIAL OILS TO HELP RELEASE UNEXPRESSED ANGER

Tuberose	Black Pepper
Ginger	Cedarwood
Patchouli	Clove
Ormenis Flower	

RELEASING UNEXPRESSED
ANGER BLEND 1

Ormenis Flower	15 drops
Ginger	5 drops
Black Pepper	5 drops

RELEASING UNEXPRESSED
ANGER BLEND 2

Patchouli	15 drops
Tuberose	5 drops
Clove	1 drop

Anxiety is, in a sense, the heightened awareness of things that can go wrong. It is a normal component of the human being and serves to keep us on our toes. But for whatever reason, and there may be more than one, our sense of impending doom balloons out, so to speak, inside us, filling us with unease, and even fear. In some instances the impending doom is a real event — a forthcoming exam, driving test or, for authors, a deadline. For others, it's just a daily generalized feeling of unease — mild to intense — about everything: the safety of the family, the state of everyone's health, financial problems, etc., brought on by years of actual hard life experience. We can only take so much.

You can guess you're pretty anxious if you find yourself sighing a lot, gasping for breath or needing to take in large chunks of air. It might even be that you're running to the toilet all the time, getting headaches or back pain, or just can't relax. Yet a sense of tiredness is common, or restlessness, even tremors. Anxiety can make you dizzy, perspire, or blush, and it can raise your blood pressure. One can feel dry in the mouth, or belch a lot, feel nauseous, get diarrhea, vomit. The stomach muscles can tighten up in a spasm, causing terrible pain. Anxiety causes stabbing pains in the chest, and stronger, faster heartbeats. It can make a person feel so unwell they seriously wonder if there isn't something physically wrong — which causes more anxiety, of course. So then you can't sleep well at night. These

ESSENTIAL OILS TO HELP RELIEVE GENERAL ANXIETY	
Bergamot	Lavender
Mandarin	Sandalwood
Vetiver	Cedarwood
Neroli	Rose Otto
Melissa	Geranium
Juniper	Frankincense
Patchouli	Clary Sage
Chamomile Roman	

are just some of the symptoms.

The real cure for anxiety is to win the lottery, get a guarantee from an angel that no member of your family will have an accident or get ill ever again, and hear on the news that all wars have stopped. But frankly, I don't think that's going to happen. Somehow we'll just have to continue coping as best we can. Fortunately, however, nature's little helpmates, the essential oils, can do a lot to help.

Because there are so many symptoms of anxiety, I am breaking this section into four different types, with blends for each. But we start with a general list of essential oils that can deflate the anxiety, and bring it down to a normal level.

The following blends relate to the four anxiety types above. The quantities given here could be blended with 30 mls (1 oz) base oil to make a massage oil, or use these proportions to make a synergistic blend that can be used in the bath, or in a diffuser or other room method, or inhaled from a tissue. See Chart 5.1 for quantities to use.

TENSE ANXIETY — TYPE 1

Symptoms: bodily tension, muscle pain, aches, sore body

Essential Oils: Sandalwood, Lavender, Clary Sage, Chamomile Roman, Patchouli

RESTLESS ANXIETY — TYPE 2

Symptoms: overactivity, sweating, palpitations, dizziness, lump in throat, frequent urination or diarrhea (overactivity of the autonomic nervous system), upset stomach

Essential Oils: Vetiver, Cedarwood, Juniper, Chamomile Roman, Frankincense

APPREHENSIVE ANXIETY — TYPE 3

Symptoms: unease, apprehension, worrying, brooding, overanxious, paranoia, sense of foreboding

Essential Oils: Bergamot, Lavender, Neroli, Rose Otto, Melissa, Geranium

REPRESSED ANXIETY — TYPE 4

Symptoms: feeling on edge, irritable, difficulty in concentrating, insomnia, feeling exhausted all the time

Essential Oils: Bergamot, Melissa, Neroli, Rose Otto, Sandalwood, Vetiver, Cedarwood

TENSE ANXIETY — TYPE 1 SYNERGISTIC BLEND	
Clary Sage	10 drops
Lavender	15 drops
Chamomile Roman	5 drops

RESTLESS ANXIETY — TYPE 2
SYNERGISTIC BLEND

Vetiver	5 drops
Juniper	10 drops
Cedarwood	15 drops

APPREHENSIVE ANXIETY — TYPE 3
SYNERGISTIC BLEND

Bergamot	15 drops
Lavender	5 drops
Geranium	10 drops

REPRESSED ANXIETY — TYPE 4
SYNERGISTIC BLEND

Neroli	10 drops
Rose Otto	10 drops
Bergamot	10 drops

Apathy

The word "apathy" derives from the Greek word for feeling, *"pathos,"* and means to be without feeling — without joy, passion, excitement, and without sadness, hurt, and pain. It can be brought on by various emotional situations including romantic heartache, depression, worthlessness, and guilt, as well as by illness, and pain. Apathetic people are difficult to get motivated. They watch the news and say, "so what?" Nothing moves them. They don't care about their appearance, or whether they're going to lose their job, or what they're going to eat tonight. Apathetic people slump around, with an air of weariness and listlessness around them, like a little gray fog. Worse than this,

ESSENTIAL OILS TO HELP FIGHT APATHY

Cardamom	Lemon
Ginger	Black Pepper
Bergamot	Orange
Jasmine	Rose Otto
Rose Maroc	Peppermint
Ormenis Flower	Basil

they're like emotional zombies — scarily half-dead.

Essential oils can certainly help in cases of apathy, but the person needs to examine why they are feeling so isolated, and ask what could have caused it in the first place. Counseling may be required, or a physical examination because apathy can have an underlying physical cause.

Choose from the following blends that seem most appropriate and use these quantities diluted with a base oil to make a massage oil, or make up a synergistic blend using these proportions and use it

GENERAL APATHY

Basil	5 drops
Bergamot	10 drops
Cardamom	15 drops

APATHY WITH EXTRA
INDIFFERENCE

Cardamom	15 drops
Ginger	10 drops
Orange	5 drops

APATHY WITH DEPRESSION	
Black Pepper	15 drops
Basil	5 drops
Bergamot	10 drops

diffused in the atmosphere, at home or at work, or sniffed from a tissue.

Bereavement

The people we love are our only true security in this life and it is they who make life loving and worth living, and help it make sense. When they go, a part of us goes too — perhaps a very large part, but all the structures of our life go as well — the security, the love, and the sense of it all. Whatever the circumstances of the death, bereavement is the most profound loss, a wrenching away of a part of us, and of course it hurts terribly.

I can't imagine the pain of losing a child, but thousands of parents must go through this ghastly fate each year, while tens of thousands of us will lose a parent, our anchor in life. As each death is such an individual experience, no person can be expected to react in a predictable way. I've known people who throw themselves into work trying to blank out the pain, and others who sit in a chair for months not saying a word. Everyone has to work it through their own way. Sometimes bereavement counseling can help and in the Addresses section of this book you can find the contact addresses for the *National Associations of Widows, Stillbirth* *and Neonatal Death Society,* and *Age Concern,* who may all be able to put people in touch with services in their area. Perhaps the worst experience is for those who have unfinished emotional business with the deceased, and who never had the chance to say "good-bye" and "I love you." For sure, around the experience of death there are many emotions aside from the sheer, awful, empty grief — there could be guilt and remorse as well.

Clearly, essential oils can only soften the terrible blow of bereavement and they cannot fill the gap. But many people have found them a tremendous support and comfort during these terrible times, and through the lonely times ahead. They are particularly effective in baths or massage oils. Also, gently diffused in a room, they can help provide a calm and comforting atmosphere in which the mourning process can take place.

You can make up individual blends from the above list, or by choosing oils from other sections in this chapter — such as those in Grief, Loss, Sorrow,

ESSENTIAL OILS TO USE IN BEREAVEMENT	
Benzoin	Rose Otto
Neroli	Lavender
Melissa	Vetiver
Patchouli	Cypress
Mandarin	Rose Maroc
Linden Blossom	
Chamomile Roman	

Depression, Anger, Anxiety, and Insomnia, depending on the emotions you are going through at any particular time, which will probably change with the process of mourning. Alternatively, use one of the comforting ones below. Blend these quantities with 30 mls (1 oz) base oil to make a massage oil, or use these proportions to make a synergistic blend of oils that can be used in any of the other methods. See Chart 5.1 for quantities to use.

COMFORTING BLEND 1	
Benzoin	5 drops
Rose Otto	12 drops
Chamomile	
Roman	2 drops
Mandarin	2 drops

COMFORTING BLEND 2	
Mandarin	15 drops
Geranium	8 drops
Patchouli	7 drops

COMFORTING BLEND 3	
Neroli	12 drops
Linden Blossom	5 drops
Melissa	8 drops

COMFORTING BLEND 4	
Vetiver	5 drops
Geranium	20 drops
Patchouli	5 drops

Research has shown that some people find smells such as cinnamon, clove, and pine comforting. It may be that these aromas remind them of happy situations such as Christmas or their mother cooking. Aroma is a very individual experience and you will need to find what is appropriate for you in these circumstances. The particular aftershaves, perfumes, or fragranced products that were used by the departed soul may be of comfort, due to the smell association.

Breakdown

If you haven't suffered a breakdown it can be very difficult to understand just how that person might feel, and identify with the torment they are going through. They, meanwhile, may not be able to express all the fears and emotions they are feeling. For the sufferer, it is a very lonely business, and for the family a very bewildering one. Breakdowns happen to all kinds of people — smart and stupid, old and young, fat and thin. I heard of a woman recently — the head of department at a university, juggling her work with two children — who recently had a breakdown. She seemed to be fine and was calmly going about her job with her usual efficiency and good natured outlook but at home she was building huge edifices on the kitchen table, out of anything and everything, and taking it all rather too seriously — as if this were her real job. She had cracked, but it took her family a few days to fully realize what was going on. Eventually, after some high trauma, she was led away, as they say, by the men in white coats, with her husband pleading with her to sign the paper saying she was booking herself in for treatment. This dramatic scene would have been quite unthinkable to the family just a short week earlier. The woman seemed to be coping. She was her usual laid-back, smiling self, a master at covering up what anguish was going on beneath — like so many of us. In fact, this breakdown will probably force her to face the real problem in her life.

"Nervous breakdown" is a vague, nonmedical term for the onset of a wide variety of problems usually related to our situation and circumstances, and our ability to cope with them. With the vast majority of people, the breakdown is just a hiccup in an otherwise normal life — a break caused by mental stress that can in time heal. "Mental breakdown," on the other hand, can take away all mental reasoning, all sense of self, of the world and reality and, sadly, some people never really recover. Many others, of course, do.

Any kind of breakdown requires professional help, comfort, care, and attention. Gentleness and compassion are the order of the day. Once the crisis is over and the recovery period has begun, essential oils can be used in a massage oil for use on the hands, feet and, possibly, the neck, shoulders, and forearms, using gentle stroking movements known to masseurs as "effleurage." Essential oil baths are particularly welcoming and help the person tremendously in the return to full mental health. Also, diffusing essential oils in the atmosphere is very beneficial.

Psychiatric units and hospitals are often unwelcoming places, certainly the ones I have visited, and if the management budget can't stretch to a lick of paint, a pleasant ambiance can be created quite cheaply by using essential oils.

Ideally, commercial size diffusers could be installed, but if not, use the Landel™ diffuser — one that involves no fire or electricity. See Appendix III for the supplier.

People who have undergone a breakdown often experience a heightened sense of smell, or have smell hallucinations. These effects may sometimes be related to the drugs being used. Clearly then, using aroma in these circumstances has to be done with sensitivity, and consultation with the patient(s). Essential oils can be chosen from appropriate lists, according to the symptoms, or taken from the lists below.

For quantities to use, and methods, see Chart 5.1.

ESSENTIAL OILS FOR USE IN CASES OF GENERAL BREAKDOWN	
Lavender	Clary Sage
Lemon	Orange
Geranium	Neroli
Helichrysum	
Chamomile Roman	

ESSENTIAL OILS FOR USE IN CASES OF EMOTIONAL BREAKDOWN	
Lavender	Cypress
Geranium	Sandalwood
Rose Otto	Mandarin
Benzoin	Neroli
Chamomile Roman	

Burnout

Burnout is usually thought of as a physical thing, but burnout can relate to the emotional and mental processes, which then affect the physical. You can get burnout when there are no more tears to cry, no feelings anymore, just emotional exhaustion. And the thing is, when the emotions shut down, so does the body.

Someone could get burnout, for example, after caring for a sick partner or relative with a terminal illness, perhaps over a long time. This can use up all of one's reserves of compassion in coping with the person's needs, plus there is the distressing experience of watching the loved one die. After this, emotional burnout is, understandably, quite common. But there are many other situations that might cause emotional burnout, after a lost love perhaps, or even during particularly deep times of self-examination or thinking emotionally about close family members. We are emotional beings, and sometimes our emotions come in for excessive use, leaving a state of emptiness or numbness.

Burnout can paralyze a person, leaving them a dead-weight in a chair, or simply feeling exhausted and depressed — to greater or lesser degree. All the feelings that go to make up a human personality seem missing, disappeared somewhere. Also, people can have a sense of being in a vacuum, or a glass bubble — unable, as the song goes, to reach out and touch somebody's hand. The feelings are there, of course, but the emotional side has closed

ESSENTIAL OILS TO HELP LESSEN THE EFFECT OF EMOTIONAL BURNOUT	
Vetiver	Bergamot
Rose Otto	Neroli
Linden Blossom	Melissa
Patchouli	Sandalwood
Hyacinth	Marjoram
Lavender	Benzoin
Clary Sage	Helichrysum
Sandalwood	Lemon
Frankincense	Petitgrain
Ginger	Jasmine
Chamomile Roman	

down for a while, to recharge the batteries. The following essential oils would be a good choice for those with all types of emotional burnout, including that experienced by those caring for the terminally ill.

The following two blends are for general emotional burnout and they are half measures because, with burnout, it is better to start softly, using only 15 drops of essential oil to the usual 30 mls (1 oz)

BURNOUT NO. 1	
Vetiver	2 drops
Bergamot	10 drops
Lavender	3 drops

BURNOUT NO. 2	
Lavender	3 drops
Clary Sage	2 drops
Marjoram	3 drops
Lemon	7 drops

base vegetable oil for a massage oil, and if you make a synergistic blend only use 1-2 drops in the bath or 1-2 drops diffused in the atmosphere.

As time goes on you can add to the number of drops of essential oils in the blend, up to the usual 30 drops of essential oil to 30 mls (1 oz) base oil — which is a general rule of 1-1 (1 drop essential oil to 1 ml (.03 oz) vegetable oil). You can refer to other sections in this book and choose which essential oils to add, those that seem appropriate for you, or look at the chart at the back of the book.

ESSENTIAL OILS THAT MAY HELP WITH CONFUSION	
Cardamom	Ginger
Black Pepper	Bergamot
Geranium	Petitgrain
Helichrysum	Grapefruit
Basil	Rosemary
Peppermint	Cypress
Thyme Linalol	Lavender
Ormenis Flower	Pine
Juniper	

Confusion

The symptoms of confusion are not remembering places, being unable to finish or even start simple tasks, giving the wrong or inappropriate answers to questions, and not being able to make sense out of anything. Confusion can be caused by stress, overwork, physical or mental illness, by head injury, or senile dementia. The morphine given for pain relief can sometimes produce confusion, while certain medical conditions may lead into confusion and then dementia. Confusion can also be caused by epileptic fits, drug overdose, drug addiction, depression, and schizophrenia. Sometimes loss of memory and confusion go together, but not always.

If the confusion has been caused by something physical, there is often an associated high temperature and a general feeling of being unwell. Although such confusion can come on rapidly and be alarming, it might only last a few days. However, it might indicate a developing serious condition and medical attention should be sought immediately.

If there is a high temperature you can help to bring it down by removing the clothing and sponging the body down with a solution of 2 drops of essential oil of eucalyptus in 1 liter (2 pints) of cool water. If the confusion has been caused by a head injury, drug overdose, or insulin deficiency, again, a doctor should be called immediately. Clearly, however, in the elderly, senile dementia may be progressive.

The essential oils are, here, being recommended for situations in which there is no clinical reason for the confusion, when they can help us focus and concentrate.

For the kind of confusion that hits us all at some point in our lives, perhaps as a result of overwork, or of stress and anxiety, the following blends should help. These quantities can be added to 30 mls (1 oz) base oil to make a massage oil, or

CONFUSION BLEND 1

Cardamom	13 drops
Black Pepper	5 drops
Ginger	4 drops
Grapefruit	8 drops

CONFUSION BLEND 2

Basil	7 drops
Helichrysum	5 drops
Grapefruit	10 drops
Ginger	8 drops

make a synergistic blend using these proportions for use in the diffuser or inhalation methods. See Chart 5.1 for quantities to use. Do not use these synergistic blends, basil, or peppermint, in the bath.

Dejection

To be dejected is to feel disheartened and dispirited, possibly as a result of being rejected in some sense — not appreciated at work, cast away by a lover, even perhaps profoundly disappointed by the negativity one experiences in life in general. Dejected people are weakened by their experience and seem to have had the sparkle taken out of them — a result of the spirit and emotional heart being damaged. People can have an "air of dejection" about them that seems to permeate the things they do, objects they make, and even meals they cook. One can practically taste the dejection in the food.

One of the best things for dejection is sunshine — lots of it! Also, bright colors really help — so pull out those old Hawaiian shirts. Or if that's too much, at least wear a bright, colorful scarf or tie. These are the essential oils that can help, use them in all the usual ways.

ESSENTIAL OILS THAT CAN HELP DISPEL FEELINGS OF DEJECTION	
Bergamot	Frankincense
Grapefruit	Mandarin
Geranium	Nutmeg
Mimosa	Orange
Linden Blossom	Rose Maroc
Jasmine	Petitgrain
Neroli	Ylang Ylang

Delirium

Delirium is a state of acute mental confusion and to suggest it can be controlled with essential oils would be totally wrong. Essential oils can, however, help bring down the temperature often associated with delirium, and reduce the restlessness. Delirium can be precipitated by the use of alcohol over long periods, by drugs, and certain poisons. It can also develop after major surgery — notably in children and the elderly. Most importantly, it can give evidence of serious physical disorder and a doctor must be called right away. Shortage of oxygen and brain damage can both cause delirium, while many elderly people also sometimes get delirious as a consequence of dementia.

In delirium, all normal conscious

thought is disrupted, there is memory loss and mental confusion. Disorientation and restlessness are classic symptoms; anxiety and mood swings are common; shakes and tremors a possibility. In severe cases, there could be illusions or hallucinations that are often monstrous and terrifying. Panic and shouting are not uncommon.

ESSENTIAL OILS TO USE IN CASES OF DELIRIUM

Peppermint	Lavender
Eucalyptus Radiata	Marjoram
Eucalyptus Globulus	

After calling a doctor, take the temperature. If it is too high, try to help bring it down by sponging the person with 2 drops of eucalyptus mixed in with 1 liter (2 pints) of cool water. You could also diffuse a cooling essential oil in the atmosphere—such as peppermint or eucalyptus. If there is no temperature and the person is restless, diffuse lavender essential oil in the room as this may calm them down.

Delirium Tremens

The "DTs," as they're known, affect those going through drug withdrawal and chronic alcoholics — especially after a period of abstinence. A classic picture of DTs is of someone brushing imaginary insects off their sleeves, terrified. The DTs sufferer is in a frightening world of confu-

sion, and they're shaking. Disorientation, sleeplessness, restlessness, and agitation is usual, as is fever, sweating, and a faster heartbeat. Vivid visual and sometimes auditory hallucinations make life a nightmare. Not surprisingly, the person sometimes gets aggressive.

Dehydration is a problem, and an attack of the DTs might require a stay in the hospital to rehydrate, as well as to sedate and rest. If someone suffers an attack, the doctor must be called immediately. It may help to overcome the effects of withdrawal by giving soothing hand and foot massages, and for them to use essential oils in the bath. Alcoholics have a severe shortage of thiamine, which is helped by giving vitamin B-complex. Calming essential oils can be diffused in the atmosphere, used in a bath, or in a massage oil, or a drop can be placed on a pillow or cushion. Use the essential oils singly, on their own, not in mixes, and make sure the person with delirium tremens likes the fragrance. Lavender and lemon have been found particularly useful in cases of alcohol withdrawal and the DTs (see Addiction), but all the following oils are useful.

ESSENTIAL OILS TO USE IN CASES OF DELIRIUM TREMENS

Lavender	Petitgrain
Lemon	Marjoram
Valerian	Geranium
Chamomile Roman	

Dementia and Alzheimer's Disease

Dementia used to be thought of as a disease of old age but, because of the HIV virus, many young people are now experiencing dementia — which perhaps fills them with more dread than any other symptom of their illness. To slowly loose one's mental capacity is bad enough at an old age, but when a person is in their thirties, it is really tragic. Dementia can also affect people who have suffered strokes, both young and old, and those who have Alzheimer's. For anyone looking after a loved one with dementia, the whole experience is terribly upsetting as the person becomes a shadow of their former selves — not remembering recent events, getting lost in familiar surroundings, losing sense of time, and not even recognizing the caring family and friends who are offering their support. It is appalling to watch a loved one literally lose their mind, slowly day by day, but for the person suffering from dementia, who must be at least occasionally aware of themselves slipping mentally away, it must be horrific, like slipping into a black hole.

Unfortunately, there is no cure for dementia unless is it caused by encephalitis, syphilis, anemia, or several other conditions that can be treated. Most cases get worse. The best we can do for them is care in a practical sense, by way of feeding, cleaning and so forth. Because of the powerful olfactory link with memory, aromas might be the last link between the real experienced world, and the mind which is now hidden within. Aroma may be the last thing the sufferer can hold on to. Plus essential oils have other benefits too. Aroma preference is a very powerful thing, however, and the person should be consulted if essential oils are to be used. A choice of aromas could be offered — if they sniff in deeply and nod their heads, you can guess they like it, and if they turn up their nose and grimace, they don't.

Essential oils can be used diffused in the atmosphere, dropped in warm baths, or made into a massage oil, which is very effective in hand and foot massages. There is no need to do a body massage and if you are the caretaker, perhaps temporary, you are a stranger, essentially, and a body massage could be seen as an invasion. But a regular hand massage from a caring person would be very welcome, and the aroma would provide a continuity link with regular care, which would be beneficial. What I mean by that is that the person suffering from dementia will come to associate the aroma with a particular person — the caretaker — and "recognize" them by smell, if not by face. Choose oils from the Concentration, Confusion, and Memory sections, or from the lists below. We start with a general list for

ESSENTIAL OILS TO HELP IN CASES OF DEMENTIA	
Basil	Cardamom
Ginger	Black Pepper
Rosemary	Rose Otto

oils that are helpful.

The following floral oils are particularly appreciated by women and they are generally good in massage oils for restlessness and tremors.

GENTLE ESSENTIAL OILS TO HELP IN CASES OF RESTLESSNESS AND TREMORS	
Rose Otto	Neroli
Lavender	Geranium
Chamomile Roman	Jasmine

Appetite can be stimulated by diffusing the following fruit and spice essential oils in the atmosphere, and these aromas tend to bring back memories, which is a good thing.

APPETITE STIMULANT AND MEMORY-EVOKING ESSENTIAL OILS	
Lemon	Orange
Lime	Grapefruit
Nutmeg	Cinnamon
Clove	Ginger
Coriander	Cardamom
Black Pepper	

One thing that might be helpful in the fight to hold off dementia is ginkgo biloba, a plant widely used by naturopaths all over the world, and available from health food stores. An excellent review of gingko's effectiveness against

ADDITIONAL MEMORY-EVOKING ESSENTIAL OILS	
Basil	Rosemary

"cerebral insufficiency" appeared in *The Lancet*[2] and should be referred to by all who care for those suffering with dementia. "Cerebral insufficiency" is defined as "absentmindedness, anxiety, confusion, decreased physical performance, depressive mood, difficulty in concentrating, difficulty in remembering, dizziness, head- ache, lack of energy, tinnitus, and tiredness." A great deal of research has now been carried out on ginkgo, all over the world, and its benefits are well established. Also, there have been no reports of any side effects. It's said that the ginkgo biloba tree is the oldest tree known (possibly 160 million years old), and clearly it still has much to offer mankind. Vitamin supplements are also useful, such as a vitamin B-complex, vitamins C and E, plus a multimineral.

Dementia – the Caretakers

Caretakers of people with dementia often have to endure a great deal. Aside from the physical work, there is the fact that it can make the person uncharacteristically difficult — they can make unreasonable demands, and accusations. The caretaker is tormented by the sadness of watching and feeling the loved one slowly lose touch, and on top of that, they may feel guilty — probably for no good reason.

Choose gentle oils that help deal with the anxiety, stresses, and strains of dealing with delirium on a regular basis; and those which help with the sadness inevitably felt as someone experiences a loved-one mentally and emotionally drifting away. Use the oils in all the usual methods. The following quantities can be blended with 30 mls (1 oz) base oil, or make a synergistic blend using these proportions. For quantities to use, see Chart 5.1.

CARETAKER'S GENTLE COMFORT 1	
Geranium	7 drops
Patchouli	5 drops
Bergamot	8 drops
Rose Maroc	10 drops
CARETAKER'S GENTLE COMFORT 2	
Benzoin	10 drops
Rose	7 drops
Orange	6 drops
Jasmine	7 drops

Depression

"The Black Dog," as Winston Churchill called it, hits between 5-15% of people in Britain at some time in their lives according to various estimates, although the figure may be higher than this because it's thought that men don't always go to the doctor and report their symptoms, (i.e., feelings). Some 1-2% of depressed persons are classified as bi-polar or manic depressive because they have sharp mood and activity swings.

The main symptoms of depression are as you would expect — feelings of sadness, hopelessness, and pessimism. Another classic symptom is no longer having a positive interest in life's pleasures, including sex. Sufferers may additionally experience the slowing down of physical or mental actions, tiredness, loss of concentration, indecision, and impaired memory. Sometimes the depressed person finds themselves crying for no apparent reason, and they're unable to control the tears. Worthlessness and guilt — excessive and/or inappropriate — often accompany depression, making it easy for someone to say to themselves, "Oh, they'd be better off without me," and this is the biggest danger of depression — suicide — which is why it must be taken seriously, and why help must be sought.

We all get depressed sometimes but we can usually be brought out of it by a vacation or even a good evening out with friends. These measures don't help the depressive at all — and is further evidence that they need help. People do react to depression in different ways, particularly in their eating and sleep patterns — which can be to either overeat or not to eat, and either to oversleep or not be able to sleep.

In 1989 clinicians in America carried out a survey among 1800 managers and engineers at the huge Westinghouse™ Electric corporation, to try to establish the degree of depression experienced by them. Psychiatry professor Evelyn Bromet of New York University, who carried out the research, found that 23% of people interviewed had experienced an episode of major depression in their life, a result she called "astounding." Depression often hits people who are particularly ambitious or hardworking, both young and old. In an article about depression among executives, *Fortune* magazine included an interview with one man who had been at the top of his career, who had never been ill but who suddenly couldn't eat or sleep. He said, "I could barely think. I'd stare at six pairs of identical white underwear in the morning and couldn't decide which pair to put on." For him, and for many others, the depression came on without apparent cause. This is known as endogenous depression, while depression that results from an identifiable event is called exogenous depression. Strangely perhaps, depression can stem from both good and bad life changes, from a promotion or being laid off, and from a birth as well as a death. However, depression usually has no one identifiable cause and just comes, appropriately, "from the blue," because that's what it is — a major case of the blues.

Anyone who feels depressed, for whatever apparent reason, should certainly seek medical advice because there is a chance that there is an underlying physical disorder at fault, possibly involving the thyroid gland, and making depression a form of hormonal imbalance (which we are aware of also in postnatal depression). In one unconfirmed press report I saw that a study by the University of Miami School of Medicine has shown

that nearly half the people in their sample diagnosed as having severe depression actually had thyroid problems. They were treated with thyroid hormones for two months, and their depression began to lift after the fourth week. Another interesting study by psychologists David Roth and David Holmes at the University of Kansas showed that students suffering from the blues were not helped by relaxation training but were helped by aerobic exercise, so if you're too depressed to get up and go to aerobic classes, buy a workout video for home.

This might sound like too much effort, however, for most depressives, who can get so low they can hardly get out of bed. As one sufferer so eloquently put it: "Depression should have a blacker name. It is a disease which shrinks the spirit and sucks the color from life."[3] How do you get out of that? The man who wrote that was helped by antidepressants, as many people have been. There does, however, seem to be some disagreement over how long the drugs should be used, and at what dose. And although the dosage doesn't have to be increased over time to achieve the same effectiveness, they are still addictive, and one has to come off them very slowly (See *Addiction*). The old generation of antidepressants, the tricyclics, and enzymatic MAO (monoamine oxidase) inhibitors have been put in the shadow recently by the new generation of "selective seratonin re-uptake inhibitors." Since the introduction in America of the first of these drugs, Prozac in 1988, at least seven separate seratonin receptors have been identified by scientists. This illustrates that this whole area of neurotransmitter research is extremely new, and as I discussed earlier, we have much to learn.

As for the natural pharmacopoeia, some interesting research comes from Dr. Tanaka, et al., at Kyoto University, Japan. They found that the root of *Glycyrrhiza uralensis*, a species of licorice widely used in Chinese medicine, has MAO inhibiting effects. One derivative of the plant extract is 450 times as effective as a standard MAO inhibitor. [4] Another natural antidepressant is the amino acid tryptophan, which is converted into an intermediate product known as 5-HTP, from which it becomes seratonin. Studies of dieters have shown them to have lower levels of tryptophan, which may explain why dieters get depressed. In some countries tryptophan can be bought over the counter as a food supplement, but it was taken off the market in Britain in 1990 for some unknown reason, which the regulatory bodies may be able to explain. If it's any consolation, bananas are packed with tryptophan.

Depression, then, might be caused by tryptophan deficiency (probably not treatable with a bunch of bananas), by thyroid problems, by a genetic factor, by problems in life — either specific or cumulative, by changes in life — either good or bad, or for no apparent reason at all. Probably, not all these people can be helped by psychotherapy, but certainly some can, especially if they've been through a bad life experience. Drugs clearly have a place in the treatment of depression, and the first point here is to make sure the doctor doesn't give you tranquilizers, which are likely to slow you down further. At least, there have been

many reports in the press about misdiagnosis in depression. You know your feelings best. Refer to the Anxiety section, and see the difference in symptoms.

Antidepressants don't have a street value as illicit drugs because they don't do anything to you unless the body needs it — that's the theory anyway — so they are being recommended as a diagnostic tool. If the person responds favorably to the seratonin uptake inhibitor, they were depressed and needed it. If they were "normal," they wouldn't need it and the drug will do nothing for them. What all the antidepressants do is alter the uptake of a variety of brain chemicals.

The "tricyclics," which have a common core chemical structure, work in different ways: one drug will block the re-uptake of norepinephrine and seratonin, but not dopamine; another blocks the re-uptake of serotonin; while another has an effect on the uptake of norepinephrine, and so on. We're talking about a lot of fine-tuning going on here, and it helps to have a doctor who knows the in's and out's of antidepressant drugs (and advises on their side effects). Balance is all. There are now a dozen seratonin-related drugs available, some increasing the level of it — sometimes at specific receptor sites, and others lowering the level at specific receptors. With all these options, it is possible there's a drug that can suit a depressive's requirements; the trick is finding it and staying on it only as long as absolutely required. Addiction can become a problem and the new drugs are by definition untested by time and may hold some surprises in terms of long-term effect. We just don't know.

Having said that, I would not recommend anyone stop taking antidepressant medication without medical advice.

If you can, as a therapy complementary to medical care, I recommend you visit an aromatherapist who can offer support and encouragement, as well as the benefits of therapeutic touch and essential oils. As depressives often have trouble receiving loving touch, an aromatherapy treatment can be a great help in overcoming that barrier. Also, friends of depressives should seek them out and lend a listening ear. Time and love are the greatest gifts and although the depressive will not be able to express their thanks, your concern will be a vital component in their recovery.

Essential oils can help in cases of depression brought about by trauma — reactive or exogenous depression as it used to be called, although there are usually many different elements to depression and each case should be treated differently. The symptoms can also be cross referenced with the charts on pages 223 and 230-236. Following this general section there are additional recommendations for types of depression classified as "Weepy," "Agitated," or Anxious," "Lethargic," and "Hysterical" — please refer to them also. "Manic Depressive Psychosis" is another type of depression altogether and is discussed at the end. However, there follows here a list of essential oils that could be called "General" oils for depression, which have been traditionally shown in aromatherapy to be effective in the treatment of depression. They will not provide a magic cure but will definitely support and complement any other ther-

ESSENTIAL OILS USED TRADITIONALLY IN AROMATHERAPY FOR DEPRESSION	
Mandarin	Lemon
Bergamot	Grapefruit
Orange	Jasmine
Ylang Ylang	Rose Otto
Rose Maroc	Neroli
Geranium	Petitgrain
Helichrysum	Sandalwood
Clary Sage	Marjoram
Lavender	Frankincense
Chamomile Roman	
Eucalyptus Citriodora	

apy or help in which the depressed person may be engaged.

The quantities in the following blends can be diluted with 30 mls (1 oz) of base oil to make a massage oil to use on yourself, or make a synergistic blend of oils using these proportions and use the synergistic blend in room methods, in baths ,and inhalation methods, using the quantities recommended in Chart 5.1.

CLASSIC BLENDS OF ESSENTIAL OILS TO USE IN CASES OF DEPRESSION

BLEND 1	
Benzoin	10 drops
Black Pepper	5 drops
Geranium	15 drops

BLEND 2	
Clary Sage	15 drops
Lavender	5 drops
Bergamot	10 drops

BLEND 3	
Rose Otto	10 drops
Sandalwood	15 drops
Lemon	5 drops

BLEND 4	
Ylang Ylang	5 drops
Nutmeg	10 drops
Coriander	15 drops

BLEND 5	
Neroli	20 drops
Petitgrain	10 drops

Weepy Depression

The weepy depressive will appear normal, carry out their work as usual, function at home, tend to everyone's needs, and then burst into tears. Out and about in the street, this type of depressive can be set off into a tearful episode by the words in a song played through the music system of a supermarket, or the sight of a couple in loving embrace in the park, or by a child trustfully grasping its mother's hand — anything, in fact, can spark off the tearful response, even the smallest gesture of concern or thanks. This tearful response might not be classified as "depression," but something is clearly wrong, and the person involved often feels desperate — they don't smile as much, they feel unwanted, and often wonder "why bother living?" Because they usually function so well on a superficial level, few people around them realize what agony they're going through until suddenly they snap and end up in the hospital (because they were found cuddling a lost kitten in the gutter, crying their eyes out). Worse still, they might try to kill themselves. Although this person feels depressed all the time they may not visit a doctor, and may shrug off the crying episodes as being "out of sorts," not telling those around them how often they occur. Because they may seem to cope with life's stresses and strains so well, unless one actually witnesses these crying episodes, it's quite easy not to suspect that the person is really very depressed. Obviously, some people cry more easily than others, and we all occasionally cry with pain, rage, temper, frustration, and sadness, but the weepy depressive finds that crying is the only way they can react, and that is a different thing altogether. Quite often, the weepy depressive person has been through an emotional trauma, or a series of traumas, and nobody, including themselves, has realized just how deeply it has affected them. Essential oils that may comfort and bring a sense of relief should be used.

Whatever the degree of weepy depression, start with the "Light" blend. If things don't improve after three days, progress to the "Moderate" blend. If things improve, stay on the "Moderate" blend until you feel better, and then slowly return to the "Light" blend. (When

ESSENTIAL OILS TO USE IN CASES OF WEEPY DEPRESSION	
Rose Otto	Neroli
Sandalwood	Patchouli
Geranium	Ylang Ylang
Chamomile Roman	

using the "Moderate" blend, you can substitute 2 drops of an essential oil of your choice, relative to your condition, for the chamomile roman.) If, after a week on the "Moderate" blend things do not improve, go on to the "Deep" blend.

The quantities in the blends below

WEEPY DEPRESSION — "LIGHT"

Sandalwood	15 drops
Geranium	10 drops
Ylang Ylang	5 drops

WEEPY DEPRESSION — "MODERATE"

Geranium	24 drops
*Chamomile Roman	2 drops
Benzoin	5 drops

*This chamomile can be substituted with an oil suitable for the person

WEEPY DEPRESSION — "DEEP"

Rose Otto	10 drops
Neroli	2 drops
Sandalwood	3 drops

can be diluted with 30 mls (1 oz) of base oil to make a massage oil, or make a synergistic blend of oils using these proportions and use a quantity of it in room methods, in the bath and inhalation methods, using the guidelines in Chart 5.1.

Agitated or Anxious Depression

The agitated depressive can never sit still for long. They're constantly moving, fidgeting, or twiddling with something — with their hair, or fingers, pens on the desk — anything. Although they're very busy, they're not really bothered whether a job has been done properly, so long as it's been done and they can move on to the next job. They'll have long faces, tired and drawn, but their minds will be racing ahead to all the plans and jobs they've got to get through. This type of depression causes symptoms such as pressure headaches, eye problems, twitches, ticks, jumping muscles and a feeling as if a tight band was being gripped around the skull. The head may feel like it's about to explode.

Agitated or anxious depression causes deep anguish that expresses itself as anger over the slightest thing. The person will despair if a little mark has been made on the furniture, as it were the end of the world, and there could be rapid mood swings. The constant fretting will be covering up deep feelings of worthlessness and fear. There may be palpitations, and unexplained tears, and thoughts of suicide — "just to get some peace." The

ESSENTIAL OILS TO USE IN CASES OF AGITATED OR ANXIOUS DEPRESSION	
Melissa	Cedarwood
Lavender	Bergamot
Marjoram	Nutmeg
Valerian	Lemon
Ormenis Flower	Orange
Chamomile Roman	

AGITATED DEPRESSION "MODERATE"

Cedarwood	20 drops
Orange	10 drops

AGITATED DEPRESSION "DEEP"

Cedarwood	5 drops
Lemon	15 drops
Ormenis Flower	5 drops
Nutmeg	5 drops

person suffering this type of depression usually throws themselves into work, as a means of covering up the underlying feeling of inadequacy.

Whatever the degree of agitated depression, start with the "Light" blend. If things don't improve after three days, progress to the "Moderate" blend. If things improve, stay on the "Moderate" blend until you feel better, and then slowly return to the "Light" blend. If, after a week on the "Moderate" blend things do not improve, go on to the "Deep" blend.

The quantities in the above blends can be diluted with 30 mls (1 oz) of base oil to make a massage oil, or make a synergistic blend of oils using these proportions and use in room methods, in baths, and inhalation methods, using the quantities

AGITATED DEPRESSION "LIGHT"

Lavender	15 drops
Ormenis Flower	5 drops
Bergamot	10 drops

recommended in the chart in *How To Use Essential Oils*.

Lethargic Depression

A lot of people have been struck with the depression that basically makes them want to stay in bed all day, with their head under the pillow. The lethargic depressive doesn't want to go anywhere or do anything. Everything is an effort, even switching on the TV. It's difficult to concentrate on books and papers. It can get very difficult to get out of bed in the morning, wash, and get dressed. Sleep beckons like welcoming arms. Important phone calls are ignored, vital letters never get written. Everything is overwhelming, including washing the hair. The sleeping causes more tiredness, more sleep, more tiredness, and when they're awake, they're asking everyone else to do things for them.

Lethargic depressives are not friendly — not at the moment anyway. Aside from

---

ESSENTIAL OILS TO USE IN CASES OF LETHARGIC DEPRESSION

Grapefruit	Cypress
Rosemary	Melissa
Helichrysum	Peppermint
Clary Sage	
Eucalyptus Citriodora	
Eucalyptus Peppermint	

---

the fact that they won't meet you in town for a social engagement, when you go to visit they're so unpleasant, you'd think they were trying to drive you away, which they are, of course, but it isn't personal. Anyone can get depressed like this. It might be a creative person being too critical of themselves, or a timid person who has been deeply hurt and emotionally wounded, even a selfish, dominating person — criticizing everyone for not being able to do things properly, but having no energy for doing it themselves. However, many people have been diagnosed with (a lethargic form of) depression when they in fact had ME — myalgic encephalomyelitis — and vice-versa, people with depression are diagnosed as having ME. The difference between them can be detected in the depressive's hopelessness and overwhelming desolation.

Whatever the degree of lethargic depression, start with the "Light" blend. If things don't improve after three days, progress to the "Moderate" blend. If things improve, stay on the "Moderate" blend until you feel better, and then slowly return to the "Light" blend. If, after a week on the "Moderate" blend things do not improve, go on to the "Deep" blend.

In the "Moderate" blend, you can substitute another essential oil, relevant to the situations and difficulties that led to the depression. If you do substitute, reduce the cypress and eucalyptus citriodora to 10 drops each, and add another 10 drops of your chosen essential oil, making the usual total of 30 drops to 30 mls (1 oz) base oil.

The quantities in the blends below can be diluted with 30 mls (1 oz) of base oil to make a massage oil, or make a synergistic blend of oils using these proportions and use in room methods, in baths and inhalation methods, using the number of drops recommended in Chart 5.1.

LETHARGIC DEPRESSION "LIGHT"

Grapefruit	5 drops
Rosemary	10 drops
Eucalyptus Citriodora	15 drops

LETHARGIC DEPRESSION "MODERATE"

Cypress	15 drops
Eucalyptus Citriodora	15 drops

LETHARGIC DEPRESSION "DEEPLY"

Helichrysum	15 drops
Clary Sage	5 drops
Eucalyptus Citriodora	10 drops

Hysterical Depression

It's sometimes difficult to know whether someone is suffering hysterical depression or having a bout of bad moods and temper. The hysterical depressive will exaggerate everything, want to be noticed, and will let everyone know they are suffering. They will heave great sighs, shout, scream and cry. They might be vivacious one minute and suicidal the next. Nobody will be able to do anything right. If you tread quietly, you'll be "creeping about," and if you carry on normally, you'll be told you don't care, especially if you're cheerful.

Shy, introverted people can become hysterical depressives, just as the naturally exuberant personality can. It often affects people who have become depressed through circumstances such as job loss, bereavement, financial problems, relationship failure, misunderstandings, and loneliness. The person may start having nightmares, and/or may become paranoiac, talking of evil spirits and the like. Their rapid mood changes make one wonder if they aren't two people in one skin. They often become suspicious and jealous, and are constantly moaning, and feeling miserable — to the point of crying. Shaking and trembling can be signs of hysterical depression — a most unpleasant state to be in. Above are some of the essential oils that may help.

Whatever the degree of hysterical depression, start with the "Light" blend. If things don't improve after three days, progress to the "Moderate" blend. If things improve, stay on the "Moderate" blend until you feel better, and then slowly return to the "Light" blend. If, after a week

on the "Moderate" blend things do not improve, go on to the "Deep" blend.

The quantities in the above blends can be diluted with 30 mls (1 oz) of base oil to make a massage oil, or make a synergistic blend of oils using these proportions and use in room methods, baths, and inhalation methods, using the quantities recommended in Chart 5.1

ESSENTIAL OILS TO USE IN CASES OF HYSTERICAL DEPRESSION

Valerian	Mandarin
Vetiver	Bergamot
Neroli	Narcissus
Lavender	Marjoram
Linden Blossom	Spikenard
Chamomile Roman	

HYSTERICAL DEPRESSION "LIGHT"

Lavender	10 drops
Chamomile Roman	15 drops
Mandarin	5 drops

HYSTERICAL DEPRESSION "MODERATE"

Neroli	15 drops
Mandarin	15 drops

HYSTERICAL DEPRESSION "DEEP"

Vetiver	15 drops
Bergamot	10 drops
Chamomile Roman	5 drops

Manic Depressive Psychosis

Extreme mood swings and behavior patterns mark manic depressive psychosis, which is much rarer than the other forms of depression. During the "mania" stage, a person will be at the peak of positivity — more talkative, their thoughts will be racing, they'll get involved in many projects, take on too much work — with unrealistic projections, and too many commitments all round. At this stage, the person often has an inflated self-esteem (which is why they think they can do so much), but they lose their power of judgment and even self-control. It is not unusual to find a manic depressive drinking to excess or spending money like it was going out of style. If they don't have money to spend, the manic depressive will use their credit cards, or borrow. They appear bright and cheerful, although perhaps laughing a little too loud or playing a little too hard. Anger can be quick to surface if the person is wronged, and even when they are not. They can become violent if denied something they want.

Then, as if by magic overnight, the manic depressive cannot get out of bed. They feel miserable, wretched, guilt-ridden, shameful, worthless, and full of despair. Self-esteem is extremely low, and they blame themselves for everyone's troubles, and the world's troubles too. During this depressive stage of sadness and self-hatred, the sufferer also has a variety of physical symptoms, including insomnia or strange sleeping patterns, weight loss or gain, no appetite, or constipation. Because of the risk of suicide, if this depressive stage continues for a long time, the person is often hospitalized and put on lithium salts and other drugs (which may have severe side effects during the manic stage).

Then, just as suddenly, the pendulum swings, and the person is rushing through life at a speed that's hard to catch up with. It's not known why these mood swings should happen, or are so severe, and many theories have been put forward. In some people, the condition may be caused by a defective gene (on chromosome 11), and changes in the level of the brain chemical dopamine may be involved. Intolerance to certain chemicals in modern life has also been suggested as a cause.

Complementary to medication, aromatherapy has helped many people through this condition, and in others, made life more tolerable. If the manic depressive is on any type of drug therapy, the usual number of essential oils used

---

ESSENTIAL OILS TO USE IN CASES OF MANIC DEPRESSION

Frankincense	Geranium
Grapefruit	Mandarin
Rose Otto	Lavender
Lemon	Neroli
Patchouli	Sandalwood
Chamomile Roman	
Chamomile German	

DEPRESSIVE STAGE 1

Mandarin	5 drops
Geranium	4 drops
Lavender	6 drops

DEPRESSIVE STAGE 2

Lavender	6 drops
Chamomile	
Roman	2 drops
Frankincense	4 drops
Geranium	3 drops

should be reduced by half — i.e., use a maximum of 15 drops of essential oil in 30 mls (1 oz) base oil for massage oils, and no more than 4-6 drops of a synergistic blend of oils in a bath. In a sense it's difficult for a manic depressive to treat themselves because they don't recognize that they need help when in the manic stage, and can't be bothered to do anything when in the depressive stage. However, if something can be done, start off with chamomile roman, lavender, geranium, mandarin, rose otto, and neroli. They are included in this larger list of useful oils for this condition.

During the manic stage, it's best to use a single oil — a maximum of 15 drops to 30 mls (1 oz) base oil for a massage oil, or 4 drops in a bath. Use lavender, chamomile roman, neroli, or rose — alone. Rose is also helpful during the depressive stage — use 10 drops to 30 mls (1 oz) base oil. Alternatively, try one of these blends.

The quantities in the above blends can be diluted with 30 mls (1 oz) of base oil to make a massage oil, or make a syn-

ergistic blend of oils using these proportions and use in room methods, in baths and inhalation methods, using half the quantities recommended in Chart 5.1.

The essential oils can be varied, choosing from the list above, but cross referencing with the symptoms mentioned throughout this book, and pages 223 and 230-236. For example, for feelings of unworthiness or self-hatred, choose rose otto or geranium.

Vitamins are useful in this condition — especially those in the B Group, 1, 3 and 6, vitamins C and E, and also zinc, magnesium, and calcium — which help sleep. There is an excellent calcium supplement called Cal-Calm that has been found helpful in cases of insomnia — see Suppliers, Appendix III.

Doubt

Doubt is a useful feeling, part of intuition. Being doubtful may prevent us entering a disastrous business deal, or prevent us making a mistake that could affect our future, or our relationships. When some-

---

ESSENTIAL OILS TO HELP BALANCE DOUBTFULNESS

Coriander	Basil*
Litsea Cubeba	Frankincense
Benzoin	Angelica Seed
Ylang Ylang	

Should not be used in baths

one says, "I have my doubts" about something, they are usually right to steer clear . Doubt can flood over into inappropriate areas, however, so a person is in a state of uncertainty as to the truth or reality of anything. Trust, of course, goes out the window. Although it may be hard not to doubt people if you have been crossed or put at a disadvantage by someone, this only blanks out your intuition, of which doubt is only a part.

Diffuse the essential oils gently in the room, use them in the bath or give yourself a massage. Also see Chapter 7, Emotional Healing, *Confidence*.

FEELING DOUBTFUL 1

Frankincense	15 drops
Benzoin	5 drops
Ylang Ylang	10 drops

FEELING DOUBTFUL 2

Coriander	20 drops
Basil	5 drops
Angelica Seed	5 drops

The quantities in the following blends can be diluted with 30 mls (1 oz) of base oil to make a massage oil, or make a synergistic blend of oils using these proportions and use in room methods, baths, and inhalation methods. See Chart 5.1 for quantities to use.

Emotional Violence

Emotional violence is probably far more widespread than anyone realizes. It can happen in the home, at school, at work, and can even come from so-called friends. Some people suffer emotional violence every minute of their lives, growing up in a house with antagonistic parents, perhaps, and then marrying someone with the same disposition — where, if the verbal abuse isn't constant, the dread and anxiety of knowing it will start again is.

Emotional violence is not simply verbal abuse, but also malicious, purposeful violation of the emotional state. It is when someone knows our most vulnerable and sensitive emotional points and goes for them, viciously trying to put us down or hurt us. It could come in the form of words that cut through to the very soul, or a look that says, "You are dirt." Emotional violence is the tool of the tyrant. And the sad thing is, it is usually perpetrated by the very people we love — our parents, partners, siblings, even children. So called "friends" are good at this too — especially if they know your secrets (and are threatening to tell your entire world).

Emotional violence is invisible — there are no black eyes or bruises to tell the tale — but it hurts far more and lasts much longer. The end result can be hopeless despair, anxiety, tension, and a lifetime of terror. The simple answer to the problem is to get away from the person who is doing it, but that is more easily said than done, especially if they are a parent, the mother or father of your children, or the girl you've been sitting next to in school. Counseling can help, as can classes in being assertive, but the real solution is to get out of the person's orbit, to "erase them out of your life," as one friend puts it. But this isn't always possible, and for every person daydreaming about winning the lottery, I bet another is planning their escape from some perpetrator of emotional violence.

Essential oils appear to help by cushioning the emotions, and the bathroom could become your refuge — particularly if you use the correct essential oils. Use the oils in the bath, lock the door, breathe the aroma in deeply, and practice a relaxation exercise. This escape may help you cope, and perhaps give you confidence to remove yourself from the emotional violator.

The essential oils can be used in all the usual methods but it is a good idea to make up a synergistic blend of oils that you can carry with you everywhere. Get a small bottle from the drug store and make up one of the following synergistic blends, using these proportions, or make up your own from the list above. Then sniff from the bottle whenever you feel the need, or put a couple of drops from the bottle onto a tissue and carry that in your pocket, and sniff from it when needed.

ESSENTIAL OILS TO HELP THOSE SUFFERING FROM EMOTIONAL VIOLENCE

Frankincense	Juniper
Geranium	Rose Otto
Neroli	Jasmine
Carnation	Hyacinth
Benzoin	Melissa
Chamomile Roman	Lavender

EMOTIONAL VIOLENCE 1

Frankincense	10 drops
Jasmine	5 drops
Melissa	5 drops

EMOTIONAL VIOLENCE 2

Chamomile Roman	5 drops
Carnation	5 drops
Neroli	10 drops

EMOTIONAL VIOLENCE 3

Frankincense	5 drops
Juniper	10 drops
Geranium	5 drops

The above blends can each be diluted with 30 mls (1 oz) base oil for a massage oil. Also use in the room methods, in baths, and inhalation methods.

Facing Death

In recent years there has been a growing awareness of "near-death experiences," when people invariably talk about a tunnel of light and being met on the other side by dear departed friends and relatives, all of whom are extremely happy. Other people are convinced there is an after-life because of their religious beliefs. Scientists even talk of a "holographic universe" in which death doesn't happen, you move on. This is reassuring, but not all beliefs make facing death so acceptable.

I can think of one 85-year-old lady who had spent her entire life doing volunteer work for the church, and who strongly believed in heaven and hell, lying fearful in her hospital bed at the thought of going to hell. One might think she had nothing to worry about, but that's old-fashioned indoctrination for you.

On the other hand, one hears stories about small children who are dying and seem well-adjusted to the idea, philosophical even, and who give counseling and support to their parents, who are of course devastated by the situation in which they find themselves. These remarkable children may not have had the time to comprehend death and they have no trouble believing that Jesus, the angels or Mohammed will meet them and take care of them until they can see mommy and daddy again. Telling a child they are dying is not an easy thing to do. One woman told me she had said to her son, "Perhaps you will get well, miracles do happen," but he didn't, and later sadly said, "I guess God doesn't love me enough for a miracle." What can one say to that? And children, simply by watching a certain amount of TV, see death associated with gory blood and boxes being put in the cold ground. For many children, teenagers and adults, death can be an unknown, frightening experience, however a brave face one puts on it.

It must be very irritating to be facing death and have people say things to you like, "We all have to go through it," or "It'll happen to me too someday" or "Now you can have some rest" or some such thing that somehow aims to negate the experience. Death is the biggest transition we make in this life. It's not like moving across

town. Let's not belittle the experience.

I would certainly recommend books on near-death experiences to anyone who is facing death, as well as the surviving relatives. They are very reassuring. However, giving them to someone facing death and saying, "Here, look, it's not so bad. What are you so worried about?" can be in danger of minimizing what they are going through. Death is not a minimal thing to experience. To grieving parents I would particularly recommend *Children of the Light* (Bantam), which documents the near-death experiences of children. It may also be that at this time books about religion and philosophy can offer a new insight into the subject of life, death, and the meaning of it all.

If we could think of death as a life cycle completed, rather than a life cycle cut short, the anguish may be easier to

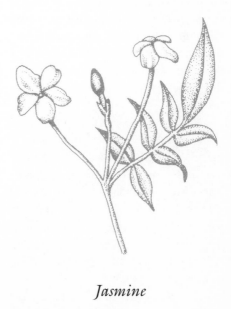

Jasmine

bear because a long list could be drawn up of accomplishments including, perhaps, children. But what does one tell a teenager who is too old to believe in Santa Claus, but too young to have had a working, exploring, life of their own? Standing on the threshold of a whole new life, the loss must be particularly great for them to bear. Why shouldn't they ask, "Why me?" and rant and rave in anger? Let them do it, and give plenty of time to listen, in great compassion, because they are right — it isn't fair. If they want to revert to childhood as a means of avoiding their present condition, let them, and if they say, "No, I won't let it happen to me," support them because with mind over matter being the powerful thing it is, they might just pull off a miracle.

Because dying is a lonely experience, having people around you who are loving and caring must be the greatest comfort of all. To pass over to the other side holding the hand of someone you love, or with their arms around you, must be the gentlest way to leave this world. It is this love that is the greatest gift we can receive at this time, and to die pain-free in dignity and peace.

Throughout known time people have been burning incense around the dying in the belief that the aroma will take the soul as it rises to heaven. The word "perfume" comes from per fumin — by fire. We also give flowers at funerals, and it was once traditional to give strong smelling flowers, herbs, and spices, so the aroma could lift the spirit to the other side. Essential oils continue this tradition.

The best essential oils now are the ones that you love, the ones that give you a lift and make you feel good about yourself. And use them for any state of mind or emotion that you may be feeling. A collection of essential oils seems to be commonly chosen when facing death, but that might only be because they are easily available. These are listed below, and may not include your personal favorite oils. If so, just choose other oils that appeal to you.

ESSENTIAL OILS USED WHEN FACING DEATH

Rose Otto	Jasmine
Frankincense	Neroli
Bay	Geranium
Benzoin	Carnation
Sandalwood	Cedarwood
Bergamot	Juniper
Lemon	Hyacinth
Linden Blossom	Rose Maroc
Tuberose	
Chamomile Roman	

All the oils above blend well with each other and can be made into combinations. Use however many drops of each essential oil you want, up to 30 drops of essential oil to 30 mls (1 oz) base, vegetable oil. Just as the life cycle is individual, so is the journey ahead, so be as individualistic as you like, or not. Essential oils are pure pleasure, and now is a good time to explore them. Life is for living, now more than ever, and the fragrances of essential oils are fabulous additions to any life and are there to be enjoyed. Use them in all the usual methods.

Some people ask for fragrance to be used at the funeral ceremony, to comfort the mourners and also give them an aromatic signature to remember them by. Then, as they go about their lives later, they'll smell that same aroma on the airwaves and say, "Oh yes, so-and-so. I wonder where they are now." — gone but not forgotten. And it is the good things we remember about people, especially the people we love.

Fatigue, Tiredness, and Exhaustion

You may not be surprised to see the headlines in the papers saying, "Nearly half the population suffer from unexplained exhaustion..."[5] You may feel exhausted yourself. A new term has appeared, TATT, tired all the time, to identify the biggest complaint doctors hear. There may be some underlying physiological reason, including low blood pressure; hypothyroidism, an underactive thyroid gland; thyrotoxicosism, an overactive one; anemia, or iron-deficiency; rheumatoid arthritis; the totally debilitating myalgic encephalomyelitis (ME); and many other things. You need to establish that you're not just tired from overwork, depression, drinking too much, or insomnia, and that you're not in the recovery period from a viral or bacteriological infection, which would inevitably leave you tired.

It's estimated that about 40% of tiredness cases are caused by psychological or lifestyle reasons, which, if they were recognized, could be worked on. The working environment is a good place to start . Are you sitting too close to photocopiers, fax machines, computers, or airvents for the air-conditioning system? Or are you hunched over in a taut position all day on a factory assembly line, with noise banging in your ear? The answer to this is a nice long vacation in the sun, but unfortunately we can't go for fifty-two weeks of the year.

Essential oils have a long tradition of helping in the many different kinds of tiredness, fatigue, or exhaustion. This section has been arranged under the headings of Exhaustion, Nervous Exhaustion, General Mental Fatigue, Intellectual Fatigue and Mental Tiredness. Each has suggested oils and one or two blends. Use the oils in all the usual ways, adding the quantities given in the blends to 30 mls (1 oz) base oil to make a massage oil, or mix the essential oils into a synergistic blend.

ESSENTIAL OILS TO HELP IN CASES OF EXHAUSTION	
Bergamot	Marjoram
Rosemary	Ginger
Eucalyptus Globulus	Grapefruit
Lemon	
Eucalyptus Radiata	Pine
Frankincense	
Cypress	Litsea Cubeba
Black Pepper	Cardamom

See Chart 5.1 for quantities to use and methods.

It may seem strange to use essential oils that are traditionally used to calm, but in tiredness, to overstimulate can sometimes result in increased tiredness, not relief from it.

ESSENTIAL OILS TO HELP IN CASES OF NERVOUS EXHAUSTION

Rosemary	Petitgrain
Juniper	Neroli
Lavender	Marjoram
Clary Sage	Orange
Chamomile Roman	

ESSENTIAL OILS TO HELP IN CASES OF GENERAL MENTAL FATIGUE

Lemon	Petitgrain
Basil	Peppermint
Rosemary	
Eucalyptus Piperata	
Eucalyptus Citriodora	

ESSENTIAL OILS TO HELP IN CASES OF MENTAL TIREDNESS

Clary Sage	Lavender
Marjoram	Rosemary
Litsea Cubeba	Grapefruit
Peppermint	

EXHAUSTION BLEND 1

Lemon	10 drops
Frankincense	5 drops
Pine	15 drops

EXHAUSTION BLEND 2

Eucalyptus Globus	15 drops
Rosemary	10 drops
Grapefruit	5 drops

NERVOUS EXHAUSTION BLEND 1

Petitgrain	18 drops
Neroli	10 drops
Lavender	2 drops

NERVOUS EXHAUSTION BLEND 2

Juniper	10 drops
Lavender	15 drops
Rosemary	5 drops

GENERAL MENTAL FATIGUE BLEND

Basil	15 drops
Lemon	15 drops

TIREDNESS BLEND

Litsea Cubeba	15 drops
Peppermint	5 drops
Marjoram	10 drops

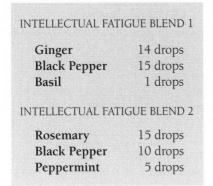

ESSENTIAL OILS TO HELP
IN CASES OF
INTELLECTUAL FATIGUE

Ginger	Black Pepper
Rosemary	Basil
Cypress	Grapefruit
Peppermint	Lemon

INTELLECTUAL FATIGUE BLEND 1

Ginger	14 drops
Black Pepper	15 drops
Basil	1 drops

INTELLECTUAL FATIGUE BLEND 2

Rosemary	15 drops
Black Pepper	10 drops
Peppermint	5 drops

Fear

Fear is a life-saver — it puts us on alert so the "flight/fight" hormones can swing into action and give us that extra impetus we need to get out of a fix. It's fear of a large, crazed dog that'll make you leap a ten-foot wall to escape — and on a normal day you couldn't jump a three-foot wall. That's fear for you. It gives you extra strength, sharpens the senses, makes reactions quicker, and makes your body do things you didn't know it could do.

Fear makes the adrenal glands release adrenaline, which stimulates the sympathetic nervous system, causing an increase of heart rate and perspiration, the drying up of the saliva glands (making the mouth dry), and stopping the digestive system working. There are of course degrees of fear and it's quite common for people exposed to a sudden, terrifying experience to urinate or defecate without control. Soldiers, exposed to fearful situations day after day, can become suddenly paralyzed, unable to move a muscle.

There's plenty to be frightened about. Burglars and rapists can break into the house at night and the streets are full of people who act in strange, unpredictable ways. According to a report in the *Los Angeles Times* [6], one person in seventy-five suffers from fear attacks of sufficient severity to make them think they're having a heart attack or about to go mad, and the attacks don't relate to actual frightening experiences but to the possibility that something could go seriously wrong in their lives — as a result of financial troubles, work, or relationship problems, for example. And I don't suppose the fear quotient there is helped by the violent crime statistics, which are high enough to put anyone into a permanent state of fear.

There is so much fear, we now have a wide vocabulary to deal with it. General fear is known as "panic disorder." Then there's "stropophobia," the fear of moving or making changes; "gamophobia," the fear of marriage; "decidophobia," the fear of making decisions; "sciophobia," the fear of shadows; and, among other phobias, "triskaidekaphobia," the fear of the number thirteen. (See Phobias.)

"Topophobia" is better known as stage fright and it even affected that best known of actors, Sir Laurence Olivier, who suffered with sweating, trembling, and a constricted throat before each performance. Another well-known actor avoided live performances for fourteen years, and a famous singer was kept away from the stage for eight years. Birmingham University's Neuropsychiatry clinic is now advising actors to use aromatherapy to dispel the fear, by choosing a relaxing essential oil, having a massage with it while a hypnotist suggests the actor feels relaxed, then sniffing that same aroma before going on stage. It's certainly a better option than giving up your profession or lying down on the stage to do relaxation exercises during a performance.

Normal fear is the reaction you feel when threatened, while abnormal fear is fear out of all proportion to the scary object or event. Pathological fear, however, is a permanent state of mind that continues long after the fearful event has passed. Fear is accompanied by an intense feeling of apprehension or dread and is often felt in the "pit of the stomach," and frequently accompanied by nausea and cold sweats. Outside the normal circumstances where one would expect a person to feel fear, exaggerated fear or chronic fear have no benefits whatsoever. It is an incapacitating and limiting feeling, which essential oils can help dispel. As there are so many types of fear, this section is arranged under several specific headings. However, we start with the essential oils that can help in cases of fearfulness and dread with no apparent cause (apart from life itself).

ESSENTIAL OILS FOR USE IN CASES OF FEAR

Sandalwood	Cypress
Vetiver	Lemon
Bergamot	Orange
Cedarwood	Neroli
Ormenis Flower	Basil
Frankincense	Clary Sage
Lavender	Galbanham
Chamomile Roman	

In addition to these oils, there are those that are very appropriate for particular types of fear, as follows.

FEAR OF FAILURE
Fennel, Coriander, Ylang Ylang, Frankincense, Basil

FEAR OF MADNESS
Fennel, Cedarwood, Ylang Ylang, Frankincense

FEAR OF CHANGE
Ylang Ylang, Frankincense, Lavender, Ormenis Flower

FEAR OF LOVE
Rose Maroc, Neroli, Carnation, Hyacinth, Benzoin

FEAR OF GOSSIP
Cypress

FEAR OF FEELINGS

Fennel, Frankincense, Neroli, Sandalwood

FEAR OF SEXUALITY

Rose Maroc, Ylang Ylang, Patchouli,
Vetiver, Galbanham

FEAR OF LOVE

Rose Maroc, Neroli, Carnation,
Hyacinth, Benzoin

FEAR OF LOVING

Neroli, Ylang Ylang, Carnation,
Benzoin, Rose Maroc

FEAR OF BEING UNLOVED

Rose Otto

FEAR OF LETTING GO

Rose Maroc, Frankincense,
Galbanham, Cypress

The essential oils can be used either singly or made into blends and used in baths, diffusers, and other room methods, inhaled from a tissue or direct from the bottle, or inhaled as a steam vapor. The quantities of the following blends should either be diluted with 30 mls (1 oz) base oil, or made into a synergistic blend using these proportions. For quantities to use see Chart 5.1.

FEAR OF CHANGE

Lavender	5 drops
Ylang Ylang	15 drops
Frankincense	5 drops

FEAR OF FEELINGS

Sandalwood	20 drops
Fennel	3 drops
Frankincense	7 drops

FEAR OF SEXUALITY

Rose Maroc	16 drops
Ylang Ylang	10 drops
Patchouli	2 drops
Galbanham	2 drops

FEAR OF LOVE

Benzoin	10 drops
Carnation	5 drops

FEAR OF LOVING

Neroli	15 drops
Benzoin	10 drops
Ylang Ylang	5 drops

FEAR OF BEING UNLOVED

Rose Otto	30 drops

FEAR OF LETTING GO

Cypress	10 drops
Galbanham	5 drops
Rose Maroc	15 drops

ESSENTIAL OILS FOR THOSE PRONE TO EMOTIONAL FITS AND OUTBURSTS

Lavender
Marjoram
Eucalyptus Citriodora
Litsea Cubeba
Chamomile Roman

Fits (Emotional) or Outbursts

In psychological terms, fits are thought of as outbursts — like "a fit of jealousy" or "a fit of anger" — something that comes on suddenly. Someone who is prone to explosions of emotions could consider counseling or see an aromatherapist who can both offer support and use the oils to help diffuse the build-up of tension. Essential oils can be diffused in the room, inhaled from a tissue, used 8 drops in a bath, or made into a massage oil. Consider the essential oils that have a calming and soothing effect but look at the situation holistically and refer to other sections in the book.

Forgetfulness

Forgetfulness can happen to us all. Sometimes it doesn't matter and at other times it matters a lot. To try not to forget things we need concentration and focus, which essential oils may help with. Gently diffuse them in the atmosphere during the time you are trying to collect your thoughts, or sniff them from a handkerchief.

ESSENTIAL OILS TO CHALLENGE FORGETFULNESS

Cypress	Lemon
Ginger	Black Pepper
Cistus	Frankincense
Rosemary	Peppermint
Basil	

EMOTIONAL FITS OR OUTBURSTS BLEND 1

Lavender	10 drops
Marjoram	5 drops
Litsea Cubeba	15 drops

EMOTIONAL FITS OR OUTBURSTS BLEND 2

Chamomile Roman	8 drops
Eucalyptus Citriodora	14 drops
Lavender	8 drops

FORGETFULNESS BLEND 1

Rosemary	15 drops
Peppermint	5 drops
Lemon	10 drops

FORGETFULNESS BLEND 2

Black Pepper	10 drops
Frankincense	5 drops
Cypress	10 drops

Grief
(Intense Sorrow)

Although the word "grief" is usually associated with bereavement, it encompasses all kinds of intense sorrow, which may include the death of a loved one, but may equally include the sorrow one feels when a loving relationship breaks down and the loved one leaves not the world in general, but you in particular. The grieving that takes place after such a loss can be intense, and last for years. One can grieve for pets, as well as people, and for objects too. People have been intensely sad when, for example, an object of deep sentimental value is lost or stolen, or when the family's collection of photographs are destroyed in a fire. Some people may grieve the loss of a job, or home, or lifestyle while others may even grieve the loss of a much-loved car. Many women grieve in silence over a miscarriage, abortion, or hysterectomy, sometimes for the rest of their lives. Others may grieve the loss of a limb. Poets have eloquently grieved for the fate of a nation, and spiritual masters have long grieved for the sad state of the human race.

Grieving goes beyond sadness or sorrow — etching itself onto every cell of our body and making a deep impression on our soul. It's felt as a deep sinking feeling in what's called "the pit of the stomach," a feeling that never seems to go away. Immediately after the loss, one can feel numb and disbelieving, hoping it's all been a bad dream. This is a form of shock and the sufferer may experience uncontrollable shaking and have nausea and an overwhelming sense of hopelessness. Often it's accompanied by feelings of loneliness and isolation. Then comes a preoccupation with how you feel, as the sadness fills your mind and your time. Despondency and despair set in, as we feel we shall never be able to experience happiness again.

Then comes the anger and guilt — "If only I'd done this (or that);" "I should have said this (or that)." One may have vivid memories of the good times and the bad times, and find yourself running over in your mind the good times that will never be, making you irritable. If the loss is of a person, there is often rage or jealousy, regret, blame, and lots of tears. You can lie in bed, tossing and turning, churning over every detail of the loss, over and over again. Aches and pains are common with grief, as is stress and anxiety, loss of appetite or overeating.

Grief can last a few weeks or for years on end — when it is called atopic grief. It's often accompanied by a sense of failure or worthlessness and, if the emotional pain becomes too great to bear, it can lead to suicide. Perhaps the only way to avoid grief is never to become involved with another person again, or so attached to a thing, but to be alive is to feel love, and to feel love is to sometimes feel the pain of loss. Grieving is, then, an inevitable part of life that we must all at some time try to get through as best we can. To deny it is potentially dangerous, both psychologically and physiologically and so grief must be allowed to take its course. If you feel rage, beat the walls. If you feel like screaming, do it. If you feel like crying, let those tears roll. We all have our own ways of coping. One friend, after a broken relationship, locked herself away at home where she sobbed uncontrollably as she listened to love songs and watched sad love movies all day and all night for months on end. People said to her, "Snap out of it, there's plenty of fish in the sea," which didn't help at all and, had this advice been taken, it could have been dangerous in the long run because she needed to express her sorrow. Eventually,

she emerged, weak and listless, and slowly picked up the pieces of her life. Now she's fine!

Grieving is a process that has to be gone through, no matter how long it takes. If you don't feel you can unload your problems onto a friend, seek out some counseling. If you can, visit an aromatherapist, as the gentle massage combined with the essential oils, chosen individually for you, will certainly help release some of the grief.

Essential oils have long been used to comfort and console but they will not stop the grieving process. That is not what they are there for. What they can do, however, is help you express the grief and come to terms with it. Choose an essential oil from the lists below, or choose several to make into a blend. Use them in the bath, diffused in the atmosphere, inhaled as a vapor, sniffed from a tissue, sniffed straight from the bottle, or made into a massage oil. See Chart 5.1 for quantities to use.

The following blends can each be diluted with 30 mls (1 oz) base oil to make a massage oil, or you can make up a synergistic blend using these proportions and use that blend in all the methods mentioned above. Also, please see the *Bereavement* section.

ESSENTIAL OILS TO HELP EXPRESS GRIEF

Hyacinth	Rose Maroc
Rose Otto	Neroli
Melissa	Helichrysum
Benzoin	Mimosa
Vetiver	

ESSENTIAL OILS TO HELP DISSIPATE GRIEF

Cypress	Rose Maroc
Rose Otto	Helichrysum
Frankincense	Narcissus
Bergamot	Carnation
Vanilla	Nutmeg
Ormenis Flower	Spikenard
Chamomile Roman	

GRIEF-INDUCED NUMBNESS, SHOCK AND DISBELIEF

Cypress	5 drops
Helichrysum	5 drops
Frankincense	10 drops
Bergamot	5 drops

GRIEF-INDUCED DISTRESS

Carnation	7 drops
Rose Maroc	4 drops
Chamomile	
Roman	1 drops

GRIEF-INDUCED DEPRESSION

Ormenis flower	10 drops
Benzoin	10 drops
Nutmeg	10 drops

CONTINUED DEEP SADNESS

Cypress	5 drops
Rose Maroc	15 drops
Hyacinth	10 drops

Guilt

There is so much to be guilty about — the library books that haven't been taken back, the "thank-you's" that haven't been said, the sick relatives we haven't visited, the money we shouldn't have spent, the bills we are ignoring, and the jobs that haven't been done. We've all felt guilty eating chocolate bars, and some of us feel guilty for buying books when the teenager wants a new pair of shoes. Some people are guilty because they have hurt someone, or lied, cheated, or stolen. People with children have a whole stack of more guilt: leaving a child with a baby sitter or taking it to the hated piano lessons. Everyone has some kind of guilt or other, we just don't go around talking about it all the time. If you are feeling guilty, you are not alone.

Aside from the guilt we devise for ourselves there is the guilt we inflict on other people — particularly children — and on this subject I recommend *Cutting the Ties that Bind* by Phyllis Krystal. Then there is the guilt other people put on us, in the form of a parent who says, "You never phone," for example, a teenager who says, "You never buy me nice clothes," or the partner who says, "You never dress up any more." All the little bits of guilt can add up — those little jobs you forgot to do for someone, the time you can't spend with the children. These outside demands can create a general atmosphere of guilt, but if there is someone close constructing their sentences so they instill you with guilt, that is a more grueling experience to have to deal with. Many partners use illness, unhappiness, or financial issues to make the other feel guilty. It's like you can't do one thing right. However, none of this inflicted guilt is as bad as the guilt of having killed someone, perhaps as a soldier, and deep guilt such as this should be discussed with a counselor, to try and come to terms with it.

For normal, everyday guilt that gets out of hand, strange as it may seem, essential oils and aromatherapy may be able to help. Aromatherapy treatments are also helpful in all kinds of guilt because the massage techniques allow emotional release. As you will see from the Massage section in Chapter 9, deep-seated emotions are often felt in our bodies and are effectively released by trained therapists. As not everyone can afford professional help, guidance can be sought from the illustrations on pages 202 and 203 that show which areas of the body tend to hold emotional tension. Relaxation exercises will be able to help further.

For normal, everyday use choose essential oils from other sections of this book that seem relevant to you. The following list is of oils which have traditionally been used for guilt. Use them in a massage oil, in the bath, or diffused or inhaled.

ESSENTIAL OILS TO HELP COPE WITH GUILT	
Linden Blossom	Vetiver
Jasmine	Pine
Rose Otto	Juniper
Clary Sage	Ylang Ylang
Nutmeg	

The quantities in the following blends can be diluted with 30 mls (1 oz) of base oil to make a massage oil, or make a synergistic blend of oils using these proportions and use in baths, room methods,

EVERYDAY GUILT	
Ylang Ylang	12 drops
Nutmeg	10 drops
vetiver	8 drops

DEEP-ROOTED GUILT	
Juniper	15 drops
Clary Sage	5 drops
Pine	10 drops

and inhalation methods. For quantities to use see Chart 5.1.

If you feel guilty about indulging yourself, this blend will help you enjoy your guilt.

INDULGENCE GUILT	
Linden Blossom	5 drops
Jasmine	5 drops
Rose Otto	5 drops

Hypochondria

If a hypochondriac has palpitations, they think they have heart disease, if they get a twinge or cramp in their bottom, they've got bowel cancer, if they have a bout of indigestion, they've got angina, and the bad back they got gardening will be kidney trouble. Hypochondriacs have fixations about their bodies, and a real fear of illness or dying. (Although there is another type of hypochondriac who just uses potential ill health to gain sympathy, visits, or attention, who usually reports vague feelings of being unwell). All this is to be distinguished from *Psychosomatic Illness*, in which there are real physical disorders brought on by certain mental activity.

Not all hypochondriacs are well. Doctors undoubtedly sometimes diagnose "hypochondria" in the person sitting in front of them, just because they can't find what is wrong — which may be depression or some other mental illness. Unfortunately, once you admit to being even mildly depressed, there's a good chance that henceforth everything physical you complain of will be dismissed as hypochondria.

Sometimes nothing can be done for the hypochondriac, no matter how many times the doctor is visited. Therapists can help as they have more time to give, and can listen to the troubles. Reflexologists often have success with hypochondriacs because they can give the equivalent of an "X-ray" diagnosis on each visit, and reassure the person. (Reflexology is the manipulation of the soles of the feet, in which all the functions of the body are supposed to be mirrored). Essential oils may help, as can homeopathy, and they are usually harmless when administering treatment to oneself on a first-aid basis, but if the hypochondriac recognizes they have a problem, counseling may be an answer.

If you have a hypochondriac in the family, buy them *The Complete Book of Essential Oils & Aromatherapy* — my book on using essential oils on physical problems; a family treatment book for homeopathy; another on Bach flower remedies; any other books you can find on self-help, plus a set of essential oils. The person might become so busy looking up the various treatments, they'll forget they had a problem. Often, when a hypochondriac uses essential oils and starts administering to themselves it deflects the dependency on others and shifts responsibility to themselves, thereby often clearing up the problem.

Use the oils singly or in blends — in all the usual methods.

ESSENTIAL OILS FOR HYPOCHONDRIACS	
Marjoram	Rosemary
Valerian	Hops
Basil	Peppermint
Ormenis Flower	Thyme
Tea Tree	Manuka
Oregano	Galbanham

Hysteria

Although, as a word, "hysteria" is becoming less used by the medical profession in favor of a variety of terms that more accurately describe the range of emotional problems people have to deal with, we all know what it is for someone to be "hysterical" — to display unusual, emotionally-excited behavior, such as screaming and shouting loudly, with perhaps crying, sighing, temper, or rage. It is often the way a person finds they can attract attention to themselves, to a problem they face, or a situation they find themselves in, and hysteria also releases some pent up anxiety. Hysteria is medically classified as a neurotic behavior disturbance, and immortalized on film by the black and white images of hysterical actresses getting a slap across the face.

Mass hysteria is when a group of people all get hysterical together, setting each other off — as among a large group of young women at a rock concert, for example. And clever individuals can set off

---

ESSENTIAL OILS TO USE IN CASES OF HYSTERIA

Mandarin	Vetiver
Bergamot	Rosemary
Neroli	Peppermint
Narcissus	Lavender
Marjoram	Valerian
Spikenard	Hops
Chamomile Roman	
Linden Blossom	

HYSTERIA 1

Marjoram	8 drops
Lavender	14 drops
Valerian	8 drops

HYSTERIA 2

Spikenard	8 drops
Chamomile Roman	17 drops
Bergamot	5 drops

---

group hysteria at business meetings, for example, disrupting the proceedings.

If a person is known to have hysterical tendencies they could carry a bottle of essential oil to use when the anxiety starts. The oils will help to calm them down. But each case is different and some people get hysterical because they think they can make an advantage out of it, and in this case nothing will stop the hysteria starting. After an hysterical outburst, when things have calmed down, essential oils are very good in a bath or massage oil. They can also be used on a more regular basis, in all the usual ways.

The quantities in the following blends can be diluted with 30 mls (1 oz) of base oil to make a massage oil, or make

SHOCK-HYSTERIA

Peppermint	10 drops
Rosemary	15 drops
Lavender	5 drops

a synergistic blend of oils using these proportions and use in baths, room methods, and inhalation methods. See Chart 5.1 for quantities to use.

Insomnia

We've all had the occasional night when we couldn't sleep. We go to bed and shut our eyes, but nothing. We don't drift off, we're awake. So we toss and turn for an hour, then sit up and read a book. An hour later we turn off the light and try again. Again, nothing. We're beginning to feel very heavy and agitated. We try relaxation techniques and counting sheep, plump up the pillow, get in a comfortable position, but nothing. We begin to think of all the things we've got to do tomorrow for which we are going to be too exhausted. Time passes. The birds begin to sing. By now we feel like lead. The sun rises, the alarm clock goes off, another day begins. And for the insomniac, the day begins like that almost every day.

Millions of people have a sleep

problem. Insomnia is caused by worry, anxiety, tension, stress, pain, fear, over-tiredness, caffeine, eating late at night, shift-work, stimulants, excitability, and noise, among other things. Certain mental states also affect the sleeping pattern — depressives tend to have trouble getting to sleep and wake early; people with dementia are afraid of the dark and that makes them confused, restless and noisy; schizophrenics can be tortured by voices and pace up and down all night; people with mania are hyperactive and don't sleep much at all. Apparently there are as many as eighty classifications of sleep disorder, and new scientific fields are being created to deal with them all, including somnologists (sleep experts), and chronobiology (the science linking natural body rhythms with physiology and psychology).

During a good night's sleep, research shows we go through periods of nonrapid eye movement (NREM) interrupted by about five episodes of rapid eye movement (REM), presumably indicating dreaming. There is "delta sleep," which is more refreshing, and "alpha sleep," which is lighter and can be easily interrupted. During sleep, our temperature fluctuates. Some researchers think our natural pattern of sleep would be to have a short nap in the afternoon, and a sleep at night. Apparently, our body rhythms are at their slowest between 3 a.m. and 6 a.m. in the morning.

Nobody really knows why we sleep but it's during this time that the body shuts down functions such as digestion, and concentrates on repair and healing. Missed sleep can affect concentration and efficiency and bring on irritability, ner-

vousness, sleepiness, tiredness, exhaustion, and aches and pains of which we would not normally be aware. I've known women who became insomniac after having their sleep pattern interrupted by babies and worry about the children, and men who could never return to a normal sleeping pattern after spending years on shift-work. DJs and other night workers have a very difficult time finding a good, long sleep, yet alone on a regular basis. Essential oils can help all these situations, and please refer to the blends to see which seem most appropriate to you.

Warm baths, relaxation exercises, and hypnotherapy tapes could all help with insomnia, as could switching to de-caffeinated coffee or tea. Have a night-time routine, use a comfortable bed, shut out noise and read a book or have sex. Warm calcium drinks (such as Cal-Calm — see Suppliers) or malt drinks can help. The homeopathic tablets arnica, aconitum, ignatia, kali-phosphoricum, or coffea might be useful too, or herbal tablets such as valerian. If nothing works, just get

---

ESSENTIAL OILS TO HELP IN CASES OF INSOMNIA

Lavender	Mandarin
Clary Sage	Marjoram
Cistus	Valerian
Hops	Vetiver
Sandalwood	Lemon
Linden Blossom	
Chamomile Roman	

up and read *The Mind-Map Book* by Tony Buzan[7], and draw yourself up a mind-map and see what's keeping you awake.

Any of the listed oils can be used singly or in combinations. Use 10 drops in a warm bath before bed. A massage oil also helps to calm and relax. Gently diffuse the essential oils in the room, or place the essential oils on a tissue or cotton ball and place under the pillow.

The quantities in the following blends can be diluted with 30 mls (1 oz) of base oil to make a massage oil, or make a synergistic blend of oils using these proportions and use in baths, room, and inhalation methods.

Irritability

We all get irritable sometimes, at various stages of our life, or just during some stage of a normal day. There are possible underlying factors that should be addressed because irritability can be caused by an illness or by an emotion, such as unhappiness, sadness, worry, stress, and tension. Pre-menstrual syndrome (PMS) also causes irritability.

Irritability is enshrined in the expression, "I got up on the wrong side of the bed today," and it's definitely within the normal range of human emotions. It may have a place as a means of expressing dissatisfaction — and let's face it, there is plenty in this life — so it is expressed outward rather than inward. But, as ever, it is a question of degree. It's one thing to get irritated listening to a politician being interviewed, but another thing to want to

INSOMNIA NIGHTMARES WAKE YOU

Lavender	15 drops
Chamomile	
Roman	5 drops
Mandarin	10 drops

INSOMNIA NOISE WAKES YOU

Lavender	10 drops
Lemon	15 drops
Vetiver	5 drops

INSOMNIA RESTLESSNESS

Vetiver	10 drops
Clary Sage	10 drops
Lemon	10 drops

INSOMNIA FITFULNESS

Marjoram	5 drops
Lavender	15 drops
Lemon	10 drops

INSOMNIA ANXIETY

Chamomile	
Roman	10 drops
Sandalwood	15 drops
Lemon	5 drops

INSOMNIA WORRY

Cistus	5 drops
Lavender	15 drops

INSOMNIA EXHAUSTION

Valerian	5 drops
Lemon	10 drops
Mandarin	10 drops

actually kill the person. Children can get irritable if they are tired, but if it happens on a regular basis, they should be checked over by a doctor. Rational people will recognize that one day a thing that would normally pass unremarked can the next day become an irritation, and it all depends on our mood. But when we're getting irritated over everyday events on a regular basis, flying off the handle over minor problems, sensitive to suggestions, remarks and even touch, then it is time to do something about it.

Clearly, if there is something to be said, and the irritability is just covering up that fact, then say what it is you have to say. It is not the job of essential oils to "cover up" what underlies irritability — you must express yourself and let the cause of irritability pass, not linger. Having said that, the essential oils can certainly help reduce irritability. Use them singly, or in blends, cross referencing with the lists elsewhere in this book.

The quantities in the following blends can be diluted with 30 mls (1 oz) of base oil to make a massage oil, or make

IRRITABILITY 1	
Cypress	10 drops
Coriander	10 drops
Lavender	10 drops

IRRITABILITY 2	
Ylang Ylang	15 drops
Coriander	10 drops
Chamomile	
Roman	5 drops

a synergistic blend of oils using these proportions and use in all the usual methods — particularly in baths. See Chart 5.1 for quantities to use.

Loneliness and Aloneness

People who are alone are often thought by other people to be depressed or lonely. This isn't always the case. Sometimes people yearn for aloneness and even devise daily stratagems so they can get a bit of it. Being alone can be an energizing, fortifying experience, drawing on the peace within, but it can also mean feeling isolated and out of touch with other people, especially people you love.

Essential oils can help in both extremes, strange as that may seem. When you've been working with essential oils as long as I have, you can practically see the loneliness cloud lift from people after their regular use of them. It is not simply the "you are never alone with essential oils" factor, but something else,

ESSENTIAL OILS TO USE IN CASES OF IRRITABILITY

Cypress	Coriander
Litsea Cubeba	Neroli
Ylang Ylang	Melissa
Narcissus	Lavender
Chamomile Roman	
Chamomile German	

as if something has been added, making the person complete, and strong — alone or in a crowd.

The very fact that someone can feel alone in a crowd illustrates that the problem is not to do with physically having people around, as such, but with how a person feels about themselves in relation to other people. In a sense then, advice about going out and meeting people or getting a new hobby is not going to help — all it means is one will be lonely in a crowd instead of lonely alone at home. More is required to shift the consciousness, away from non-peace to peace. When we are at peace, people are much easier to handle and they do not have to be shunned.

There is nothing wrong with being alone. When alone we can reorientate ourselves and go forward, or come to terms with particular feelings or actions. And the views can be amazing when one wanders lonely as a cloud, exhilarating even, untouched by other people's wants, needs, and expectations. Being alone only becomes a problem when one feels loneliness, and then essential oils can help by giving comfort, the ability to cope, and enjoyment. Use the oils singly or in blends, in all the usual methods.

The quantities in the following blends can be diluted with 30 mls (1 oz) of base oil to make a massage oil, or make a synergistic blend of oils using these proportions and use in baths, room, and inhalation methods. For quantities to use see Chart 5.1

ESSENTIAL OILS TO USE WHEN FEELING (NEGATIVE) LONELINESS

Bergamot	Helichrysum
Narcissus	Neroli
Chamomile Roman	Benzoin

ESSENTIAL OILS FOR (POSITIVE) ALONENESS

Orange	Neroli
Rose Otto	Rose Maroc
Jasmine	Melissa
Frankincense	Neroli
Chamomile Roman	

MELANCHOLIC LONELINESS

Benzoin	10 drops
Helichrysum	5 drops
Bergamot	10 drops
Chamomile Roman	5 drops

PEACEFUL ALONENESS

Neroli	10 drops
Orange	5 drops
Rose Otto	10 drops

Misery

We all feel miserable at times, but some people feel more misery than others. I have a friend who once shared an apartment with a woman, Betty, who came back from work each evening and complained about the journey, about her workmates, the poor quality of the food in the shop she stopped at, her lack of money, the fact that the laundry needed doing, the fact that nothing was on TV, the fact that there was nowhere to go out, and so on. My friend tells me that she used to hear the key go in the lock, look at the clock, and time how long it would take Betty to make the first complaint about her (inevitably) miserable day. It was usually under two minutes — and it went on all evening! Betty was the roommate we all dread having!

People who are miserable usually know they are miserable, even if they don't put their plethora of complaints down to it. They would dearly like to shake their misery off, but just can't. The unhappiness and wretchedness just cloaks them, like a second skin. It is distressing to be miserable, because it is not the intended human state, and it can lead to serious emotional discomfort and, ultimately, depression. Therefore, help should be sought before things get too bad. If the feelings of misery only come during the autumn and winter months it could indicate a degree of seasonal affective disorder (SAD), which affects to some extent as many as one person in twenty, and is caused by a lack of light. Help is available for this disorder in the form of a light-box.

Using essential oils will not magically dissolve the problems that caused the misery, but they may alleviate the negative feelings that have arisen as a consequence of them, which ultimately leaves the

ESSENTIAL OILS TO USE WHEN FEELING MISERABLE

Narcissus	Petitgrain
Benzoin	Orange
Neroli	Rose Maroc
Jasmine	Clove
Cinnamon	Ginger
Carnation	Pimento Berry

person free to deal with those problems.

The following blends can be diluted with 30 mls (1 oz) of base oil to make a massage oil, or make a synergistic blend of oils using these proportions and use in baths, and all room and inhalation methods. For quantities to use see Chart 5.1.

WARMING AND COMFORTING	
Clove	5 drops
Pimento Berry	10 drops
Orange	15 drops
CUSHIONING	
Benzoin	10 drops
Cinnamon	5 drops
Rose Maroc	15 drops

Moodiness and Mood Swings

Moods can swing *really* fast. We can feel all bright and happy and then the final demand arrives from the mortgage company

ESSENTIAL OILS TO USE WHEN FEELING MOODY

Lemon	Geranium
Neroli	Lavender
Ylang Ylang	Patchouli
Eucalyptus Citriodora	
Ormenis Flower	

ESSENTIAL OILS TO HELP BALANCE MOOD SWINGS

Geranium	Cardamom
Lavender	Coriander
Angelica Seed	Cypress
Linden Blossom	Cedarwood
Helichrysum	

We seem to have an innate ability to harmonize our moods with other human beings — a strong force for social cohesion. Mood synchronization can also be seen as a form of communication. Some people are particularly responsive to "emotional contagion," as psychologists now call it. These are the "good listeners" who have great empathy with other people and pick up on all their moods, often not expressing their own.

Moodiness is not uncommon in teenagers, and during the premenstrual days of a woman's cycle, and there may well be a hormonal factor involved. More generally, moodiness is brought on by particular events during the day, or by life in general. Moody people can be fed-up, or frustrated, bored, isolated, repressed, irritable, or bad tempered, and usually think nobody understands them. (Well, in this frame of mind, who would want to?)

The essential oils can be used in all the usual methods.

The quantities in the following blends can be diluted with 30 mls (1 oz) of base oil to make a massage oil, or make a

and, bang, our mood is foul. Then the doorbell rings and a delivery man is standing there holding a big bunch of flowers. "Oooh," we say, excitedly, "I wonder who they're from?"

Like most other things in this world, moods are under the scrutiny of scientists, who are coming to the conclusion that moods are catching. In one piece of research, tiny electrodes were attached to different facial muscles of the subjects, who were shown pictures of people in different moods — happy, sad, angry, etc. The subjects responded to the photos by subtly moving their muscles to mimic the expressions of the faces in the pictures.

MOODINESS

Eucalyptus Citriodora	12 drops
Ormenis Flower	8 drops
Geranium	10 drops

MOOD SWINGS

Cedarwood	15 drops
Helichrysum	5 drops
Cypress	15 drops

synergistic blend of oils using these pro-portions and use in baths, and all room and inhalation methods. For quantities to use see Chart 5.1.

Obsessions and Compulsions

This is a true story, only the names have been changed: a man named George went with his friend, David, to visit David's mother. The house was spotless. David's mother went out and George and David went into the kitchen to make coffee. In the cupboard George noticed some home-made mincemeat waiting to be put in the Christmas pies and, being a gourmet and cook, he took half a teaspoonful out of the jar and ate it. David went mad saying "If mother sees that! . . . and got a clean spoon and started rearranging the top layer of mincemeat in the jar so it wouldn't look as if it had been touched. Obviously, mother didn't miss a trick. George went to the toilet and, standing there, he had a thought. He flushed the toilet, put the seat down, stood on the toilet seat and ran his finger across the top of the cistern. He couldn't believe it — not a speck of dust!

Some people are just obsessive about a particular thing — washing hands, checking doors, dressing in a certain way, and so on. In a sense, these are just sensi-ble things done to extreme — washing hands is hygienic, checking locks is a pro-tective measure, and dressing in a certain way can even be thought practical. But when a person washes their hands five times, or checks the locks five times, that is orderliness gone to extreme.

Anxiety and fear are usually at the root of obsessions. It could be that the obsession keeps the person so busy that helps them shut out what the anxiety is about. Psychotherapy often helps, as do such things as art therapy, behavioral ther-apy, and autogenic training. Certainly, help must be sought from a professional because the obsession can easily lead to depression, as well as a disrupted life. Obsessions very often lead to being unable to function well with other people because they can never come up to the obsessive's standards of orderliness (unless they become obsessive themselves). The family, of course, suffers most.

Essential oils are no substitute for therapy, but they can have a beneficial role in managing obsessions. The obses-sive could choose an essential oil, or make a blend, from the anxiety-relieving essen-tial oils, or the following list (or any other favorite and relevant oil) and sniff from the bottle, or tissue, each time they felt the obsessive behavior coming on. They should sit down, close their eyes, breathe the aroma deeply and let the thought pass. This approach has one advantage in that it provides an alternative ritual that can be dealt with later, and another advantage in that it relieves the anxiety that can often be the cause of the obses-sive behavior (which, hopefully, won't be around later to have to deal with). These diversionary aroma tactics would work best with people who are committed to changing their behavior. Many people, of course, do not accept they are obsessed.

Treatments from an aromatherapist

who has also trained as a counselor would be particularly helpful, although the essential oils can also be used at home in all the usual methods — massage oils, baths, diffused in the atmosphere, or inhaled from a tissue. Use the oils singly, or in blends.

ESSENTIAL OILS TO USE IN CASES OF OBSESSION

Sandalwood	Vetiver
Cedarwood	Narcissus
Clary Sage	Orange
Lemon	

OBSESSIONS RELAXING

Clary Sage	5 drops
Orange	15 drops
Cedarwood	10 drops

OBSESSIONS ANXIETY RELIEVING

Lavender	5 drops
Orange	10 drops
Sandalwood	15 drops

Compulsions are more or less the same as obsessions, although they are rather more related to unhappiness, rather than anxiety. Anorexia and bulimia develop from compulsions, as can overeating. Anorexia, refusing to eat food, is said to be the expression of the unconscious desire to be childlike. It usually affects teenage girls, with only 1 in 15 anorexics being male. Anorexia is life-threatening and help must be sought. Bulimia is the compulsion to binge on food, which is vomited up to prevent weight gain. It also gives the feeling of being in control. Bulimia is often associated with deep unhappiness and guilt.

Compulsions sprout from a thousand scenarios, all true and heart-felt. There's Joanne who overeats because she wants to punish her husband for having an affair, and subconsciously refuses to be attractive to him; and Denise who had to look after her elderly mother who sabotaged her romantic connections, so made herself feel unattractive by getting overweight. Then there's Rachel who found being overweight put her in a non-woman category, which helped in the sexist business world; and Annette, who became overweight to stop herself having affairs — not because she was worried about losing the husband she didn't love, but because she didn't want to lose the children. Lisa, constantly chided as a child, became overweight because she didn't think she deserved to be happy. All these women are unhappy — about the faithless husband; the manipulative mother; the sexist environment; the loveless marriage; and the negative parents. But their stories show that overeating is more than oral gratification or "comfort eating." It is a strategy of life, and for the compulsion to change, the circumstances of the life have to change too. At least, they should be discussed, and dealt with, perhaps in therapy — with or without other family members or partners.

Essential oils can help compulsive behavior in the areas of *Self-Esteem, Self-Blame*, and *Confidence*, among others, and they are discussed elsewhere. Coriander, geranium, and lemon are three oils that people have said they find most helpful, and they would work very well in a blend.

Pain

Wouldn't it be nice to be a baby again and able to cry out loud with pain? We could open our mouths wide and wail and howl, tears rolling down our faces, and everyone would run toward us, concerned. When you're a grown up, though, you're expected to deal with the pain without making too much fuss — which can be a bit difficult, especially when it sucks up all your energy, so you can't even think. People don't understand that, inside, you are fighting a violent battle with a monster that threatens to leave you with nothing left.

The pain of toothache, which we all get sometimes, is like a pebble compared to the mountain of pain some people have to deal with each and every day and night. The amount of pain going on in the world is mind-boggling, and a constant reminder to those of us not in pain how lucky we are. Yet we never see pain so, actually, we don't often think about it. Unless, of course, we have it and then we think about it all the time. Even when we're not in pain, we wonder when it will come again.

Pain can be caused by disease, accident, swelling, inflammation, or degeneration. It affects people with arthritis, osteoporosis, cancer, lower back pain, pain in the neck and shoulders, tension headaches, and many other conditions. Childbirth is a painful experience, but people do experience it differently. I remember one midwife telling me that when she worked in the north of a particular African country she found the women went through childbirth without hardly a word — still and quiet, yet in the south of the country the women went wild — throwing themselves around the walls of the room (along with their many loud and supportive female friends and relatives), wailing and screaming at the tops of their voices. To a certain extent then, the experience of pain is cultural. Presumably their potential for pain was the same, the women just approached it differently. As to which group felt the least pain, I'm afraid I do not know.

It is well known that feeling happier and better in yourself can reduce the experience of pain, if not the pain itself. This link between emotion and pain occurs in endorphins — morphine-like substances produced by the human body, which also play a part in determining mood; and in enkephalins, protein molecules with an analgesic (painkilling) effect, which also have sedative and mood-changing effects. The action of these chemicals may explain why the mood can affect the pain.

The ability of the human mind to lessen the experience of pain is now well-documented, especially due to the good work of the pain-relief clinics that have been set up around the country. By counseling, teaching relaxation techniques, and encouraging an outgoing attitude, the person coping with pain can certainly learn to manage the pain better. Everything is worth trying. Acupuncture has been extremely effective for many people, as have hypnotherapy and healing. Tension headaches happen to twice as many women as men because, it is thought, they have the extra and conflicting demands of family as well as work. For them, a possible rearrangement of lifestyle is the only answer. At the end of this chapter I briefly explain some techniques that may help the relief of pain, including *Visualization* and *Relaxation*.

Essential oils may help ease the tension and stress that come with pain, and so bring relief. They can be used in all the usual ways and it would be particularly useful to diffuse them in the atmosphere when doing relaxation exercises. A massage oil will help relieve the tension and a warm bath at night will aid sleep. Some essential oils do have analgesic value but it takes a skilled therapist to help in this

area as it is so individualistic. Choose from the following list of oils classically used in the area of pain relief.

If the pain is associated with inflammation, use chamomile roman. The tension relieving oils include marjoram, lavender, clary sage, and vetiver. To relax, use lavender or neroli. Also check the lists elsewhere in this book and choose oils that suit you best.

Panic and Panic Attacks

Panic sometimes follows trauma of some sort — such as an accident or bereavement — or is brought on by fear, anxiety or phobias. In some cases the panic is expressed as panic attacks, which reinforce the fears of phobics. Phobias are discussed in a later section because not everyone who has a panic attack has a phobia.

The mind-body connection is very obvious in the case of panic attacks — a thought in the mind can set off a whole range of physical sensations such as hyperventilation, perspiration, dizziness, fainting, nausea, shaking, trembling, and feelings of being very hot or cold. The heart can start to race, the breath can be difficult to catch, there may be choking, and pains in the chest. Not surprisingly, people sometimes think they are dying. This thought is heightened by the terror of some imaginary impending disaster. Another symptom is to have feelings of stepping outside oneself, depersonalization, and feelings of being in a state of

ESSENTIAL OILS USED FOR PAIN

Nutmeg	Clove
Rosemary	Lavender
Sage	Clary Sage
Helichrysum	Peppermint
Basil	
Betula Alba (Birch)	
Chamomile Roman	

perceptual distortion, like in a dream, known as derealization. If someone has four or more of these symptoms, it is classified as a panic attack, although many people have these symptoms with more long-lasting generalized feelings of panic unrelated to any particular thing, person, or environment.

Panic attacks can cause hyperventilation in some people and the best remedy I know for this is to breathe into a brown paper bag. This was one of the first things I learned as a student in Switzerland. It ensures the intake of carbon monoxide, which is lost during the process of over-breathing. Over the years the paper bag trick has come in very handy. I remember once on a transatlantic flight the call went out for a doctor because a passenger seated nearby had started hyperventilating, sweating, and trembling. He was refusing oxygen from the crew and was clearly distressed. His girlfriend said he was frightened of flying. The doctor who had come forward from among the passengers had no remedy and immediately agreed that we should try the paper bag method for the hyperventilation, and lavender oil to relax. The man was perfectly fine after five minutes, and continued the flight panic-free.

It is essential for anyone prone to panic attacks to learn deep breathing techniques, which can be utilized immediately when the sensations begin. Use deep, slow breaths from the abdomen. This technique works wonderfully well to relax in times of stress. It would also be sensible to learn a relaxation technique for regular practice at home.

ESSENTIAL OILS FOR USE IN PANIC ATTACKS	
Lavender	Frankincense
Helichrysum	Marjoram

PANIC ATTACK CALMING BLEND	
Lavender	10 drops
Frankincense	5 drops
Helichrysum	10 drops
Marjoram	5 drops

Luckily, panic attacks do not last long and gradually the body's metabolism adjusts to withstand the onslaught, and the blood and hormone levels return to normal. However, they can be socially debilitating, and physically very unpleasant and worrying.

The oils above are among the best that someone can use if having a panic attack, which, if severe, might require medical help. If you feel a panic attack coming on, use lavender essential oil neat (undiluted) on the chest and neck area, and in view of this effective remedy it would be worth carrying a bottle around with you. After an attack, a warm relaxing bath will be helpful — add 8 drops of lavender. Also, add 5 drops of lavender to a teaspoon of vegetable oil, mix well, and massage across your abdomen, shoulders, and neck. If you are prone to attacks, make up a panic-attack blend using the proportions given below. For quantities to use see Chart 5.1.

Add the quantities above to 30 mls (1 oz) base oil to make a massage oil or blend the essential oils together in these proportions and make a synergistic blend of oils that can be used in baths, and in all room, and inhalation methods. For a synergistic blend, multiply the quantities of the formula above by three and put those undiluted essential oils in a small bottle to carry around with you at all times. You can simply sniff from the bottle, or put a drop on a tissue and inhale from that.

Passivity

If you feel you cannot complain to the chef when he prepares you a terrible meal, or feel that you shouldn't bother the shopkeeper who sold you dud goods, or if you get pushed around by other people, you may be too passive for your own good. Passive people hang around on the fringes of conversations, feeling unable to join in. They might even pretend to agree with people, so they are liked, and keep their own opinions to themselves, so there isn't an argument. Passivity can even extend to feelings of love, worth, caring and sharing, so one finds oneself "accidentally" involved with someone romantically, almost by default.

It is inviting to think that passivity is always good in so much as it doesn't cause much harm. Pacifists, after all, don't start wars. But passivity is not innocent. By *allowing* things to happen, by not interrupting the course of events, one is involved. And if it is in something you don't like — change it! These days passivity is not encouraged in the work situation, managers want proactive people around them, and many people are going to assertion classes to address that issue. Women too have traditionally been encouraged to be passive (which has gotten them into all kinds of trouble) and there are many classes available for them to change that attitude. Passivity can cause frustration, stress, tension, feelings of worthlessness, helplessness, loneliness, anger, and depression — all of which is bottled up, of course, and then eats away inside. Clearly, it takes time to shake the passivity off and come into one's own, but it is well worth the try and it gets easier by the day. The essential oils can help overcome passivity and encourage you to become more assertive, used in all the usual ways.

The quantities in the following blends can be diluted with 30 mls (1 oz) of base oil to make a massage oil, or make a synergistic blend of oils using these proportions and use in baths, and all room, and inhalation methods. For quantities to

ESSENTIAL OILS TO HELP COUNTERACT PASSIVITY	
Rose Maroc	Ylang Ylang
Cedarwood	Pine
Jasmine	Tuberose
Orange	Patchouli
Bay	

PASSIVITY 1	
Rose Maroc	10 drops
Orange	10 drops
Patchouli	5 drops
Tuberose	5 drops

PASSIVITY 2	
Jasmine	8 drops
Cedarwood	5 drops
Ylang Ylang	7 drops
Bay	5 drops

use see Chart 5.1

Both the above blends are, unfortunately, rather expensive. The following are less expensive.

PASSIVITY 3	
Patchouli	10 drops
Ylang Ylang	5 drops
Bay	5 drops
Orange	5 drops
Cedarwood	5 drops

Phobias

To have a phobia is to have an ongoing, irrational fear of a particular object or situation. The most common fear is of open spaces or public places (agoraphobia). People are also afraid of heights, flying, or enclosed spaces (claustrophobia). The most common so-called "specific" phobias are the fear of dogs, snakes, spiders, and mice. "Social" phobias, which are much rarer, are concerned with interactions with other people in some way. So a person may be generally frightened of people and excessively shy, fearful of eating in front of other people, or speaking, fearful of using cups and cutlery in restaurants, or using public toilets, or fearful of getting crushed and stamped on.

Phobias have been described as a fear that is out of all proportion to the situation, which logic and discussion cannot dispel, is not under voluntary control, and leads to avoiding the feared situation. This makes phobias a psychological reaction, an emotional reaction, a behavioral reaction and, if panic attacks are involved, a physiological reaction. The whole person is involved, and their lifestyle, and, possibly, the lifestyle of their family and friends.

Phobias may be related to a major change in earlier life — perhaps a house move, or a traumatic incident, bereavement, or accident. Or they may have developed from a particular incident — being bitten by a dog as a child, for example. Some kind of therapy is probably needed to work through the phobia, and success rates at specialist clinics are good. It is even possible that the phobia will resolve itself. Mary was an animal lover with many pets, but terrified of spiders. A group of her young friends decided to go on a camping vacation in Greece. Everyone was going but Mary immediately thought about the spiders that might be crawling in the tent. It was a very tough decision, but her friends insisted she come. The amazing thing was, when they got there, there *weren't* any spiders. Mary slowly relaxed and by the end of the first week she was wondering where all the spiders had gone. By the end of the second week she was *looking* for them. She never found one. But, when she got back home, she looked for a spider again, and found one, which she put in a box and looked at occasionally. They became friends, then she let him go, to roam her house again.

Further information about phobias can be obtained from the *Phobics Society* and *Phobic Action* (see Appendix IV), and there is specialist help. There is even a company that takes people who are afraid of flying up in the air. I would suggest reading *Living With Fear* by Professor Isaac Marks or some other literature on the subject. Phobias can be overcome. If you have a phobia it is wise to seek professional help in the form of counseling, psychotherapy, or whatever. Relaxation exercise (see page 207) can also be of use, as can aromatherapy treatments. Behavioral therapy will encourage you to recognize the fear and may help you to face the fear in a controlled way. Hypnotherapy can help too, as can homeopathy. If you have therapeutic treatments, ask your therapist if he or she would mind diffusing an oil while they give the positive messages of reassurance. This same aroma can then be taken out, on a handkerchief for example, and sniffed whenever required. Diffusing the oils while doing relaxation exercises would be helpful too, and the same essential oil can be used in the same way later, sniffed for reassurance when feeling phobic, so possibly bringing relief. Choose an oil you really like the

smell of, from the list of calming and relaxing oils. Then carry that same oil with you, especially when possibly facing the feared object or situation. The oil can be put on a tissue or handkerchief and just sniffed. Today there are even necklaces being sold with little bottles for a pendant that can hold essential oils, and of course bottles of essential oils are tiny enough to fit into even the smallest evening handbag. There is no need to be without nature's helpmates. If you're not worried about the material, a few drops of essential oil could even be put on a jacket or shirt sleeve and sniffed when needed. Just by running your fingers through your hair, reassuring aroma molecules will waft into your nose. The memories of the therapy will flood back, the fear may hopefully dissipate — and nobody need ever know.

Used in phobias, essential oils can help in panic attacks, build up confidence, allay anxiety, help a person come to terms with the phobia and also develop the balance needed when, for example, having to face up to the problem. Plus, the essential oils can help overlay good memory patterns over bad. Some people might say it's bad to encourage a dependency on something, an oil in this case, but smell/ memory/behavior patterns can easily be overlaid. If there is a psychologist or psychotherapist involved, it will help them do their job better if you are relaxed, perhaps by the anxiety-relieving essential oils that are listed on page 222. Also, looking at the chart section will help you decide what your symptoms are and which oils are best suited to your situation. There are of course many more calming and relaxing essential oils than those listed below, but these have been reported as being the most useful for this situation.

CALMING, RELAXING ESSENTIAL OILS

Linden Blossom	Lavender
Clary Sage	Neroli
Ylang Ylang	Marjoram
Ormenis Flower	Sandalwood
Chamomile Roman	

There are no general blends that help with phobias as so many systems are involved and the phobia expresses itself so differently in different people. It is best to write a list of all your symptoms and make up your own personal oil.

Psychosomatic Illness

Psychosomatic illnesses *feel* real but aren't. The symptoms are real enough, but they are not caused by anything, other than the mind. It's all very confusing — to the patient and doctor alike. Headaches, nausea, irritable bowl syndrome, peptic ulcer, and asthma sometimes have a psychosomatic cause, or are made worse by psychosomatic factors. This connection between the mind and body is well known but difficult to diagnose and treat. No doubt there are many people going to their doctor and being treated for something

which could be better treated by counseling, and no doubt there are people diagnosed by their doctor as having psychosomatic illness when they do not. Those of us in the complementary fields have seen many such patients over the years, and often a problem is found and the person is told to go back to their doctor again. Clearly, the biggest danger is to miss an actual symptom of real disease because the psychosomatic factor makes diagnosis a problem. It's the old "crying wolf" syndrome and it can get one into trouble.

There are no specific oils for this problem. As the symptoms are real — the pain is actually felt — there is no reason not to treat them with essential oils, and I refer you to my book *The Complete Book of Essential Oils and Aromatherapy*. Please also refer to other sections of this book that may be relevant, including *Anxiety*.

Quarrelsomeness

Quarrelsome people are difficult to be with because everything you say, every opinion you have, is twisted and turned around into an argument. If you have a quarrelsome person in your family they can make life unbearable. Some people react by saying nothing. I know of at least one woman who has learned to skip over any event she knows may provoke her partner, who must watch her tone of voice, who looks at everything in a split second, evaluating the trouble it could cause, and arranging things so it doesn't. But of course, her quarrelsome partner

ESSENTIAL OILS FOR QUARRELSOMENESS

Clary Sage	Lavender
Lemon	Sandalwood
Patchouli	Cistus
Clove	

QUARRELSOMENESS 1

Lemon	20 drops
Clove	8 drops
Cistus	2 drops

QUARRELSOMENESS 2

Sandalwood	10 drops
Patchouli	5 drops
Lemon	15 drops

still finds things to set him off.

Trying to change somebody else's attitude isn't really what *The Fragrant Mind* is about, but if you yourself feel that you are perhaps overdoing the way you get your point across, maybe it's time to look at things from a different perspective. (If you really enjoy being antagonistic, that is a different matter, and perhaps you should join a debating club and give the family some peace.) Use the essential oils in all the usual methods.

The quantities in the following can be diluted with 30 mls (1 oz) of base oil to make a massage oil, or make a synergistic blend of oils using these proportions and

use in baths, and in all room and inhalation methods.

Rage

Unlike normal anger, rage is a violent form of intensive anger, often completely uncontrollable. People can go "blind with rage" and become violent, even kill, giving loss of reason as a defense. Rage is an outburst that wells up from somewhere deep inside, usually in response to an intensely provoking incident.

There are no specific essential oils for rage but some people could undoubtedly benefit from them by using oils for aggression, stress, and tension. However, in the rage type of personalities the stress and tension does not easily dissipate but remains lodged in the muscles and it would be best to visit an aromatherapy practitioner who can, through specialist techniques, release the tension.

Choose essential oils from the stress and tension lists or from the one below; use in all the usual methods. For quantities to use see Chart 5.1.

ESSENTIAL OILS TO HELP LESSEN RAGE

Ylang Ylang	Clary Sage
Vetiver	Lavender
Marjoram	Galbanham
Chamomile Roman	
Ormenis Flower	

RAGE 1	
Vetiver	8 drops
Chamomile	
Roman	10 drops
Lavender	12 drops

RAGE 2	
Ylang Ylang	8 drops
Ormenis Flower	12 drops
Galbanham	10 drops

Regret

It is amazing how many people say they don't have any regrets, despite the fact that they may be terminally ill or have had, to the outside eye, a pretty miserable life. Edith Piaf sang the immortal song "Je ne regrette rien," and her life was no picnic. We seem instinctively to realize that in bad experiences there are lessons to be learned, and that, in fact, we gain insight from bad experiences. How can one regret that? Even so, we probably all have one or two regrets kicking about somewhere that, with the benefit of hindsight, we can identify. But we don't dwell on them. The thing we regret just flickers quickly through the mind occasionally, perhaps when things are particularly bad, and then is forgotten. At least, it should be. However, there are some people who cannot rid themselves of thoughts of regret and who let it overcome their life so they are no longer living present-day life to the fullest. If this is you, use the following essential oils singly or in blends in all the usual methods.

ESSENTIAL OILS FOR REGRET	
Hyacinth	Cypress
Pine	Rose Maroc
Mimosa	

REGRET 1	
Rose Maroc	5 drops
Hyacinth	5 drops
Mimosa	3 drops

REGRET 2	
Rose Otto	10 drops
Cypress	2 drops
Mimosa	4 drops

REGRET 3	
Cypress	20 drops
Pine	10 drops

The quantities in the following blends can be diluted with 30 mls (1 oz) of base oil to make a massage oil, or make a synergistic blend of oils using these proportions and use it in baths, and in all room and inhalation methods.

Rejection

The dictionary definition of "to reject" is "to throw away as useless or worthless" — and that's just about how it feels. To feel rejected in love is perhaps an essential requirement in the "to have experienced life" department and I doubt that one could claim to be an artist until you could identify with the depths of that despair. Or perhaps that is being dramatic and it would be fabulous to be the "golden" boy or girl who manages to go through life getting everything and everyone they want. For most of us, however, it isn't like that. It isn't a question of *if* rejection will come but a question of how much and in what form. Professionally, the recessions bring a trail of rejections in the form of people who have been told they've lost their job.

Some very sensitive souls often feel rejected because they can "sense" the underlying rejection of one of their ideals, or the unwillingness of someone else to accept a situation, a kind of rejection of their plans and desires. This is hurtful because it is disrespectful, as if we were useless and worthless. But also, some people feel rejected when it is not actually the case, they are misreading the situation — being too sensitive.

I can think of dozens of people who have rejected tricky or uncomfortable

REJECTION FORMULA 1	
Carnation	5 drops
Ylang Ylang	5 drops
Sandalwood	15 drops

REJECTION FORMULA 2	
Tuberose	5 drops
Benzoin	15 drops
Cypress	2 drops

changes, usually by doing and saying nothing — playing dead, refusing to accept that a situation has changed, that they are being asked to move on. This is rejection of reality and it can have a profound effect on us and even lead to depression and stress. The only answer is to come to terms with the truth and the inevitability of the situation.

Rejection needs comfort and understanding. Try to talk your situation through with someone, perhaps an outsider. Rejection is definitely distressing, but it doesn't last forever, or doesn't have to. These would be the essential oils to try, either singly or in blends, in all the usual methods.The quantities in the following blends can be diluted with 30 mls (1 oz) of base oil to make a massage oil, or make a synergistic blend of oils using these proportions and use in baths, and in all room and inhalation methods. For quantities to use see Chart 5.1.

ESSENTIAL OILS TO USE IF FEELING REJECTED

Pine	Cypress
Sandalwood	Benzoin
Neroli	Rose Otto
Ylang Ylang	Hyacinth
Tuberose	Carnation
Chamomile Roman	

Repression

Just as repression can stunt the growth of a people or nation, repression can stunt the growth of individuals. Repression by a person or situation can often be dealt with by becoming assertive, although this is easier said than done, especially in the home or workplace. We may feel unable to speak out, tell our truths, be who we are. There is repression too in feeling unable to fight against injustice, as if our views are ineffectual because of the largeness of "the system," and our feelings of anger and dismay can never be heard where they are intended. It isn't *everyone* who gets a private conversation with the president.

Once you can shake off the feelings of repression it will be as if a heavy winter coat and hat have been lifted from you. Again, talking helps. Many writers took up the pen as a way of being able to speak out and break free of repression, and you can do it too. Keep a diary, make lists, draw up brain maps — anything to express what you are feeling inside.

Watch out too for self-repression — keeping uncomfortable feelings, actions or situations away from our conscious mind. It is a safety mechanism to protect our emotional state, but it is of limited value. There should come a time when it is no longer required.

To help shake off repression, use the following essential oils in all the usual methods, especially in baths, diffused around the home, or in a massage oil.

The quantities in the following blends can be diluted with 30 mls (1 oz) of base oil to make a massage oil, or make a synergistic blend of oils using these proportions and use in the bath, and in all room, and inhalation methods. For quantities to use see Chart 5:1.

REPRESSION 1	
Patchouli	5 drops
Frankincense	15 drops
Jasmine	10 drops

REPRESSION 2	
Cedarwood	14 drops
Pine	8 drops
Juniper	8 drops

ESSENTIAL OILS FOR REPRESSION	
Hyacinth	Jasmine
Frankincense	Ylang Ylang
Cedarwood	Pine
Patchouli	Vetiver
Juniper	

Schizophrenia

The word "schizophrenia" conjures up images of "mad" behavior, like hearing voices, talking nonsense and jumping in the lion's den. Symptoms include having incorrect beliefs, for example that people are conspiring against you, or believing that you are another person, perhaps a dead one, or being controlled. The senses are very much affected, in that voices can be heard, and tastes, smells, or sights imagined. Schizophrenics also tend to have confused thinking, a loss of interest in and affection of other people — even to the point of laughing at their misfortunes — self-absorption and self-neglect. But these are generalizations because each schizophrenic experiences the illness in a different way. Schizophrenics do *not* have a split personality. They are suffering changes in perception which are affecting their thinking, behavior, and feelings.

One young man described the nightmare like this: "I had never felt so terrified. I was confused and helpless, trapped in a menacing world where everyone and everything conspired against me."[8] And this is a nightmare one in every hundred people in the U.S. will suffer before they reach forty-five, perhaps as a one-time incident or as a series throughout life. Each attack might last a few weeks or longer and in-between times, the person appears perfectly normal. Usually, schizophrenia develops for the first time when people are in their twenties.

Why it should do this is a mystery. Certainly the chemical messenger dopamine is involved and by regulating it more effectively the new generation of drugs is having tremendous impact on treatment, which is much improved (unless you are one of the unlucky few who develop agranulocytosis, a serious condition of the bone marrow).

Bearing in mind the drug treatment schizophrenics should be on and should continue to take, they should reduce by half the usual number of essential oils used, in massage oils, baths, diffusers, inhaled or whatever, or use less still. Only use these gentle oils.

ESSENTIAL OILS TO USE IN CASES OF SCHIZOPHRENIA

Lavender	Mandarin
Geranium	Lemon
Chamomile Roman	Rose Otto

When choosing your essential oils, bear in mind your condition at the time, which may vary. The two blends below, for example, are more appropriate for different times of the day. For quantities to use see Chart 5:1.

DAYTIME	
Geranium	5 drops
Lavender	5 drops
Lemon	5 drops
NIGHTTIME	
Lavender	8 drops
Lemon	4 drops
Chamomile Roman	3 drops

To make a massage oil, blend either of the above with 30 mls (1 oz) vegetable oil, or make a synergistic blend by mixing the essential oils in these proportions. Use a maximum of 4 drops in a bath — geranium is particularly useful. Lavender is excellent in diffusers — use 4 drops, three times a day, with 2 drops of lemon also each time. If the feel of oil on the skin is unpleasant, benefit can still be obtained by applying the massage oil and showering or bathing a short time later. The oils could also be diffused during any therapy sessions.

It is well worth exploring the link between allergies and schizophrenia, and it may be worth keeping a diary of what was eaten and drunk, and when the attacks occurred. There may be no link, but it's worth a look. Allergy tests are available and a nutritionist may also be able to give advice as to which foods may cause an allergic reaction, such as glucose and gluten for example. A high-protein, low-carbohydrate diet is often recommended, along with no caffeine. Vitamins that might be taken are those of the B group — B12, B3, B6, along with vitamins C and E; also thiamine, biotin, folic acid, zinc, or PABA (para aminobenzoin acid). A group of psychiatrists called orthomoleculists use vitamins as part of the treatment, along with conventional methods. Homeopathy may be able to help too.

Self-blame

We all blame ourselves at some time for things we should have done, situations that shouldn't have been. They can range from the minor, as when we knock over an ornament and say, "Oh, I am stupid," for example, to the major, as when we drive carelessly and harm someone. Self-blame is occasionally justified and shows that we are human, compassionate, and aware. But sometimes it goes too far and people blame themselves for everything

ESSENTIAL OILS WHEN FEELING SELF-BLAME	
Rose Otto	Lemon
Geranium	Bergamot
Orange	Ylang Ylang
Carnation	Tuberose
Benzoin	Melissa
Chamomile Roman	
Eucalyptus Citriodora	
Ormenis Flower	

— including the weather. "Sorry, sorry, sorry, sorry," they say, rather like a crowd of English people bumping into each other on the sidewalk.

Self-blame can develop if a child is made to feel that everything is their fault, and the guilt gets carried forward into adulthood. This is particularly sad because children do in any case blame themselves for all sorts of things that are not their fault, including domestic strife or divorce and shortage of money. Their little shoulders carry all sorts of self-blame that we can probably not imagine, but it pops out occasionally and makes us aware.

For young and old alike, it is very helpful to discuss self-blame, to try and get a realistic perspective on the subject. Words are powerful things and if you can just hear the sentence that self-blames, and re-word it in your head, things might start to be different. Having the courage to say they are different would be even better. The crucial thing with essential oils is to choose those that make you feel good about yourself. You might find them on lists in other sections of this book or among those below. Use in all the usual methods.

SELF-BLAME FORMULA 1

Lemon	10 drops
Bergamot	10 drops
Orange	8 drops
Ormenis Flower	2 drops

SELF-BLAME FORMULA 2

Eucalyptus Citriodora	15 drops
Chamomile Roman	5 drops
Ylang Ylang	10 drops

The quantities in the following blends can be diluted with 30 mls (1 oz) of base oil to make a massage oil, or make a synergistic blend of oils using these proportions and use in the bath, and in all room and inhalation methods. For quantities see Chart 5.1

Sorrow

Deep sadness can be caused by grief, loss, disappointment, suffering, and regret. It can last a long time depending on the person and the cause. Some people never get over sorrow and carry it with them always. See also Bereavement and Grief. The following oils have been found to be helpful; use in all the usual methods.

ESSENTIAL OILS TO HELP ALLEVIATE SORROW

Cypress	Hyacinth
Melissa	Benzoin
Frankincense	Sandalwood

SORROW 1

Sandalwood	15 drops
Frankincense	10 drops
Benzoin	5 drops

SORROW 2

Hyacinth	5 drops
Sandalwood	10 drops

Can be used at half-strength

Stress

Psychologists talk about three types of stress: *Normal Stress, Distress*, and *Eustress*. *Normal Stress* is what one would feel after narrowly escaping a car accident — short of breath and with a racing heart. This physical reaction is caused by the release of chemicals from the adrenal "gland," which has two distinct parts — the central *adrenal medulla* and an outer *adrenal cortex*. This is a mechanism for survival, a sudden and immediate shot in the arm, so to speak, to get us out of a fix, to sharpen reactions so we can move faster and use all our wits. It may be that we have to decide which way to turn the car steering wheel to best avoid an accident, or which way to jump in front of an oncoming herd of buffalo — it's all stress. This emergency system is chemical and involves *epinephrine* and a smaller amount of *norepinephrine*, which are released directly into the bloodstream. The heart begins to pound immediately. Metabolic changes take place that cause energy immediately to be supplied where required, especially to the brain. The adrenal cortex releases the stress-related hormone *cortisol* which, among other things, increases the level of glucose in the blood and redirects it to the brain and causes hypertension — which are handy physiological back-ups when looking a tiger in the eye.

Stress isn't meant to be an everyday occurrence. What happens is that we get overloaded on the natural chemicals because we're stimulated by stressful situations too much and it gets bottled up. This chronic situation is called, appropriately, *Distress*. It is dangerous because it can lead to a hardening of the arteries, heart attacks and strokes, and lesser problems. One way people find to off-load their stress is to work it off with exercise and I know several New York high-flyers who say they simply wouldn't survive without their hour workout at the gym each day. Another answer is to rearrange your life or job so there isn't so much stress to deal with. Most especially, look at the degree of control in your life. One study found that the people who suffered most stress were those who had high demands made of them, but little control

— such as waiters, cooks, firemen, and cashiers. Another interesting piece of research from Sweden tested commuters at journey's end for their level of stress and found that those who boarded early, and had choice in where to sit, were less stressed — control again. Working mothers of young children are a group who are particularly prone to stress because they have all the pressures but little control. If little Billy wets his bed in the middle of the night, you get up, you have no choice. *Eustress* is the ideal state — buzzed up over some exciting project that is under our control, the energy flowing and the work going great.

You know you've got distress if you "blow a fuse" or have a "hair trigger" with everyday annoyances — like getting caught up in a traffic jam or shouting at the kids for the smallest thing. You may have persistent doubts about being able to cope, or feel helpless and out of control. Stress can arise from mental causes, such as exam or office pressure; from emotional problems, such as a relationship break-up; from physical pressures, such as too much driving, squash, or gardening; chemical sources, such as too much caffeine or drugs; and environmental pressures, such as persistent noise on the factory floor. Symptoms of the mind include irritability, loss of sense of humor, difficulty in making decisions or concentrating, or doing jobs in logical order, feeling defensive or angry inside, and being disinterested in large areas of life. Physical symptoms include insomnia, sweating, breathlessness, fainting, loss of appetite and binging, indigestion, constipation or diarrhea, headaches, cramps, muscle spasms, eczema, and sexual disinteres. But of course the biggest symptom is heart attack or stroke, by which time stress-management will be too late.

Until relatively recently, "stress" wasn't taken very seriously and was pigeon-holed as a thing that only affected powerful executives with a thousand telephone calls to make. We now know that isn't true. It's as likely to be the secretary being ordered around by her tyrannical boss that has the stress, especially if she's juggling child-care arrangements as well as her job. The government certainly takes stress seriously, with an estimated 100 million days lost each year through it, to the cost of $2.25 billion a year. This is a massive financial loss to the nation and an inestimable loss in terms of human happiness.

Essential Oils and Stress

Potentially, all essential oils can help combat stress because they are used in massage and baths, which are themselves therapeutic procedures. Of course, essential oils go much deeper than this, and some essential oils work particularly well on stress. Indeed, they are so effective that essential oils may provide the most successful way of coping with the problems associated with and caused by stress. They certainly strengthen the immune system, which gets considerably weaker during stressful periods, whereas people who lead stress-free lives have a better

ESSENTIAL OILS TO HELP ALLEVIATE STRESS	
Bergamot	Frankincense
Geranium	Grapefruit
Lavender	Lemon
Mandarin	Marjoram
Melissa	Neroli
Rose Otto	Sandalwood
Vetiver	Clary Sage
Ylang Ylang	Bay
Jasmine	Benzoin
Osmanthus	Tuberose
Hyacinth	Yarrow
Linden Blossom	Narcissus
Nutmeg	Hops
Spikenard	Valerian
Ormenis Flower	Litsea Cubeba
Chamomile Roman	
Eucalyptus Citriodora	

ability to fight off disease.

Each aromatherapist has their own favorite oils to use in the fight against stress and the ones listed above consist of those in common use and easily available. They all blend well with each other and can be successfully interchanged, each having medical properties that are useful in treating stress.

Of the above, one of my favorites is the much-neglected eucalyptus citriodora (eucalyptus lemon). Not only does it have antibiotic, antifungal, and slightly antiviral properties, it appears to boost the immune system, has electrical properties akin to our own energetic force, and is adaptogenic, which basically means it's subtle and bends to our needs. All these properties make it a must for anyone who is dealing with stress and its harmful effects.

The following oils could be considered the "essential stress kit" oils because various combinations of them would be suitable in most situations. They have been selected from the recommended lists drawn up by aromatherapy organizations, and they are reasonably priced. All will work well, singly or in combinations, and have been the basis for aromatherapy relaxation and stress-relief treatments for a considerable length of time.

THE ESSENTIAL STRESS KIT

Lavender	Geranium
Ormenis Flower	Clary Sage
Ylang Ylang	Sandalwood
Petitgrain	Mandarin
Eucalyptus Citriodora	
Chamomile Roman	

If resources were unlimited, I would choose as my personal stress kit the essential oils of rose otto, rose maroc, hyacinth, carnation, linden blossom, neroli, and jasmine, each of which has proven its worth in the treatment of stressful disorders time and time again. These highly emotional essential oils can be added to your personal stress kit, as and when funds allow. By choosing your additions to the essential stress kit carefully you can build up a set of oils that will suit all types of stress and problems that are incurred because of it. Using only the original stress kit oils, many formulations can be made.

STRESS LEVEL ONE
tiredness, irritability, aches and pains, occasional depression

STRESS LEVEL ONE BLEND 1

Eucalyptus Citriodora	10 drops
Geranium	15 drops
Lavender	5 drops

STRESS LEVEL ONE BLEND 2

Mandarin	15 drops
Ylang Ylang	5 drops
Petitgrain	10 drops

STRESS LEVEL TWO
anxiety/depression, food allergies, persistent infection, sub-acute disease, hidden weaknesses (such as otherwise dormant viral infections)

STRESS LEVEL TWO BLEND 1

Clary Sage	10 drops
Chamomile Roman	5 drops
Lavender	5 drops
Geranium	10 drops

STRESS LEVEL TWO BLEND 2

Ormenis Flower	10 drops
Ylang Ylang	5 drops
Petitgrain	5 drops
Sandalwood	10 drops

STRESS LEVEL THREE

complex pattern of symptoms (anything from suicidal tendencies to stomach pain), fear, withdrawal from society, despair

STRESS LEVEL THREE BLEND 1

Chamomile	
Roman	5 drops
Clary Sage	15 drops
Ormenis Flower	5 drops

STRESS LEVEL THREE BLEND 2

Geranium	6 drops
Eucalyptus	
Citriodora	14 drops
Mandarin	10 drops

The blends have been designed for general use with stress. The quantities can be diluted with 30 mls (1 oz) of base oil to make a massage oil, or make a synergistic blend of oils using these proportions and use in the bath, and in all room, and inhalation methods.

Stress Management

Write up a list of all the activities you have in your life and order them in terms of priorities. Get rid of those things that come at the bottom of your list, the nonessentials, by delegating responsibility for them to someone else or simply deleting them from your life. Ask yourself, as you look at your list, who am I doing this for — me or someone else?

Then reevaluate them again. Are they really necessary? Make time for yourself, so you can do something you enjoy in peace. Talk to people about your problems and see what solutions they can come up with. Think laterally — do you enjoy your job, and are you good at it? If not, change it. Do ten minutes relaxation each and every day. Take vitamins, cut caffeine, get some exercise, laugh, cry, and then go out and enjoy yourself!

Trauma

Many emotional problems start during a traumatic situation, whether this is a crisis or a tragedy that changes a whole life, or a deeply personal event. Many therapists believe that a traumatic birth can lead to emotional wounding later in life, particularly if the following events in life give no comfort. We know that physical and environmental trauma — caused by accidents, having an illness, being in an earthquake, — affects the body's structure, causing blockages, stresses, and tensions in the way the body functions. Emotional trauma — such as leaving home, changing a job, losing a loved one — can do the same thing. Vibrational trauma can come when the electromagnetic patterning around us, our aura, gets disturbed by outside factors. Our etheric state can also have an effect on our mind and body.

Clearly, trauma is an intensely personal thing, with many sources, and how much it affects us depends on how we view it. But traumas do have an affect on us all in some way, whether we like it or not.

ESSENTIAL OILS TO USE IN CASES OF TRAUMA	
Thyme Linalol	Lavender
Geranium	Lemon
Marjoram	Petitgrain
Clary Sage	
Chamomile Roman	

Human beings are mind/ body/spirit complexes, walking, talking electrical energy, and we cannot separate these three, especially in the case of trauma. Therefore all three must be considered when using essential oils for this condition.

If you have suffered from trauma look at the lists and charts throughout this book to find your symptoms and choose oils from there. Trauma victims need to release the tension and stress to stop further complications happening. If you can, visit an aromatherapist who may be able to help you further.

Withdrawal from Life

Withdrawal from life is very common. People hide themselves away or seem to withdraw inside themselves. This may happen gradually in a series of small steps toward solitude, such as not going out any more, not making phone calls, or visiting friends, not buying clothes, and not paying attention to themselves.

Withdrawal from life may follow a trauma or deeply felt emotion or event, but it is not normal and most people are dreadfully unhappy with the situation in which they find themselves. Withdrawal of emotional feelings is another aspect of withdrawal, for example, to no longer give freely of love, compassion, understanding, and even anger. Again, this is not right and often goes hand in hand with withdrawal from life.

Another kind of withdrawal is the kind yogis do, sometimes for years in a cave — contemplative withdrawal. This is

WITHDRAWAL FROM LIFE	
Narcissus	Orange

WITHDRAWAL OF EMOTIONS	
Bergamot	Rose Otto
Hyacinth	Neroli
Mandarin	Geranium
Chamomile Roman	

WITHDRAWAL FOR PEACE	
Rose Otto	Neroli
Carnation	Bergamot
Frankincense	Geranium
Cypress	Cedarwood
Juniper	
Chamomile Roman	

the kind of withdrawal that gives us insight, peace, and strength. Some people withdraw for periods of meditation, to feel near God, to look deep inside themselves, or perhaps to create a masterpiece.

The quantities in the following blends can be diluted with 30 mls (1 oz) of base oil to make a massage oil, or make a synergistic blend of oils using these proportions and use in the bath, and in all room and inhalation methods. For quantities to use see Chart 5.1.

EMOTIONAL WITHDRAWAL 1

Chamomile	
Roman	1 drops
Neroli	10 drops
Geranium	1 drops

EMOTIONAL WITHDRAWAL 2

Bergamot	15 drops
Hyacinth	5 drops

WITHDRAWAL FOR PEACE

Frankincense	5 drops
Juniper	5 drops
Bergamot	5 drops

To the above blend you could add another 15 drops of essential oil. Use essential oils to which you feel particularly attuned. Spend some time meditating and then use your intuition to guide you to the right ones for you.

Worthlessness

Feeling that you have no worth or are without value, that you are despicable, and not fit to walk this planet, may seem alien to some. But many people have to live with these feelings every day. It is crucial to talk these feelings through, if only with yourself. Write down who said you were worthless, when and why, what are you worthless at exactly, and what are you good at? Try to trace when you began to feel worthless, and write down what was going on at the time. If you can't figure out where these feelings of worthlessness came from, take your notes to a counselor or psychotherapist and see if they can figure it out. Perhaps hypnotherapy can reveal a cause you hadn't thought of. At least find a friend to talk to, even a stranger. A professional aromatherapist will be able to tell a great deal from seeing which muscles tense and stress as you speak and will be bound by ethics never to repeat your most inner thoughts. Also, relaxation techniques can help to clear your mind, and as that happens, you might just find the answer to it all.

ESSENTIAL OILS TO HELP ALLEVIATE FEELINGS OF WORTHLESSNESS

Frankincense	Sandalwood
Cedarwood	Clove
Ormenis Flower	Neroli
Juniper	Geranium
Chamomile Roman	

Essential oils can help you to sort out your feelings by working on the limbic system, helping you focus your thoughts. Use in all the usual ways.

The quantities in the opposite blends can be diluted with 30 mls (1 oz) of base oil to make a massage oil, or make a synergistic blend of oils using these proportions and use in the bath, and in all room and inhalation methods. For quantities to use see Chart 5.1.

WORTHLESSNESS 1	
Juniper	10 drops
Cedarwood	10 drops
Frankincense	5 drops
Geranium	5 drops

WORTHLESSNESS 2	
Clove	5 drops
Sandalwood	15 drops
Chamomile	
Roman	5 drops
Ormenis Flower	5 drops

CHAPTER 9

TAKING CONTROL

Autogenic Training

In the late 1920s a German neurologist named Dr. Johanes Schultz became intrigued by the possibility that the healing benefits of hypnotism could be reproduced without actually putting the patient into a trance. He developed autogenic training, which consists of a series of six mental exercises that can be done in one of three positions — lying on your back, sitting upright in a chair, or sitting on the edge of a chair with your head and shoulders slumped forward. The technique is used not only to reduce anxiety, stress, or depression and induce relaxation but, by allowing the body's natural healing mechanisms to work effectively, has a beneficial impact on many physical disorders including bronchitis, colitis, irritable bowl syndrome, high blood pressure, migraine, and ulcers.

The tremendous success of autogenic training has spawned over 3,000 research studies that can prove its effectiveness but are unable to explain why it works so well. That secret is still tied up with the mystery of the mind-body connection. Almost anyone can benefit from autogenic training, from businessmen who want to operate at their peak efficiency, and sports players who want to improve their performance and stimulate the body's healing mechanisms so injuries can heal faster, to people trying to cut down or get off drugs.

Taking one of the three positions mentioned above that is most comfortable (or appropriate, given the time of day because this technique can be practiced while sitting on a commuter train, for example), you can go through one or more of the six mental exercises, each of which are accompanied by a phrase that is silently repeated. During the first exercise, which focuses your thoughts on *heaviness* of the arms, legs, neck, and shoulders, the phrase might be "my left arm is heavy." The *warmth* exercise involves concentrating on the warmth felt in the arms and legs. The *heartbeat* exercise is simply to focus on your heartbeat. The fourth exercise is to focus on *breathing*. The fifth is to focus on a feeling of warmth in your *stomach*. The sixth is to concentrate on a feeling of coolness on your *forehead*.

Ideally, the technique should be taught by a trained therapist, a process which takes 8-10 one-hour sessions — probably within a group setting. You may be able to find books on the subject, or try it yourself. In the "slumped" position, sit on the edge of the chair with your hands on your thighs and feet about twelve inches apart. In the "reclining" position, lie flat on your back with a pillow under your head and another under your knees, arms resting at your side. Breath deeply and slowly from the abdomen. To begin, just do the heaviness exercise, concentrating on heaviness in your arms, legs, neck, and shoulders, then progress to the other exercises, adding them as you become more adept at concentrating. For each exercise, repeat a phrase that helps focus your mind on what you are doing — such as, for excercise number six, "My forehead is cool," "My forehead is cool." People do autogenic training every day, from as little as two minutes, three times a day, to twenty minutes, three times a day. If you have any physical area that is causing problems, mentally direct your healing energy to that region. One interesting aspect of autogenic training is "autogenic discharges" — fleeting but often powerful impressions of aromas, tastes, touch, and so on, which are related to events that happened in the past. This release of trapped energy causes a flow or rush of energy.

The "autogenic discharges" are perhaps a strange phenomenon, but one sees the same thing happening during aromatherapy treatments when emotions such as anger and grief are dislodged from the musculature, and many other therapies report the same releasing dynamic at work. If essential oils are to be diffused while doing the exercises, choose an oil from the relaxing list, or one that is particularly relevant to your requirements.

Breathing

Learning to breathe properly is essential to health. When we inhale, oxygen is absorbed into the blood and circulated to all organs and when we exhale, waste gases are expelled. As we all know, breathing rates change to suit the situation. If we're building a house of cards we hold our breath; and if we're anxious, we can find ourselves gasping for breath. Fear and excitement tend to make people breathe from the chest, as does aerobic exercise.

The kind of breathing that is done for relaxation and health is diaphragmatic breathing. Basically, it is a controlled and slightly prolonged variation on the old advice to "take a couple of deep breaths" before stressful situations. This uses the diaphragm muscle, which separates the chest and abdominal cavities. When you breathe from the diaphragm, the ribs expand as the lungs are filled with air and the abdominal organs can actually be massaged by the diaphragm muscles as they rhythmically move. In very stressful situations one of the easiest and quickest ways of relieving tension or coping with nerves, before public speaking for example, is a few deep, controlled diaphragmatic breaths.

Using essential oils while doing breathing can make the exercise even more effective. Essential oils are reported to help oxygenate the blood and as they may also work directly on the nervous system, the combination can help all sorts of problems. Deep breathing should be used during all relaxation exercises and is an integral part of yoga, for example. Clients are also often asked to breathe deeply several times before and after an aromatherapy massage or reflexology treatment to, first, help the energy flow and, second, to help expel any gasses that may have been released from the muscles and organs during treatment.

Massage

All over the world, and for as long as we know, people have massaged each other. They do it on Pacific Islands, in Moroccan bath houses, in Chinese shops, everywhere, in fact, where there are people. Many systems of massage have developed and they have different intents and purposes. Some are simply about relaxation, some are therapeutic, and some are designed to release blockages, which might be called "mental" because they originated in the mind, but are actually physical, because they are lodged in the body itself. The simplest form of massage is the kind done to young children who have bumped themselves. We "rub it better," not simply by giving attention and showing love, but by stimulating the area so more blood comes there, and healing can progress.

On a simple level, we can see from someone's hunched up shoulders that they are carrying tension. It doesn't stop there though. The human body holds all the traumas, pain, distress, tension, and emotional crisis within its muscular structure. Every thought and feeling we have is etched in our body, the map of our experiences. Some people can read the maps better than others and know which areas to work with special techniques to relieve some of the tension. We are not concerned with those techniques but with safe and efficient massage that can be carried out at home. One very important benefit of massage is that it increases blood circulation, which enables the body to get rid of the waste products produced by all our cells and organs. The oxygenation of massage, combined with the detoxifying, stimulating, and healing properties of essential oils is extremely effective, but is even more so in the hands of a trained aromatherapist using special massage techniques that also release the emotional blockages in the body itself.

Consider for a moment what happens when you hear a loud bang in the street. We are "startled" — our eyes blink; our body can "jump out of its skin" or at least the muscles in the head, neck, shoulders, arms, legs, and abdomen become taut; our nerves get tense; our hearts race; while our mind is calculating the danger and figuring out whether a car is out of control and we should prepare to jump out of the way. All this happens instantaneously, but the effects linger on. Some events linger longer than others, lodged in the body until something releases them. Fear, pain, anxiety, fatigue, stress, and depression can all be locked in the body, which, like the face, has a story to tell. Negative emotions tend to shorten the neck muscles, which then displaces the head and back muscles, putting more stress on the body.

Swedish Massage

The system known as "Swedish Massage" was developed by Per Henrikling as part of a medical program designed to assist in the eradication of disease. People who are bedridden are particularly disadvantaged because they don't get the exercise that allows oxygenation and the elimination of cellular waste products, and they were of particular concern to Henrikling. Some of the massage strokes were designed to be more stimulating, some more relaxing, but all strokes went toward the heart to stimulate the circulation as well as lymphatic flow. (The lymphatic system of vessels extends through the entire body and is part of the immune system; the lymph nodes are filters that trap unwanted microorganisms and destroys them with lymphocytes, white blood cells). There are five basic strokes to Swedish massage, only two of which are required for home use:

Effleurage movements are strokes — which can be long or short, gentle or hard. Do them in an unhurried way, simply stroking in long, smooth movements.

Petrissage movements are more like the action of kneading dough. Although the whole hand is involved, the two thumbs work in a circular movement (right, clockwise; left, counter clockwise) and a fair amount of pressure is exerted — but not so much that any pain is felt. The movement is like a squeezing, rolling action, involving the thumbs and fingers more than anything else, but also the flat of the hand as it comes into contact with the skin.

The other movements are *Vibrations, Frictions,* and *Tapotement,* which should not be done without further information or instruction as they're not that easy to perform correctly and may cause harm to the underlying organs. But using effleurage (stroking) and petrissage (the rolling, squeezing, kneading movement), carried out only on the muscles, is not harmful and can be done to anyone — even to oneself, to promote health and well-being.

Massage is a wonderful therapy because it relaxes, heals, and involves touch — itself a healing tool. There is one problem with it, however — it can be an excuse for people to exert power over others. Never jump up and say, "Oh, you're so tense, I'm going to give you a shoulder massage" and impose your will on another person in this way. Okay, they may be tense, but this isn't the approach

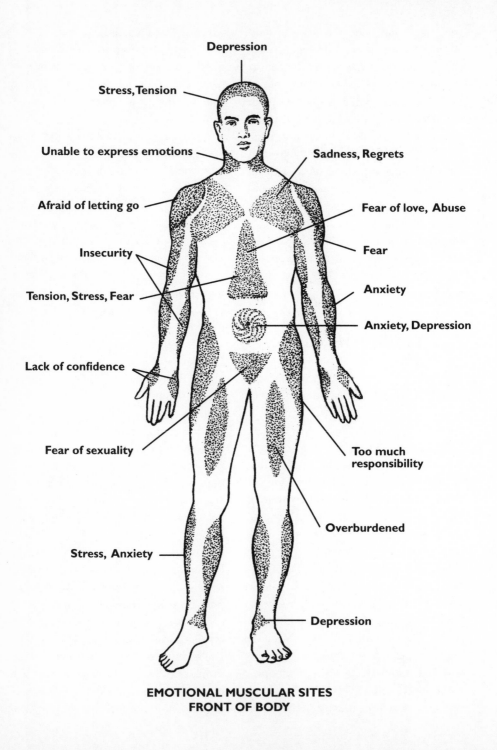

Depression

Stress, Tension

Unable to express emotions

Sadness, Regrets

Afraid of letting go

Fear of love, Abuse

Insecurity

Fear

Tension, Stress, Fear

Anxiety

Anxiety, Depression

Lack of confidence

Fear of sexuality

Too much responsibility

Overburdened

Stress, Anxiety

Depression

**EMOTIONAL MUSCULAR SITES
FRONT OF BODY**

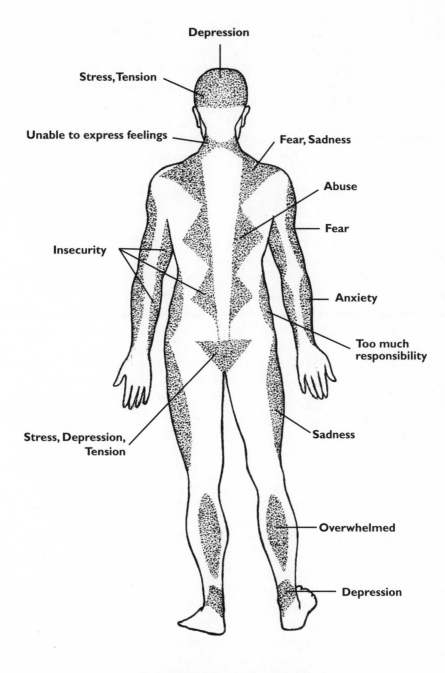

Depression

Stress, Tension

Unable to express feelings

Fear, Sadness

Abuse

Fear

Insecurity

Anxiety

**Too much
responsibility**

**Stress, Depression,
Tension**

Sadness

Overwhelmed

Depression

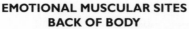

**EMOTIONAL MUSCULAR SITES
BACK OF BODY**

to take. In a way, you're saying, "Oh, you're so tense and I'm not, I'm better at coping than you are, here let me show you what a selfless, caring, giving person I am." All of which can make the person feel worse than they did to begin with! I can't remember the number of times I have seen some poor person attacked by another in this way, imposing their will. The person being massaged sits there, even more tense, as the imposer pushes and pummels their already strained muscles, with the person (trying to be polite) saying, "Yes, that's lovely, fine, yes, that's it, now I'm okay, can you stop please," just wishing the whole thing were over. Please make sure you do not fall into the category of imposer and get permission to massage, and make sure your intent is pure (and not intended to show how great you are), thoughtful, and respectful. Only then will it be a pleasure, and help, to both receiver and giver.

The diagrams on page 202 and 203 show which parts of the body are liable to hold emotional tension, both past and present. These areas can be worked on using gentle effleurage or petrissage movements, although if you find sore areas (which is not unusual and does not necessarily mean something is wrong) they should not be overworked. Throughout this book I have referred to "massage oils" and while, certainly, these can be put on the body as part of a massage, they could also simply be *put on* the body and rubbed into the skin in the same way that you apply body lotions, but particularly on those areas of the body that, you can see from the illustrations, might be holding the particular tensions you have.

We also carry tension in our faces, and this can be helped with essential oils. Use 30 mls (1 oz) of a good skin oil, such as macadamia, hazelnut, or sweet almond and a maximum of 30 drops of a single essential oil — either lavender, geranium, chamomile roman, rose otto, or ylang ylang — or blend these according to your needs. Recipes for skin care can be found in *The Complete Book of Essential Oils & Aromatherapy*.

Other Therapies

There are a great number of therapies that involve some form of massage or body-work and the sheer number of them is confusing. Instead of asking, "Which is the best?" it may be better to consider the fact that "there are many routes to the same place." They may all be "best," but one route may suit you better. One major step forward in recent years, however, is a growing appreciation of the mind-body connection and that body-work is becoming more commonly used as an integral part of talking-therapy. Today, psychologists study body-work and body-workers study psychology.

Humanistic Psychology is a new discipline that utilizes body-work and, through talking, encourages the release of emotions in a safe setting. *Psychiatric Orgone Therapy* combines the techniques of psychoanalysis and character analysis with body-work principles established by Wilhelm Reich. *Reichian Therapy* aims to make the client aware of how their posture, breathing, and muscular tension — called "body armoring" — reflect their emotions.

Physical manipulation is used to release physical/emotional tension, after which clients often report a feeling of energetic "streaming" — energy flowing through the body. Reich had a student named Alexander Lowen who took aspects of Reich's body-work theories and developed *Bioenergetics*. Again, therapists aim to make the client aware of the way their body is holding emotions and to unlock the "character armoring" so the body is able to function freely, and healthily.

For Professional Therapists

There has been a tendency in the past for therapists to ask their clients to "keep silent and relax" during treatment but this is, in a sense, a contradiction in terms. Relaxing is about "letting it all out" and one can't do that if you've been asked to keep quiet. Therapy is a time for releasing the bottled up emotions, and that involves talk, so encourage your client to chat about themselves. Don't chat about yourself — you are not the one who needs to talk, but be sensitive to the client's need to express themselves as you work on their body and release emotionally congested areas.

Meditation

Meditation used to be the preserve of New Agers and, before them, the hippy generation. Now everybody does it. Meditation is an exercise of the mind designed to calm and connect the mind, body, and spirit. Yogis have been teaching the benefits of meditation for thousands of years and now we have machines that can actually record these benefits. For example, machines that record the electrical impulses sent out by muscles show that while meditating, muscular tension drops to almost zero. Circulation is also improved, and EEG (electroencephalograph) readings have shown that brain activity during meditation is almost the same as we have while asleep — which explains perhaps why meditation is so relaxing and refreshing.

People who have practiced meditation for some time can do it anywhere, anytime. When starting out, however, find a quiet room, take the phone off the hook and get yourself into a comfortable position. It is preferable not to eat or drink anything for half an hour beforehand. Some people like to lie down but teachers do not approve of this as a rule because there's a chance the person might fall asleep. Keeping the back straight is important, whether you sit in an upright chair, or with a cushion under your bottom. Some people meditate with their eyes open, others with their eyes closed. People with their eyes open might be concentrating on a particular image — a candle, for example, or a picture of a flower, or a yantra — an abstract picture with metaphysical meaning. People with their eyes closed might be visualizing an image. These images are for a purpose — to give you something to focus on so that when distracting thoughts come into your mind they can be replaced with the meditative image, so the distracting thoughts can float away. Whether with eyes open or closed, some people have a mantra — a word or few words — which they repeat over and over again, to block out distracting thoughts and also to set up a vibration conducive to meditation. Others concentrate on their breathing. In any case, breathe deeply through your nose, expelling the breath through the mouth if you wish. Also try relaxing — mentally say to your forehead, "relax," to your clenched teeth, "relax," and so on. There are many classes, books, audio tapes and videos available, and can be very useful.

Even ten minutes of meditation each day is extremely beneficial. The essential oils are helpful in that they help to focus the mind and their aroma can even become the thing you concentrate on as a means of blocking out unwanted thoughts. The list below shows the oils that are most popular for meditation but you may prefer to use one of your personal choice, or one that will help with any particular problem you have, chosen from the lists throughout this book. If you have high blood pressure, tension, and stress, lavender would be a good oil to choose. Also see *Focus* and *Concentration* in Chapter 7. You can use essential oils singly or in blends.

Oils should be used to help the atmosphere and set the scene. No not wear them in the form of perfume or massage oil because this combination of essential oils and meditation may be too much and you don't really need it. Simply use a room method, 4-6 drops at the most. Many people make their own formulations exclusively for use in meditation.

Using essential oils can also contribute to the ritualistic element involved,

POPULAR ESSENTIAL OILS FOR MEDITATION	
Lavender	Neroli
Lemon	Juniper
Frankincense	Sandalwood
Jasmine	Rose Maroc
Rose Otto	Carnation
Chamomile	Hyacinth
Roman	Geranium
Bergamot	Cedarwood
Cypress	Ylang Ylang

MEDITATION BLEND 1	
Lavender	5 drops
Lemon	15 drops
Juniper	5 drops
Geranium	5 drops

MEDITATION BLEND 2	
Neroli	16 drops
Ylang Ylang	2 drops
Bergamot	10 drops
Frankincense	2 drops

which helps to focus your mind on the meditation to come. Calm your mind as you go about preparing the room, lighting a candle perhaps, or putting on a music tape, and preparing your diffuser.

Relaxation

Relaxation is recognized as an integral part of physical and mental health, but stress and tension prevent the type of relaxation needed for health of mind and body. Relaxation depends on good breathing techniques (see *Breathing*), among other things. A good exercise to help you recognize areas in your body where you may be carrying tension and stress is the "tense and release" exercise, a classic relaxation technique used in hospitals and by various therapists, and I have personally taught this version to many patients and people in workshops.

First of all make sure you have time to do the exercise with no interruptions. Turn off the radio, although you may play some relaxing music you particularly enjoy. Turn down any bright light and get yourself comfortable in a chair that supports your back. We start the exercise with the feet.

Tense and Relax Exercise

Feet: Some people prefer to concentrate on one foot at a time, some concentrate on both at the same time.

(A) Concentrate on your feet; totally think yourself into your feet consciously focus on your toes, and then your toenails; feel the skin on your feet; and the soles. Now feel your feet becoming very heavy.

(B) Now tense your feet as hard as you can, pointing your toes and pushing your feet away from you. Hold the tension count to five and relax. Make a point of noticing how you feel about your feet — are there any tense areas

when you relax them?

Legs: Again, some people may prefer to concentrate on one leg, some do both at the same time.

(A) Focus on your calf muscles and clench them tightly; you may want to stretch your legs out to do this more effectively.

(B) Now relax them, noticing if there are any areas that feel tense or uncomfortable. If so, tense those areas again and relax them.

Thighs: One or both

(A) Focus on your thigh muscles; relax them by making them feel heavy; then tense them as tightly as possible, pushing them into the seat of the chair.

(B) Now relax them, focusing on any areas that feel tense and uncomfortable; if so, tense them again, and relax.

Bottom: Tense the muscles in the cheeks of your bottom as tight as you can, clenching them together (which will also help you notice any tight areas that are retained in your thighs); then relax. This is an area that often holds tension, surprisingly to many people.

Abdomen:

(A) Tense the muscles of your abdomen by pulling them in really tightly, and gripping them there.

(B) Relax them, and notice if there are any areas of discomfort; if so, repeat.

Back:

(A) Tense the muscles of your back by pushing the lower back hard against the back of the chair.

(B) Relax. We all carry tension in this area and it really feels good to tense and relax here. Again, notice any discomfort or any tense areas and repeat the exercise once more.

Hands: One at a time or both together.

(A) Tense your hands by making fists as tight as you possibly can.

(B) And then let them go. Some people like to imagine they are gripping onto something — money (greed), pain, fear or guilt for example — and then, just let it go as you release your hand muscles.

Arms: One or both.

(A) Tense the muscles as hard as possible by pushing your arm downward as far as you can.

(B) Release, noticing any areas of discomfort and, as before, repeating the exercise with them.

Head: Just let your head and neck flop forward as far as they will go; and then backwards — holding it for a few seconds in each position.

Shoulders: Push your shoulders up as high as you can into your neck; notice any tight areas; then release the muscles. Repeat.

Face: Open your mouth as wide as you can; really stretch it; then just relax it. Repeat the exercise. Now, screw your face up into a ball as tight as you can; then just let it relax. Repeat. Raise your forehead as high as you can; and then let it go. Smile the widest smile you can with the lips together, pushing the cheeks upwards; then let them go. Repeat.

Screw the eyes up as tightly as you can; then let go. Repeat. Tense the scalp, and then let go. Repeat.

People are often surprised at the tension they are holding in their scalp, and by the relief they feel when they let it go.

Concentrate your thought into the solar plexus — the area in between the rib cage and diaphragm, breathe deeply several times, letting whatever thoughts come to flow through your mind. Even if they are very emotionally painful, just let them flow and let them go. This exercise can be done anywhere at anytime, once you have the hang of it.

Use plenty of essential oil diffused around the room you are sitting in. Choose oils from the relaxing and tension-relieving lists. You can combine them with other oils that may be pertinent to your mood or emotions.

Visualization

As a technique, until very recently, visualization might have been considered a bit weird, not to say bizarre. All that has changed. Not only has medical research shown that mind and body are one integrated whole, visualization techniques have been shown to work. It is well known that visualization is very much a part of the eastern philosophies but less well known that the Greeks used it and that it was part of the Western medical tradition until the mid 1600s, when the supposed mind-body dichotomy came into fashion. The first research into visualization was done by Edmund Jacobson in the 1920s who showed that a person's leg muscles would twitch involuntarily when he visualized himself running.

In visualization, the person imagines a scene or scenario they wish to occur happening. Most commonly, the technique is used to have an influence on the course of disease and the scene imagined is of the diseased cells being in some way or other destroyed or banished. The same principle applies to conditions of the mind, even love. For example, one might imagine oneself full of confidence striding up to the boss and asking for a raise and, crucially, he or she saying "yes;" or one might imagine the perfect partner — in full detail physically, mentally, and spiritually — coming into their life. This kind of imaging has to be repeated over and over again, reinforcing the reality you want to create.

It is not easy to visualize anything without practice — the practice of actually seeing, rather than passively looking. Start out by looking at a two-dimensional picture for two or three minutes and then trying to remember all the details. You won't be able to at first, but keep on practicing until you have really noticed all the details in the picture and can remember them, and as you remember them, see them in your mind's eye. Then do the same exercise with a three-dimensional object, repeatedly once a day, until you can remember all the details of that object clearly and, as you remember, again, see it in your mind's eye. Eventually progress to a living image — the garden for example, and try to train your eye to really see what is going on there. Now progress to the image on which you want to work. Is it you being a fabulous success on the opening night of the dramatic society's latest show, or you working contentedly behind your desk and efficiently processing the papers from the in-tray to the out-tray? Whatever it is you want to visualize and make happen doesn't matter, so long as you are consistent, and persevere.

Visualization is very often incorporated into meditation and relaxation techniques, and is also an integral part of autogenic training. Use essential oils during visualization that are specific to the reason for the visualization. If your image involves you being confident, use a confidence boosting oil, and so on. Refer to the charts for *Mind, Moods, and Emotions*. Depending on whether you are utilizing a stimulating or relaxing image, choose from the essential oils below.

STIMULATING ESSENTIAL OILS FOR VISUALIZATION	
Rosemary	Ginger
Black Pepper	Thyme

RELAXING ESSENTIAL OILS FOR VISUALIZATION	
Lavender	Neroli
Chamomile Roman	Clary Sage

CHAPTER 10

THE HEALING PROFESSIONS AND ESSENTIAL OILS

Professionals in both the allopathic and complementary fields can benefit from using essential oils, which can be used in conjunction with any form of healing. This book is concerned with the mind and emotions but, as we know, the mind has a powerful impact on the workings of the body. Attending to the mind, perhaps by using essential oils, can greatly benefit the well-being of the entire person — also in conditions that seem superficially to be quite unrelated to mental processes. While for those professionals that deal exclusively with the mind, such as psychotherapists, essential oils provide a marvelous tool for helping to release hidden problems and anxieties.

Doctors

Over the past five years there has been a complete shift in the attitude of doctors in general, away from ignorance and intolerance of complementary therapies and toward understanding. So much so, in fact, that doctors can now legally refer patients to complementary therapists, including aromatherapists. Also, some physicians now employ aromatherapists as part of their team. All over the world there are courses introducing doctors to the fundamentals of complementary therapies, so they can better understand what benefits they have to offer. Ironically perhaps, this new attitude has partly been driven by financial considerations. If a practice can help a patient by complementary means and their overall budget is less, in today's new reorganized money-conscious system, that is all for the good, especially for the patient.

Because prescriptions now cost so much money, the logic of using essential oils — which are cheaper, nonaddictive, effective, and harmless — suddenly makes sense to people who, just a few years ago, wouldn't have considered this option. Also, a profound shift has occurred in the public's mind toward complementary therapies because millions of people now have tried them and found that they work. The proof is in the pudding. The word travels, of course, and attitudes change. Meanwhile, the media make the public very aware of the dangers that can come with certain allopathic medications, some of which take years to become apparent. Patients now appreciate a doctor who says, "Look Mrs. Smith, I can give you a prescription for sleeping pills if you like but why don't you try taking lavender baths instead? If that doesn't work, we can then try the sleeping pills." It shows an openness of mind. Of course I wouldn't suggest that doctors give up their armory of drugs, I don't know anybody who would, but if essential oils can do as well if not better, why not try them before resorting to stronger medication? There is no longer any reason not to.

We haven't reached the point where essential oils are sold at the doctor's office or at pharmacies (and I look forward to that day) but there's no reason why doctor's offices shouldn't diffuse essential oils in the waiting room — they would certainly make the room more pleasant. Choose essential oils that could allay anxiety or, in times of "flu" epidemic, those with antibacterial and microbial action. As we all know, especially if we've attended baby clinics, waiting to see the doctor and having to sit next to someone who is coughing out germs, can actually *make* you ill. Essential oils can do away

with this problem, which keeps many people away from the doctor when they should in fact be making a visit.

Hospitals

"I hate the smell of hospitals" is something you often hear. The aroma of institutional cleaning fluids reminds people of why they were in the hospital or had to visit a hospital — because they or someone they loved was suffering. This association turns a moderately unpleasant aroma into a feared one. Hospitals are places where people are sick — literally, where they spill blood or where urine and feces are expelled behind curtains in public wards. And in crowded emergency waiting rooms people have to wait for hours, sometimes next to people who didn't have time to wash before coming in, or those who are there because they simply have no home to go to. For many reasons then, hospitals need an aromatic uplift more than most places.

The waiting areas in hospitals should be diffused with aromas that are acceptable to a wide range of people. The citrus, floral, and woody essential oils are among the best choices. The most frequently used essential oil, lavender, has an aroma that is not universally liked, although it is usually accepted as moderately pleasant and, of course, it's loved by some people. The ideal is to create a pleasant atmosphere that induces calm, using essential oils that are not too expensive. One also needs to give the impression of freshness and cleanliness, and use something that is refreshing — to take the edge off the long wait. I would suggest lemon, pine, geranium, eucalyptus lemon (E citriodora) and, in mixes, lavender. The citrus essential oils tend to evaporate fairly quickly but they are cheap and have a calming effect, and they are acceptable to almost everyone. All the above can be used on their own or blend the following oils in these proportions:

BLEND 1

**Lemon 5 parts to
Pine 1 part**

BLEND 2

**Lemon 5 parts to
Geranium 1 part**

BLEND 3

**Lemon 5 parts to
Lavender 1 part**

BLEND 4

**Eucalyptus citriodora 5 parts
to Pine 1 part**

BLEND 5

**Eucalyptus citriodora 5 parts
to Geranium 1 part**

For the partner's waiting room in the maternity ward, the lemon and geranium blend should be used because it is the most anxiety-relieving.

Obviously, in a public place such as a hospital one would not use a diffuser that involved the use of bare flame — candles — to heat the essential oil; and electric

sockets may not be installed in convenient places, or the diffuser may not be fitted with the correct fuse and runs the risk of blowing the whole electrical system — so the electrical type of diffuser may be impossible to use. There is now, however, a small, portable diffuser on the market that uses neither candles nor electricity and is very effective in small areas — please see the supplier list in Appendix III, where I also list companies that supply commercial diffusing units for larger areas.

The antiviral, antibacterial and antifungal properties of essential oils have been discussed in my previous book, *The Complete Book of Essential Oils and Aromatherapy*; however, these are very important aspects of essential oil use and their benefits within the hospital environment are obvious. Indeed, it is somewhat of a sick joke that if you don't have an infection when you go into hospital, you'll have one by the time you come out. There is a tremendous potential, then, for essential oils being diffused in hospital atmospheres, especially in operating rooms and intensive care units.

These anti-infection qualities of essential oils can be used, however, by individuals who are obliged to stay in the hospital. In my experience there's never been a complaint from other patients and, indeed, they and the nurses tend to be very interested in the whole subject. People like the idea that they — simply by being in the same vicinity — are receiving a certain amount of protection themselves and I've been requested on many occasions to bring in a bottle of this or that essential oil for other patients. As a general rule, if you're in a large ward with many people, try to stick to the citrus, floral, and woody aromas, which are the most generally acceptable.

Hospices

A marvelous woman, Elizabeth Kubler-Ross, encouraged the development of the hospice movement in the 1960s and since then it's gone from strength to strength, country to country, so that now there are hospices all over the world — usually supported by donations and in great part run by volunteers. They all deserve all the help they can get.

Hospices care for the dying, aiming to make the client's last months as pleasant and pain-free as possible. Essential oils are about uplifting the spirit and allaying stress and anxiety, and obviously have a role here and can truly help a person pass over in peace and even happiness.

It would be nice to think that each hospice could have a variety of essential oils available from which each patient could choose an essential oil or make a blend of oils to be used in their room, or that relatives might be asked if they'd like a particular aroma brought in. In the more public areas it would be best, again, to choose the citrus or floral essential oils — something light, rather than heavy. I would suggest the following oils used singly or in combinations: lemon, eucalyptus citriodora, grapefruit, mandarin, geranium, petitgrain, coriander, and lavender. Here are three blends that are light, refreshing, and acceptable to most people:

HOSPICE BLEND 1	
Coriander	1 drop
Petitgrain	1 drop
Eucalyptus	
citriodora	1 drop

HOSPICE BLEND 2	
Lemon	1 drop
Geranium	1 drop
Grapefruit	1 drop

HOSPICE BLEND 3	
Coriander	1 drop
Mandarin	1 drop
Geranium	1 drop

The odor should be only just perceptible, not very noticeable. The aim is not to perfume the area so much as to impart a subtle pleasant fragrance. This helps to make the atmosphere of the whole building happy, relaxed, pleasant, fresh, and lively. All this helps friends and relatives visiting the building, who are often more distressed than the patients themselves. Indeed, I have often heard hospice patients say of relatives, "I wish they'd relax, they're trying to put such a brave face on, they're really not themselves." By imparting a sense of relaxation into the building with essential oils it helps everyone — patients, visitors, and staff alike.

Also, if an aroma becomes associated with the patient in their last days, it can act as a reminder of them in future times. I remember one woman telling me that her mother chose to have neroli diffused in her room during her last weeks here on earth and the daughter was so grateful there was something that so easily evoked the memory of her mother. She could pick up her bottle of neroli whenever she was feeling sad, sniff deeply, and the memory of her mother would all come flooding back — not her dying, but her living, happy days. It became their final link, their special way of communicating.

Nurses

It is among the nursing professions that there has been the greatest growing interest in aromatherapy over recent years. You can see why. Working the front line, with patients, they can see that essential oils do what they say they can do. They're interested in delving further. And who can blame them when it is they who have to wipe Mrs. Jackson's tears when she cries in pain. The trouble is, many are not getting good enough and long enough training. And, unless they are professionally registered aromatherapists, they are not insured to carry out any work other than nursing.

Registered tutors of aromatherapy have to have been in practice for five years at least and have several years of experience as an assistant tutor. But nurses are often advised to go to a weekend workshop, which is often taught by someone who has little more than a weekend workshop training themselves. One weekend workshop is fine for self-help and home use, which is what they are intended for, but to work in conjunction with the medical profession, you should be a clinical

aromatherapist, and that takes training. Most "aromatherapists" work to prevent disorders. Nurses, on the other hand, are dealing with people who are already ill, often quite seriously. Another difference is that registered aromatherapists are literally hands-on, and nurses are, within the hospital environment, rather hands off. Traditionally, the doctors hand out the therapy. Nurses are certainly right to think essential oils could quite easily do away with many of the problems they see in hospitals every day, but aromatherapy is more than the application of essential oils, and to use essential oils correctly and safely, nurses may have to revise their thinking on how healing actually works.

It is very encouraging that nurses should be so excited by the possibilities in aromatherapy. It is not their fault that training is not standardized. There can't be anything wrong with more people learning more ways to care for other human beings. Of course it's fine to use a diffuser in the ward, if the other staff agree. There are more and more courses designed especially for nurses who, when properly trained, could effectively treat patients with aromatherapy.

Dentists

Some dentists are using essential oils to overcome the "Oh no, I've got to go to the dentist" factor. They can see the fear and anxiety written all over the faces seen each morning in the waiting room. It can't be a great start to the day. In some clinics, a gentle diffusion of essential oils has proven of great value in calming patients before treatment. Good essential oils to use in this situation might be lavender, lemon, geranium, clary sage, juniper, and grapefruit.

Chiropractors and Osteopaths

Although it appears that chiropractors and osteopaths deal only with the physical body, particularly the bones and nerves, they also deal with the stresses their patients undergo during the course of their day, not to mention in life. They can *feel* them, in the form of rigid, tightly contracted muscles in their hands, which make treatment more difficult. It is much easier and more effective to treat someone who is not so tense.

Using relaxing essential oils gently diffused in the treatment room may help the client and therapist alike. Even if the client isn't feeling particularly stressed, just anticipating the potential clunks and clicks when the bones are going to be manipulated is enough to make some people tense up, particularly as these people are in pain anyway. Essential oils can also be used in manipulative massage in whatever lotion or cream the practitioner usually uses, and this will help ease tense muscles further.

Caretakers

Anyone who is at home caring for an elderly or sick relative knows the strain of wanting to have their own life while feeling obliged not to leave the relative alone. Caretakers need a lot of emotional support, but it doesn't always come easily. Who cares for the caretaker? Using essential oils doesn't take away the jobs but they can help by making both caretaker and cared for calm and emotionally steady, which can lighten the work load tremendously. Use the charts for specific problems (pages 219-236), and gently diffuse the oils to help create a nice, gentle, pleasant atmosphere. The following oils are all helpful: grapefruit, juniper, geranium, lavender, mandarin, bergamot, chamomile roman, clary sage, and sandalwood.

The caretaker can also try one of these bath blends after a heavy day. Blend the essential oils together in the following proportions, then use 5 drops in a bath. The synergistic blends below are enough for four baths each.

CARETAKER'S CALMING BATH BLEND

Ormenis Flower	2 drops
Mandarin	15 drops
Geranium	3 drops

CARETAKER'S STIMULATING BATH BLEND

Cypress	2 drops
Grapefruit	15 drops
Rosemary	3 drops

Healers

Healers come into contact with all kinds of problems and they are continuously giving out healing energy to others. Diffused in the treatment room, the following essential oils protect the healing energies and can also help the healing process: rose otto, chamomile roman, neroli, frankincense, sandalwood, geranium, jasmine, bergamot, spikenard, myrrh, and petitgrain.

Counseling

Counseling is for everyone, including healthy people who find themselves unable to cope with life's problems or a particular situation. It might take time to find the right service, and the person within that service who suits you — compatibility is of prime importance. But it's worth the trouble, so keep looking. Find out what the various qualifications mean — some people might have had a few months training, while others have had years. It might seem odd to go to a stranger with your problems but it's often much easier and less embarrassing to talk them over with someone who is not involved. It's also easier to be honest about a situation to a stranger than to family and friends, who probably have their own interest in the matter.

All sorts of people go for counseling. You may need to discuss how your job is negatively affecting you or proving difficult to do, or discuss bereavement, debt, or divorce. You may just have heard you have a terminal illness, or that someone close to you is suffering. You may feel unable to cope with life's ups and downs; or be depressed, stressed, and tense; or

perhaps you suffered a loss of confidence, or feel helpless or frustrated. These are the things counseling is there to help with — problems both large and (apparently) small. There is also specialist counseling, as for people who have suffered trauma called "post traumatic stress disorder," caused by incidents such as train crashes, air or boat disasters, or trauma caused by various types of abuse. Some aromatherapists are now also training as counselors to help them in their practice.

Counselors can use essential oils in the same way as psychotherapists — gently diffusing essential oils in the waiting room or consulting room to help clients feel more at ease and more able to talk freely and confidently. Appropriate oils would be bergamot, geranium, lemon, lavender, clary sage, ormenis flower, cypress, sandalwood, and grapefruit. However, rather than using the same essential oil(s) all the time, choose oils from the charts that seem appropriate for particular clients. You might also suggest that clients use the oils diffused at home, or in the bath.

Psychotherapists

The basis of psychotherapy is talking, which is perhaps the way our ancestors dealt with the stresses and strains of life. Today, however, our family and friends are quite likely to live on the other side of the country, if not the world, and the telephone system is kept busy with people sharing their problems. Psychotherapists, are trained to help you express your feelings, problems, and experiences and they deal with problems that may have been too deeply hidden to be dealt with by a chat with a friend. To a psychotherapist, you can reveal very personal experiences and they'll help you identify what is worrying you, and help you understand your behavior. They'll give you advice, encouragement and privacy.

The idea with psychotherapy is that you can discuss your problems and look at things from a different angle, to gain a better understanding of why the problems started in the first place, thus enabling negative patterns of behavior to be broken. Psychotherapists do not prescribe drug treatment or electrical shock therapy. They talk over any kind of problem including emotional problems, anxiety, stress, tension, depression, obsession, compulsions, insomnia, fears, educational or work problems, aggression, disruptive behavior, phobias such as agoraphobia or claustrophobia, and sexual problems, among other things. There's no point in being reticent — they've probably heard it all before!

Many psychotherapists have been trained in special techniques that can be carried out within the context of individual or group sessions. They'll organize the time you spend with them rather than "simply" allowing the conversation to ramble on, and this may be a better option for some. Included among these special techniques are psychodrama, regression therapy, behavioral therapy, hypnotherapy, Gestalt therapy, autogenic training, relaxation techniques, and trans-

actional analysis, among others. It's important to pick a qualified practitioner.

Psychotherapists can use essential oils gently diffused in the waiting room or consulting room to help clients feel more relaxed and able to talk freely and confidently. Suggested oils for this are mentioned in the previous section, *Counseling*. But by using Chart 11.2 on page 221 and the personality profiles in Chapter 14, on pages 277-368, the psychotherapist will be able to pick out an essential oil that is best suited for his or her particular clients. These can be used in a diffuser in the consultation room. Aromatherapy courses are also available for psychotherapists and will give them a more comprehensive idea of the possibilities. The psychotherapist might also suggest that the client use essential oils diffused at home, or in the bath. Clients undergoing psychotherapy could choose their own oils to be used in conjunction with the sessions, but do inform your therapist if you are using them at home or would like to use them during sessions.

Psychodrama

Psychodrama was invented by Jacob Moreno, a contemporary of Freud, who was inspired by an actress into the idea that acting out emotional problems in the form of a play or drama can help solve them. It usually takes place within the context of group therapy, where everyone acts together under the guidance of a qualified professional. It might involve shouting and screaming, punching cushions or knocking foam bricks over, which might sound a bit dramatic — but that's what it's about. And it helps people to discover and express feelings they would not otherwise be able to do, and release them.

Regression Therapy

Some psychotherapists use regression therapy to release persistent stresses and problems that do not respond to treatment. One of the best regressionists is Dr. Roger Woolger, a Jungian psychologist who uses simple techniques that allow the mind to regress to past lives. [1] This process allows people to release not only mental problems, but also physical ones, as the mind-body connection re-enacts situations that troubled them in the past. This technique should only be undergone in the hands of a fully qualified practitioner as it can be very traumatic and distressing when situations are relived and re-experienced.

Dr. Woolger says that he doesn't even know if his sessions show evidence of past lives as there are no scientific methods of analysis to establish that, however, the information people come up with during these sessions is often quite alien to their present life experience and strongly suggests that there may in fact be past lives. The aim of regression therapy is to examine these past lives, which may contain what Woolger describes as "unfinished business." He encourages clients to recognize the conditions, problems, and disorders that have arisen as a consequence of this unfinished business, and leave it behind, so the personality can advance forward in life.

———

CHAPTER 11

CHARTS 1-4

CHART 11.1
Emotional Healing — Positive States

The essential oils in italics are those traditionally used in aromatherapy, the others have been adopted for these uses in more recent times.

Alertness
Basil, bergamot, black pepper, cardamom, cinnamon, coriander, eucalyptus citriodora, _grapefruit_, juniper, lime, _peppermint_, petitgrain, pine, _rosemary_, thyme linalol

Assertiveness
Basil, _cedarwood_, cypress, fennel — sweet, frankincense, ginger, patchouli, _ylang ylang_, black pepper, jasmine, _ormenis flower_, bergamot, coriander, carnation, _tuberose_, pimento berry, lime, _cardamom_, cistus, _litsea cubeba_

Concentration
Intellectual
Lemon, basil, lemongrass, _litsea cubeb_a, cardamom, bergamot, orange, cedarwood, _rosemary_, eucalyptus, peppermint, _frankincense_

Spiritual
Frankincense, neroli, _chamomile roman_, rose otto, narcissus, hyacinth

Confidence
Cedarwood, _cypress_, linden blossom, _cardamom_, sweet fennel, ginger, bergamot, _grapefruit_, _jasmine_, pine, rosemary, orange, coriander, tuberose

Contentment
Rose otto, cypress, *lavender*, neroli, *bergamot*, orange, sandalwood, patchouli, ylang ylang, chamomile roman, clove

Creativity
Bergamot, cistus, lemon, *frankincense*, geranium, *neroli*, rose, jasmine, bay, clove, *carnation*, mimosa, litsea cubeba, sandalwood, cypress, *juniper*

Focus
Thyme linalol, *lemon*, fennel, bergamot, *basil*, basil linalol, cedarwood, *cypress*, juniper, lemongrass, *litsea cubeba*, ginger, cinnamon, clove, ylang ylang, linden blossom, nutmeg, *rosemary*

Happiness
Orange, rose, jasmine, coriander, ginger, clove, cinnamon, benzoin, carnation, *pimento berry*, *geranium*

Joy
Sandalwood, frankincense, lemon, rose otto, petitgrain, orange, ylang ylang, *neroli*, chamomile roman, linden blossom, *mimosa*, *bergamot*

Peace
Everyone has essential oils that they can attune to. These are a guideline only.

Chamomile roman, neroli, juniper, frankincense, rose otto, melissa, angelica seed, spikenard, yarrow, jasmine, carnation.

Performance
Bay, bergamot, cistus, eucalyptus citriodora, *frankincense*, lemon, lavender, *grapefruit*, *helichrysum*, rose maroc, jasmine, geranium, ormenis flower, *cypress*, tuberose

Positivity
All essential oils used in aromatherapy have a positive nature and positive benefits upon the human organism. The following essential oils are only a guideline.

Basil, lemon, cedarwood, *grapefruit*, pine, vetiver, *patchouli*, juniper, myrrh,cypress, cardamom, petitgrain, *geranium*, *frankincense*, rosemary, hyssop, pimento berry, bay

Restfulness
Lavender, geranium, rose maroc, clary sage, *linden blossom*, neroli, marjoram, petitgrain, rosewood, *sandalwood*, mimosa

Self-Awareness
Clary sage, ylang ylang, *cypress*, geranium, pine, *sandalwood*, *bay*, ormenis flower, *jasmine*, clove, pimento berry, mandarin, *coriander*, angelica seed, *sage*, cistus, *myrtle*

Self-Esteem
Hyacinth, sandalwood, vetiver, *ylang ylang*, rose maroc, *jasmine*, carnation, *bergamot*, geranium, ormenis flower, *cedarwood*, tuberose

Self-Image
Orange, lavender, melissa, neroli, chamomile roman, ylang ylang, rose maroc, jasmine, sandalwood, cypress, juniper, cedarwood, pine, black pepper, frankincense, mandarin, nutmeg, myrtle, bay

CHART 11.2
Emotional Healing — Problems

The essential oils in italics are those traditionally used in aromatherapy, the others have been adopted for these uses in more modern times.

Abuse

Emotional
Ormenis flower, *chamomile roman*, melissa, *rose otto*, neroli, mandarin,

Hurt inner child
Geranium, lavender, neroli, *melissa*, mandarin, benzoin, rose otto

Addiction

General
Vetiver, narcissus, *helichrysum*, basil, frankincense, spikenard, benzoin

Alcohol
Helichrysum, *juniper*, lemon, bergamot, marjoram, *clary sage*, eucalyptus citriodora

Drugs
Vetiver, helichrysum, spikenard, *valerian*, omenis flower, *nutmeg*, juniper, *bergamot*, basil, clary sage, geranium, hyacinth, narcissus, tuberose

Hypnotics
Narcissus, jonquil, rose maroc, *hyacinth*, carnation, jasmine, hops, *valerian*, tonka bean, vanilla, osmanthus, *tuberose*, spikenard

Other useful essential oils
Marjoram, bergamot, chamomile roman, juniper, patchouli, bay, *clary sage*, *nutmeg*, cistus

Aggression

General aggression
Geranium, frankincense, sandalwood, grapefruit, cedarwood, vetiver

Soothing effect in aggression
Neroli, *lavender*, *clary sage*, chamomile roman, benzoin, *marjoram*, coriander, litsea cubeba, *valerian*, *spikenard*, *rose maroc*, tuberose, mimosa, carnation

Aloneness
Neroli, *chamomile roman*, rose otto, jasmine, melissa, frankincense

Amnesia

Confusion
Cardamom, tuberose, ginger, *black pepper*, bergamot, geranium, *petitgrain*, helichrysum, grapefruit, basil

Shock induced
Mandarin, ylang ylang, rose maroc, rose otto, neroli, melissa, peppermint, lavender

Fear induced
Sandalwood, chamomile roman, cypress, vetiver, lemon, bergamot, orange, cedarwood, neroli, geranium

Anger

Calming down
Chamomile roman, chamomile German, tuberose, lavender, linden blossom

vetiver, bergamot, rose maroc, rose otto, petitgrain, patchouli

Coping with
Black pepper, Chamomile roman, linden blossom, vetiver, ylang ylang, rose maroc, valerian, spikenard, myrtle, benzoin

Expressing unrealized anger
Tuberose, black pepper, ginger, ormenis flower, cedarwood, patchouli, clove.

Anorexia
See anxiety, obsession, self-esteem, confidence

Anxiety — General
Bergamot, *lavender*, mandarin, sandalwood, *chamomile roman*, vetiver, cedarwood, *neroli*, rose otto, *melissa*, *geranium*, juniper, basil, frankincense, patchouli

Apprehensive anxiety
Bergamot, *lavender*, neroli, rose otto, melissa, geranium

Depressed anxiety
Bergamot, melissa, neroli, *rose otto*, *sandalwood*, vetiver, cedarwood

Restless anxiety
Vetiver, *cedarwood*, juniper, chamomile roman, frankincense

Tense anxiety
Sandalwood, *clary sage*, chamomile roman, patchouli

Apathy
Cardamom, lemon, *ginger*, *black pepper*, bergamot, orange, jasmine, rose otto, ormenis flower, basil, peppermint, hyacinth

Bereavement
Benzoin, *rose otto*, neroli, *linden blossom*, lavender, melissa, rosewood, *chamomile roman*, carnation, patchouli, cypress

Breakdown

General Breakdown
Lavender, clary sage, lemon, orange, chamomile roman, geranium, neroli, helichrysum

Emotional Breakdown
Lavender, cypress, sandalwood, rose otto, mandarin, benzoin, *chamomile roman*, *geranium, neroli*

Bulimia
See rage, guilt, self esteem, confidence

Burnout — Emotional
Vetiver, bergamot, rose otto, neroli, linden blossom, *melissa*, patchouli, sandalwood, *hyacinth*, marjoram, lavender, benzoin, clary sage, helichrysum, lemon, frankincense, chamomile roman, petitgrain, ginger, jasmine

Confusion
Cardamom, ginger, *black pepper*, bergamot, geranium, petitgrain, helichrysum, grapefruit, *ormenis flower*, basil, rosemary, peppermint, cypress, juniper, pine, thyme linalol, lavender

Dejection
Bergamot, *frankincense*, grapefruit, mandarin, geranium, nutmeg, *mimosa*, linden blossom, orange, rose maroc, jasmine, petitgrain, neroli, ylang ylang

Delirium

Peppermint, *eucalyptus globulus*, *eucalyptus radiatia*, *lavender*, marjoram

Delirium Tremens

Lavender, petitgrain, lemon, chamomile roman, *marjoram*, *valerian*, geranium

Dementia

Memory

Basil, cardamom, ginger, black pepper, *rosemary*

Stimulating appetite

Lemon, orange, lime, grapefruit, black pepper, ginger, coriander, cardamom, clove, orange, lime, grapefruit, nutmeg, *cinnamon*

Gentle oil, for restlessness

Rose otto, neroli, *lavender*, *geranium*, jasmine, chamomile roman

Depression

Mandarin, chamomile roman, lemon, bergamot, grapefruit, orange, jasmine, ylang ylang, rose otto, rose maroc, neroli, geranium, petitgrain, helichrysum, eucalyptus citriodora, sandalwood, clary sage, marjoram, lavender, frankincense

Weepy depression

Rose otto, neroli, chamomile roman, sandalwood, patchouli, geranium, ylang ylang

Agitated or anxious depression

Melissa, cedarwood, lavender, chamomile roman, bergamot, marjoram, nutmeg, ormenis flower, valerian, lemon, orange

Lethargic depression

Grapefruit, cypress, rosemary, melissa, helichrysum, peppermint, clary sage, eucalyptus citriodora, eucalyptus peppermint

Hysterical depression

Mandarin, chamomile roman, linden blossom, vetiver, bergamot, neroli, narcissus, lavender, marjoram, valerian, spikenard

Depressive — Manic

Chamomile roman, chamomile german, frankincense, geranium, *grapefruit*, mandarin, rose otto, *lavender*, lemon, *neroli*, patchouli, sandalwood

Doubt

Coriander, basil, *frankincense*, benzoin, angelica seed, ylang ylang, litsea cubeba

Emotional States

Emotional Violence

Frankincense, juniper, geranium, rose otto, neroli, *chamomile roman*, jasmine, *carnation*, hyacinth, *benzoin*, melissa, lavender

Emotional exhaustion

Chamomile roman, cypress, bergamot, marjoram, *rosemary*, *eucalyptus globulus*, *eucalyptus radiata*, frankincense, litsea cubeba, grapefruit, black pepper, cardamom, ginger, lemon, pine

Facing Death

Rose otto, rose maroc, *jasmine*, linden blossom, *frankincense*, neroli, chamomile roman, geranium, narcissus, benzoin, bay, carnation, *sandalwood*, cedarwood, bergamot, *juniper*, hyacinth, tuberose

The choice of essential oils depends very much upon culture and personal preference, and may differ from those above.

Fatigue

Intellectual fatigue

Ginger, *black pepper*, *rosemary*, lemon, basil, cypress, grapefruit, peppermint

Mental fatigue

Lemon, petitgrain, *basil*, *peppermint*, rosemary, eucalyptus piperata, eucalyptus citriodora

Fear

General

Sandalwood, chamomile roman, cypress, *vetiver*, lemon, bergamot, orange, *cedarwood*, neroli, ormenis flower, basil, *frankincense*, clary sage, *lavender*, galbanham

Fear of failure

Fennel, *coriander*, *ylang ylang*, basil, frankincense

Fear of gossip

Cypress

Fear of madness

Fennel, *cedarwood*, ylang ylang, *frankincense*

Fear of feelings

Fennel, frankincense, sandalwood, *neroli*

Fear of change

Ylang ylang, frankincense, lavender, *ormenis flower*

Fear of sexuality

Rose maroc, *ylang ylang*, patchouli, vetiver, galbanham

Fear of love

Rose maroc, neroli, *carnation*, hyacinth, *benzoin*

Fear of loving

Neroli, *ylang ylang*, carnation, benzoin, rose maroc

Fear of being unloved

Rose otto

Fear of letting go

Cypress, rose maroc, frankincense, *galbanham*

Fits — Emotional

Lavender, marjoram, eucalyptus citriodora, *litsea cubeba*, chamomile roman

Forgetfulness

Cypress, lemon, ginger, black pepper, cistus, frankincense, *rosemary*, *peppermint*, basil

Grief

Dissipating grief

Cypress, *chamomile roman*, rose maroc, *rose otto*, *helichrysum*, ormenis flower, frankincense, *narcissus*, bergamot, *carnation*, vanilla, nutmeg, spikenard

Difficulty in expressing grief

Hyacinth, rose maroc, *rose otto*, neroli, melissa, *helichrysum*, *benzoin*, mimosa, vetiver

Guilt

Linden blossom, vetiver, jasmine, pine, *rose otto*, juniper, clary sage, ylang ylang, nutmeg

Hypochondria

Marjoram, rosemary, valerian, hops, basil, peppermint, *thyme*, *ormenis flower*, tea tree, manuka, oregano, galbanham

Hysteria

Mandarin, *chamomile roman*, linden blossom, *vetiver*, bergamot, rosemary,

neroli, peppermint, narcissus, *lavender*,
marjoram, *valerian*, spikenard, hops

Insomnia

Lavender, mandarin, linden blossom,
clary sage, marjoram, cistus, *valerian*,
hops, vetiver, *chamomile roman*,
sandalwood, lemon

Irritability

Cypress, chamomile roman, chamomile
German, coriander, litsea cubeba, neroli,
ylang ylang, melissa, narcissus, *lavender*

Loneliness

Bergamot, *helichrysum*, narcissus,
chamomile roman, neroli, *benzoin*

Memory — Lack of

Ginger, *basil*, *lemon*, grapefruit, *rosemary*,
thyme linalol, *cardamom*, black pepper,
coriander, pimento berry

Misery

Narcissus, petitgrain, *benzoin*, orange,
neroli, *rose maroc*, jasmine, clove, cinnamon, *ginger*, carnation, *pimento berry*

Moodiness

Lemon, *geranium*, *eucalyptus citriodora*,
neroli, *lavender*, ylang ylang, ormenis
flower, patchouli, chamomile maroc

Mood Swings

Geranium, *cardamom*, lavender, coriander,
angelica seed, cypress, *cedarwood*, linden
blossom, helichrysum

Nervous Exhaustion

Rosemary, petitgrain, *juniper*, neroli,
lavender, chamomile roman, marjoram,

clary sage, orange

Obsessional Behavior

Sandalwood, *vetiver*, cedarwood,
narcissus, clary sage, orange, lemon

Pain

Betula alba (birch), nutmeg, clove, rosemary, *lavender*, chamomile roman, *sage*,
clary sage, *helichrysum*, peppermint, basil

Inflammation and pain
Lavender, chamomile roman

Tension and pain
Lavender, clary sage, vetiver, *marjoram*

Relaxing with pain
Lavender, neroli

Panic Attacks

Lavender, frankincense, *helichrysum*,
marjoram

Passivity

Rose maroc, ylang ylang , cedarwood, pine,
jasmine, *tuberose*, orange, *patchouli*, bay

Phobias

To calm and relax
Lavender, linden blossom, *clary sage*,
neroli, ylang ylang, marjoram, ormenis
flower, *chamomile roman*, sandalwood

Quarrelsomeness

Clary sage, lavender, lemon, *sandalwood*,
patchouli, cistus, clove

Rage

Chamomile roman, ylang ylang, ormenis
flower, *vetiver*, clary sage, lavender,
marjoram, *galbanham*

Regrets
Hyacinth, cypress, *pine*, *rose maroc*, rose otto, mimosa

Rejection
Pine, *cypress*, sandalwood, *benzoin*, *chamomile roman*, neroli, rose otto, ylang ylang, hyacinth, tuberose, *carnation*

Repression
Hyacinth, *jasmine*, *frankincense*, ylang ylang, *cedarwood*, *pine*, patchouli, vetiver, juniper

Schizophrenia
Lavender, mandarin, geranium, chamomile roman, lemon, rose otto

Self-blame
Rose otto, lemon, geranium, *chamomile roman*, *bergamot*, orange, ylang ylang, carnation, tuberose, benzoin, *melissa*, eucalyptus citriodora, ormenis flower

Sorrow
Cypress, hyacinth, melissa, benzoin, frankincense, sandalwood, rose otto

Stress
Bergamot, *chamomile roman*, *ormenis flower*, frankincense, *geranium*, grapefruit, *lavender*, lemon, mandarin, *marjoram*, melissa, *neroli*, rose otto, *sandalwood*, vetiver, *clary sage*, *ylang ylang*, bay, *jasmine*, benzoin, eucalyptus citriodora, osmanthus, tuberose, hyacinth, narcissus, linden blossom, nutmeg, hops, *spikenard*, *valerian*, yarrow, litsea cubeba

Tiredness — Mental
Clary sage, lavender, marjoram, rosemary, litsea cubeba, grapefruit, peppermint

Trauma
Thyme linalol, *lavender*, geranium, lemon, *marjoram*, petitgrain, clary sage, *chamomile roman*

Withdrawal
From life
Narcissus, orange

Of emotions
Bergamot, rose otto, hyacinth, chamomile roman, neroli, mandarin, geranium

For peace
Cypress, frankincense, cedarwood, juniper, rose otto, camomile roman, neroli, carnation, bergamot, geranium, juniper

Any essential oil can be used for peace if you feel personally attuned to it.

Worthlessness
Feelings of
Frankincense, sandalwood, cedarwood, clove, ormenis flower, neroli, juniper, chamomile roman, geranium

CHART 11.3
Essential Oils Used for Positive States

The essential oils in italics are those traditionally used in aromatherapy, the others have been adopted for these uses in more recent times.

Angelica Seed
Peace, Self-Awareness

Basil
Alertness, Assertiveness, Positivity, Focus

Bay
Creativity, Performance, Positivity, Self-Awareness, Self-Image

Benzoin
Happiness, Contentment

Bergamot
Alertness, Assertiveness, Concentration, Confidence, Contentment, Creativity, Focus, Joy, Performance, Self-Esteem

Black Pepper
Alertness, Assertiveness, Self-Image

Cardamom
Alertness, Assertiveness, Concentration, Confidence, Positivity

Carnation
Assertiveness, Creativity, Happiness, Peace, Self-Esteem

Cedarwood
Assertiveness, Concentration, Confidence, Focus, Positivity, Self-Esteem, Self-Image

Chamomile Roman
Concentration, Contentment, Joy, Peace, Self-Image

Cinnamon
Alertness, Focus, Happiness

Cistus *(rock rose, labdanum)*
Assertiveness, Creativity, Performance, Self-Awareness

Clary Sage
Restlessness, Self-Awareness

Clove
Contentment, Creativity, Focus, Happiness, Self-Awareness

Coriander
Alertness, Assertiveness, Confidence, Happiness, Self-Awareness

Cypress
Assertiveness, Confidence, Contentment, Creativity, Focus, Performance, Positivity, Self-Awareness, Self-Image

Eucalyptus *(radiata/globulus)*
Concentration, Alertness

Eucalyptus Citriodora *(lemon)*
Alertness, Performance

Fennel, Sweet
Assertiveness, Confidence, Focus

Frankincense
Assertiveness, Concentration, Creativity,
Joy, Peace, Performance, Positivity,
Self-Image

Geranium
Creativity, Happiness, Performance,
Positivity, Restfulness, Self-Awareness,
Self-Esteem

Ginger
Assertiveness, Confidence, Focus,
Happiness

Grapefruit
Alertness, confidence, performance,
positivity

Helichrysum
(immortelle or Italian everlasting)
Performance

Hyacinth
Concentration, Self-Esteem

Jasmine
Assertiveness, Confidence, Creativity,
Happiness, Peace, Performance, Self-
Awareness, Self-Esteem, Self-Image

Juniper Berry
Alertness, Creativity, Focus, Peace,
Positivity, Self-Image

Lavender
Contentment, Performance, Restfulness,
Self-Image

Lemon
Concentration, Creativity, Focus, Joy,
Performance, Positivity

Lemongrass
Concentration, Focus

Lime
Alertness, Assertiveness

Linden Blossom
Confidence, Focus, Joy, Restfulness

Litsea Cubeba
Assertiveness, Concentration, Creativity,
Focus

Mandarin
Self Awareness, Self-Image

Marjoram
Restfulness

Melissa
Peace, Self-Image

Mimosa
Creativity, Joy, Restfulness

Myrrh
Positivity

Myrtle
Self-awareness, Self-Image

Narcissus
Concentration

Neroli *(orange blossom)*
Concentration, Contentment, Creativity,
Joy, Peace, Restfulness, Self-Image

Nutmeg
Focus, Self-Image

Orange
Concentration, Confidence, Contentment, Happiness, Joy, Self-Image

Ormenis Flower
Assertiveness, Performance, Self-Awareness, Self-Esteem

Patchouli
Assertiveness, Contentment, Positivity

Peppermint
Alertness, Concentration

Petitgrain
Alertness, Joy, Positivity, Restfulness

Pimento Berry
Assertiveness, Happiness, Positivity, Self-Awareness

Pine
Alertness, Confidence, Positivity, Self-Awareness, Self-Image

Rosemary
Alertness, Concentration, Confidence, Focus, Positivity

Rose Maroc
Performance, Restfulness, Self-Esteem, Self-Image

Rose Otto
Concentration, Contentment, Creativity, Happiness, Joy, Peace

Sage
Self-Awareness

Sandalwood
Contentment, Creativity, Joy, Restfulness, Self-Awareness, Self-Esteem, Self-Image

Spikenard
Peace

Thyme
Alertness

Thyme Linalol
Alertness, Focus

Tuberose
Assertiveness, Confidence, Performance, Self-Esteem, Self-Image

Vetiver
Positivity, Self-Esteem

Yarrow
Peace

Ylang Ylang
Assertiveness, Contentment, Focus, Joy, Self-Awareness, Self-Esteem, Self-Image

CHART 11.4
Essential Oils Used for Emotional Healing

The essential oils in italics are those traditionally used in aromatherapy, the others have been adopted for these uses in more recent times.

Angelica Seed
Doubt, Mood swings

Basil
Addiction — general, Addiction — drugs, Anxiety — general, Apathy, Confusion, Dementia — memory loss, Doubt, Fatigue — mental, Fatigue — intellectual, Fear of failure, Fear — general, Hypochondria, Memory — lack of, Pain, Rejection

Bay
Addiction, Facing death, Stress

Benzoin
Addiction, Aggression — soothing, Anger — coping with, Bereavement, Breakdown, Doubt, Emotional violence, Facing death, Fear of love, Fear of loving, Grief — expressing, Loneliness, Misery, Self-blame, Stress

Bergamot
Addiction, Addiction — alcohol, Addiction — drugs, Amnesia — confusion, Amnesia — fear induced, Anger — calming, Anxiety — general, Anxiety — apprehensive, Anxiety — depressed, Apathy, Burnout, Confusion, Dejection, Depression, Depression — agitated or anxious, Depression — hysterical, Exhaustion, Facing death,

Fear — general, Grief — dissipating, Hysteria, Loneliness, Self-blame, Stress, Withdrawal from life, Withdrawal — for peace

Betula Alba *(birch)*
Pain

Black Pepper
Amnesia — confusion, Anger — coping, Anger — expressing unrealized, Apathy, Confusion, Dementia — memory, Dementia — appetite stimulant, Exhaustion, Fatigue — intellectual, Forgetfulness, Memory — lack of

Cardamom
Amnesia — confusion, Apathy, Confusion, Dementia — memory, Dementia — appetite stimulant, Memory — lack of, Mood swings

Carnation
Addictions, Aggressions — soothing, Bereavement, Emotional violence, Facing death, Fear of love, Fear of loving, Grief — dissipating, Misery, Rejection, Self-blame, Withdrawal — for peace

Cedarwood
Aggression — general, Amnesia — fear induced, Anger — expressing unrealized, Anxiety — general, Anxiety — restless,

Anxiety — depressed, Depression, Depression — agitated or anxious, Facing death, Fear — general, Fear of madness, Mood swings, Obsessions, Passivity, Repression, Trauma, Withdrawal — for peace, Worthlessness — feelings of

Chamomile German

Anger — calming, Depression — manic, Irritability

Chamomile Roman

Abuse, Addiction, Aggression — soothing, Aloneness, Amnesia — fear induced, Anger-calming, Anger — coping with, Anxiety — general, Anxiety — tense, Anxiety — restless, Bereavement, Breakdown — general, Breakdown — emotional, Burnout, Delirium tremens, Dementia — restlessness and tremors, Depression, Depression — weepiness, Depression — agitated or anxious, Depression — hysterical, Depression — manic, Emotional violence, Emotional exhaustion, Facing death, Fear — general, Fits — emotional, Grief — dissipating, Hysteria, Insomnia, Irritability, Loneliness, Nervous exhaustion, Pain, Pain — inflammatory, Phobias, Rage, Rejection, Self-blame, Schizophrenia, Stress, Trauma, Withdrawal — of emotions, Withdrawal — for peace, Worthlessness — feelings of

Cinnamon

Dementia, Exhaustion — nervous, Misery

Cistus (*rock rose*)

Addictions, Forgetfulness, Insomnia, Quarrelsomeness

Clary Sage

Addictions, Addictions — alcohol, Addictions — drugs, Aggression — soothing, Anxiety — tense, Breakdown — general, Burnout, Depression, Fear — general, Guilt, Insomnia, Nervous exhaustion, Obsession, Pain, Pain — with tension, Phobias, Quarrelsomeness, Rage, Stress, Tiredness — mental, Trauma

Clove

Anger — expressing unrealized, Dementia — appetite stimulant, Misery, Pain, Quarrelsomeness, Worthlessness — feelings of

Coriander

Aggression — soothing, Doubt, Dementia — appetite stimulant, Fear of failure, Irritability, Memory — lack of, Mood swings

Cypress

Amnesia — fear induced, Breakdown — emotional, Confusion, Depression — lethargic, Exhaustion, Fatigue — intellectual, Fear — general, Fear of gossip, Fear of letting go, Forgetfulness, Grief — dissipating, Irritability, Mood swings, Regrets, Rejection, Withdrawal from life

Eucalyptus Citriodora (*lemon*)

Addiction — alcohol, Depression, Fatigue — mental, Fits — emotional, Moodiness, Self-blame, Stress

Eucalyptus Radiata/Globulus

Delirium, Exhaustion

Fennel, Sweet
Fear of failure, Fear of madness, Fear of feelings

Frankincense
Addiction — general, Aggression — general, Aloneness, Anxiety — general, Anxiety-restless, Burnout, Dejection, Depression, Depression — manic, Doubt, Emotional violence, Exhaustion — emotional, Facing death, Fear — general, Fear of failure, Fear of madness, Fear of feelings, Fear of change, Fear of letting go, Forgetfulness, Grief — dissipating, Panic attacks, Repression, Stress, Withdrawal — for peace, Worthlessness — feelings of

Galbanham
Fear — general, Fear of sexuality, Fear of letting go, Hypochondria, Rage

Geranium
Abuse — the inner child, Addiction — drugs, Aggression — general, Amnesia — confusion, Amnesia — fear induced, Anxiety — general, Anxiety — apprehensive, Breakdown — general, Breakdown — emotional, Confusion, Dejection, Delirium tremens, Dementia — restlessness and tremors, Depression, Depression — weepy, Depression — manic, Emotional violence, Facing death, Moodiness, Mood swings, Self-blame, Schizophrenia, Stress, Trauma, Withdrawal of emotions, Withdrawal — for peace, Worthlessness — feelings of

Ginger
Amnesia — confusion, Anger — expressing unrealized, Apathy, Burnout,

Confusion, Dementia, Exhaustion, Fatigue — intellectual, Forgetfulness, Memory, Misery

Grapefruit
Aggression — general, Amnesia, Confusion, Dejection, Dementia — stimulating appetite, Depression, Depression — manic, Exhaustion, Fatigue — intellectual, Fear — general, Memory — lack of, Tiredness — mental, Withdrawal — for peace

Helichrysum
(immortelle or Italian everlasting)
Addiction — general, Addiction — alcohol, Addiction — drugs, Amnesia — confusion, Breakdown — general, Burnout, Confusion, Depression — general, Anxiety — dissipating, Grief — expressing, Loneliness, Mood swings, Pain, Panic attacks

Hops
Addictions, Hysteria, Hypochondria, Insomnia

Hyacinth
Addictions, Addiction — drugs, Apathy, Burnout, Emotional violence, Facing death, Fear of love, Grief — expressing, Regrets, Rejection, Repression, Stress, Tiredness — mental, Withdrawal of emotions

Jasmine
Addictions, Aloneness, Apathy, Burnout, Dejection, Dementia — restlessness and tremors, Depression, Emotional violence, Facing death, Guilt, Misery, Passivity, Repression, Stress

Juniper

Addictions, Addictions — alcohol, Addiction — drugs, Anxiety — tense, Anxiety — restless, Confusion, Emotional violence, Exhaustion — nervous, Facing death, Guilt, Repression, Withdrawal — for peace, Worthlessness — feelings of

Lavender

Abuse — the inner child, Aggression — soothing, Amnesia — shock induced, Anger-calming, Anxiety — general, Anxiety — apprehension, Bereavement, Breakdown — general, Breakdown — emotional, Burnout, Confusion, Delirium, Delirium tremens, Dementia — restlessness and tremors, Depression, Depression — agitated or anxious, Depression — manic, Emotional violence, Exhaustion — nervous, Fear — general, Fear of change, Fits — emotional, Hysteria, Insomnia, Irritability, Moodiness, Mood swings, Pain, Pain — with inflammation, Pain — relaxing, Panic attacks, Phobias, Quarrelsomeness, Rage, Schizophrenia, Stress, Tiredness — mental, Trauma

Lemon

Addiction — alcohol, Amnesia — fear induced, Apathy, Breakdown — general, Burnout, Delirium tremens, Dementia — appetite, Depression, Depression — manic, Exhaustion, Fatigue — mental, Fatigue — intellectual, Fear — general, Forgetfulness, Insomnia, Memory — lack of, Moodiness, Obsession, Quarrelsome, Self-blame, Schizophrenia, Stress, Trauma

Lime

Dementia — appetite

Linden Blossom

Anger — calming, Anger — coping, Bereavement, Burnout, Dejection, Dementia — restlessness, Depression — hysteric, Exhaustion — emotional, Facing death, Guilt, Hysteria, Insomnia, Irritability, Mood swings, Phobias, Stress

Litsea Cubeba

Aggression, Doubt, Exhaustion, Fits — emotional, Irritability, Stress, Tiredness — mental

Mandarin

Abuse — emotional, Abuse — the inner child, Amnesia — shock induced, Anxiety — general, Bereavement, Breakdown — emotional, Dejection, Depression — general, Depression — manic, Hysteria, Insomnia, Schizophrenia, Stress

Manuka

Hypochondria

Marjoram

Addiction, Addiction — alcohol, Aggression — soothing, Burnout, Delirium, Delirium tremens, Depression, Depression — agitated or anxious, Depression — hysterical, Exhaustion, Fits — emotional, Hypochondria, Hysteria, Insomnia, Pain, Panic attacks, Phobias, Rage, Stress, Tiredness — mental, Trauma

Melissa

Abuse — emotional, Abuse — the inner child, Aloneness, Amnesia — shock induced, Anxiety — general, Anxiety — apprehensive, Anxiety — depressed, Bereavement, Burnout, Emotional violence, Depression — agitated or anxious, Grief — expressing, Irritability, Self-blame, Stress, Withdrawal of emotions

Mimosa

Aggression — soothing, Dejection, Grief — expressing

Myrtle

Anger — coping with

Narcissus

Addiction — hypnotic, Addiction — drugs, Depression — hysterical, Emotional exhaustion, Facing death, Grief — dissipating, Hysteria, Irritability, Loneliness, Misery, Obsession, Stress, Withdrawal from life

Neroli

Abuse — emotional, Abuse — the inner child, Aggression — soothing, Aloneness, Amnesia — shock induced, Amnesia — fear induced, Anxiety — general, Anxiety — apprehensive, Anxiety — depressed, Bereavement, Breakdown — general, Breakdown — emotional, Burnout, Dejection, Dementia — restlessness, Depression, Depression — weepy, Depression — manic, Emotional violence, Exhaustion — nervous, Facing death, Fear — general, Fear of feelings, Fear of love, Fear of loving, Grief —

expressing, Hysteria, Irritability, Loneliness, Moodiness, Misery, Pain — relaxing, Phobias, Rejection, Stress, Withdrawal of emotions, Withdrawal for peace, Worthlessness — feelings of

Nutmeg

Addictions, Addiction — drugs, Dejection, Dementia — appetite stimulant, Depression — agitated or anxious, Grief-Dissipating, Guilt, Pain, Stress, Tiredness — mental

Orange

Amnesia — fear induced, Apathy, Breakdown, Dejection, Dementia — appetite, Depression, Fear — general, Misery, Nervous Exhaustion, Obsession, Passivity, Self-blame, Withdrawal — from life.

Oregano

Hypochondria

Ormenis Flower (Chamomile Maroc)

Abuse — emotional, Addiction — drugs, Anger — expressing unrealized , Apathy, Confusion, Depression — agitated or anxious, Fear — general, Fear of change, Grief — dissipating, Hypochondria, Moodiness, Phobias, Rage, Self-blame, Stress, Worthlessness — feelings of

Patchouli

Addictions, Anger — calming, Anger — expressing unrealized, Anxiety — general, Anxiety — tense, Bereavement, Burnout, Depression — weepy, Depression — manic, Fear of sexuality, Moodiness, Passivity, Quarrelsomeness, Repression

Peppermint

Amnesia — shock induced, Apathy, Confusion, Delirium, Fatigue — mental, Fatigue — intellectual, Hysteria, Pain, Forgetfulness, Hypochondria, Tiredness — mental

Petitgrain

Amnesia — confusion, Anger — calming, Burnout, Confusion, Dejection, Delirium tremens, Depression, Exhaustion — nervous, Fatigue — mental, Misery, Trauma

Pimento Berry

Memory — lack of, Misery

Pine

Confusion, Exhaustion, Guilt, Passivity, Regrets, Rejection, Repression

Rose Maroc

Addiction, Aggression — soothing, Amnesia — shock induced, Anger — calming, Anger — coping with, Apathy, Bereavement, Dejection, Depression, Facing death, Fear of sexuality, Fear of love, Fear of loving, Fear of letting go, Grief — dissipating, Grief — expressing, Misery, Passivity, Regrets, Self-blame, Stress, Withdrawal — of emotions

Rosemary

Confusion, Depression — lethargic, Dementia, Exhaustion, Exhaustion — nervous, Fatigue — mental, Fatigue — intellectual, Forgetfulness, Hysteria, Hypochondria, Memory — lack of, Pain, Tiredness — mental

Rose Otto *(Bulgur)*

Abuse — emotional, Aloneness, Amnesia — shock induced, Anger — to calm, Anxiety — general, Anxiety — apprehensive, Anxiety — depressed, Apathy, Bereavement, Breakdown — emotional, Burnout, Dementia, Depression, Depression — weepy, Depression — manic, Emotional violence, Facing death, Fear of being unloved, Grief — dissipating, Grief — expressing, Guilt, Regrets, Rejection, Self-blame, Schizophrenia, Stress, Tiredness — mental, Withdrawal — of emotions, Withdrawal — for peace

Sandalwood

Aggression, Amnesia — fear induced, Anxiety — general, Anxiety — tense, Anxiety — depressed, Breakdown — emotional, Burnout, Depression, Depression — weepy, Depression — manic, Facing death, Fear — general, Fear of failings, Insomnia, Obsession, Phobias, Quarrelsomeness, Rejection, Stress, Worthlessness — feelings of

Sage

Pain

Spikenard

Addiction — general, Addiction — drugs, Addictions — hypnotic, Aggression — soothing, Anger — coping with, Depression — hysterical, Grief — dissipating, Hysteria, Stress

Tea Tree

Hypochondria

Tuberose

Addiction, Addiction — drugs, Aggression — soothing, Amnesia — confusion, Anger — calming, Anger — unrealized expression, Confusion, Facing death, Passivity, Rejection, Self-blame, Stress

Thyme Linalol

Confusion, Hypochondria, Memory — lack of, Trauma

Vanilla

Grief — dissipating

Valerian

Addiction, Addiction — drugs, Aggression, Anger — coping with, Depression — agitated or anxious, Depression — hysterical, Delirium tremens, Hypochondria, Hysteria, Insomnia, Stress

Vetiver

Addiction, Addiction — drugs, Aggression — general, Amnesia — fear induced, Anger — calming, Anger — coping with, Anxiety — general, Anxiety — restlessness, Anxiety — depressed, Burnout, Depression — hysterical, Fatigue — mental, Fear — general, Fear of sexuality, Grief — expressing, Guilt, Hysteria, Insomnia, Obsession, Pain — tension, Rage, Repression, Stress

Yarrow

Grief — dissipating, Stress

Ylang Ylang

Amnesia — shock induced, Anger — coping, Depression, Depression — weepy, Dejection, Doubt, Fear of failure, Fear of madness, Fear of change, Fear of sexuality, Fear of love, Guilt, Irritability, Moodiness, Passivity, Rage, Rejection, Repression, Self-blame, Stress

Part 3

Aroma-Genera:
Human Characteristics and Personalities of Essential Oils

"The whole earth is a thurible heaped with incense, afire with the divine, yet not consumed. This is the most spiritual of earth's joys – too subtle for analysis, mysteriously connected with light and with whiteness, for white flowers are the sweetest – yet it penetrates the physical being to its depths. Here is a symbol of the material value of spiritual things. If we washed our souls in these healing perfumes as often as we washed our hands, our lives would be infinitely more wholesome."

– MARY WEBB
The Joy of Perfume

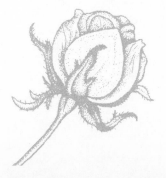

CHAPTER 12

WHAT IS PERSONALITY?

Physically, human beings are the same. We all have a skeleton, with muscles, respiratory system, cardiac and circulatory systems, and digestive organs, so that, if put under the microscope, we would look very similar. Where we differ profoundly from one another is in our brain functions — our thoughts, emotions, and behavior. In other words, our personality. Just think about your family and friends for a moment — no two people are the same in terms of their ideas, attitudes, dreams, temperament, and so on. Where does this difference come from?

Personality is not etched forever into us, like a fingerprint. It changes both depending on who we are with at any given point in time, and at different times in our lives. I can think of a little six-year-old girl, for example, who is perfectly behaved and creatively occupies herself when she is with her friend Celeste, but behaves like an obstreperous teenager when she is with her friend Mandy. She is an out-and-out brat when she plays with Miranda, and a bossy tyrant when she is with the passive Susan. She bursts into tears at the slightest thing when she plays with her next door neighbor, Peter. If she just had one person to play with all the time these differences would not be so apparent, and perhaps her mother would think that, indeed, her personality was etched into her like a fingerprint. As it is, we can see that her personality changes in relation to the people she is with. Personality also changes depending on life's experiences and so we hear people say, "His whole personality changed after he got that job," and so forth. People do change — quite dramatically sometimes — either because of an outside influence, new job or love, or because of an internal

239

influence — such as finding a spiritual home.

Psychologists have found that babies of seven to eight weeks display differences in terms of their activity levels, attention span, intensity of reaction, changeability of mood, and degree of persistence. When these babies were followed up later, these same differences could be observed, despite the social and emotional environment in which the children grew up. Clearly we are born with a unique personality but exactly how much of our adult personality is due to genetic or environmental factors is the question that has fascinated researchers. In the search to get to the root of personality, identical twins have been under a great deal of scrutiny, especially those who were bought up in different homes. Take the case of the American "Jim twins" who were adopted at birth by different families and didn't meet each other until they were thirty-nine years old. By then, both Jims had worked as part-time sheriffs, both drove Chevrolets, both regularly vacationed in St. Petersburg, Florida, both had married and divorced women named Linda, both had remarried women named Betty, both had dogs named "Toy," and both had sons named James — in one case it was James Alan and in the other, James Allen.

A review of forty studies into twins found that identical twins (with the same genes because they grew from a fertilized ovum that separated into two) reared apart from each other were more similar in their personality traits than fraternal twins (with different genes because they grew from two ovums that were fertilized by two sperm). On this basis, it could be said that *nature* has more impact on an individual than *nurture,* and we are also reminded that individuals inherit their sympathetic nervous system, which regulates blood pressure and heartbeat, from their parents, and can influence the way a person responds to circumstances, making it similar to that of their parents. But it is not that simple. Other research clearly shows that *nurture* has a powerful impact on an individual.

Any parent knows that if they have a fit of anger one day their child is liable to have a fit of anger the next. We can observe our children doing and saying what we do. It is thought that the personality traits most likely to be reactive to parental influence are bad temper, aggression, anxiety, timidity, impetuosity, and altruism. Anxiety, depression, phobias, compulsions, and obsessions are also very likely to have their roots in the high level of emotional drama in their childhood home life. And simply by growing up around our parents we could adopt their political leanings and religious beliefs, and may even go into the same professions.

Another important influence on our personality is whether we were the first-born child. Research shows that first-borns are more likely to be achievement oriented, conservative, and reserved. It is thought this is because they made themselves more acceptable to their parents as a way of overcoming the displacement they felt with the arrival of siblings. But parents are often more protective of the first child, believing all manner of harm will come to them, whereas with subsequent children the parents have learned that the child will survive. Also, older children take on responsibility for their younger siblings and even have to protect them — either from other children or from the parents. Firstborns are also given more responsibility by their parents in that they have to do jobs around the home to help out while the younger ones are just not capable.

Younger siblings, on the other hand, are never asked to help their older brothers and sisters get dressed or washed and I don't know any younger siblings who have sat for hours and helped the firstborn with their reading, unless the firstborn had learning difficulties. Younger siblings tend to be given more freedom because the parents aren't as worried as they were with the first; they have less responsibility and have not needed to develop skills in protecting others. All this can make them a little "wild," a fact usually attributed to them being rebellious because they feel they are not as loved as the older child, or to them hating their older sibling. I find this theory rather dubious because in my experience younger siblings are as likely to idolize their older siblings as to hate them.

Finding the roots of personality is not easy. Children from similar environments have very different personalities and may, in fact, have a similar personality to a child who grew up in a totally different environment. Also, two children from very strict homes may develop in different ways — one may become cautious and correct and the other may rebel and go completely the other way. The old *nature versus nurture* debate seems to have come to the conclu-

sion that it is 50% due to inborn factors, and 50% to environmental ones.

Personality, then, comes from many areas. There is a certain genetic factor, and being male or female has a powerful influence, both in terms of hormones and socially expected behavior (probably the latter being more influential). Our parents influence us, as do siblings and our age relative to them. The environment we grow up in is important (whether it is in Somalia, Sarejevo, or Surrey), as are the people available for us to play or work with. Are we then just a mish-mash of influences, clay in the hands of circumstance? The answer to this is no. We are born individuals, as research also shows, and in a sense, it is our adult prerogative to recover our individuality and shake off those influences we no longer desire.

It is easy to feel like a piece of flotsam adrift on the sea of life, sent here and there by the tides of time. Powerful eddies are created by other people imposing their ideals and behavior patterns onto us. They are forces that are difficult to fight, especially when they are our nearest and dearest. We go around and around, wondering where we are, and where we will end up. And powerful, dangerous tides are created by life circumstances such as illness, unemployment and bad relationships. Meanwhile strong forces within us — created by abuse, violence, and fear — project us onto shores where we do not really want to be.

Yet in our mind's eye we probably all have an image of the ideal place we would like to end up, the perfect person we would like to be. Among the qualifications we might aim for are thoughtfulness and sensitivity toward others, integrity, tolerance, trust and openness, professional creativity, and a concern for justice, peace and freedom in the world. Psychologists agree that conformity is not necessarily good for us, while being true to ourselves is. We need to develop control over our lives, deep personal relationships, time for reflection, the imagination to overcome problems, and a zest for living. Then, we might be happy.

But who are "we?" The answer is ever elusive. Dr. Roger Woolger, a Jungian psychologist, writes about regression therapy: "Each other life that comes to us, however brief or fragmentary, is a piece of another self. The personality is not single, it is multiple — not in the psychiatric sense of multiple personality, but in that there are many levels to the self like many skins to an onion. We peel off these selves as we look into our past lives or as we look into our own dreams." [1]

Multiple Personality Disorder (MPD) is the other aspect of complexity, and is extremely interesting from a mind-over-matter point of view because it proves, if nothing else does, that there is still much to learn. People with MPD, (known as "multiples") switch from one personality to another and have been shown to have different brain-wave patterns depending on which personality they are "in" at any given time. They can even have different physical disorders, present or not present, depending on the personality they are expressing. There are many scientifically recorded incidences of this, with people

having and then losing symptoms when the well personality takes over. Not only can allergic reactions, scars, burn marks, swollen insect stings, and cysts disappear almost immediately, even the eye color can change. A multiple with diabetes can lose all the symptoms when in a nondiabetic personality, and it has even been reported that a person with cancer can "disappear" the tumor when "in" the personality that doesn't have the cancer. [2]

Although MDP is an extreme, we are all to some extent "multiple personalities." The little six-year-old girl mentioned earlier is a different personality depending on whether she plays with Celeste, Mandy, or Peter. And we know that we ourselves can have different personalities depending on who we are with. We would not, for example, behave in the same way we do at the rugby club ball as we do when we're asking the bank manager for a business loan (unless your rugby club is *extremely* sedate). We are, in a sense, multifaceted like a diamond, throwing out different reflections and colors in response to the light coming from outside. This phenomenon is well recognized in psychology, which considers Jung's theory of a total "Self" comprised of many sub- or secondary personalities to be one of his most enduring contributions to the study of the human mind. The beauty of the human mind is that we have this complexity, fluidity, and potential, which need not merely be reactive but can be controlled to a certain extent. Let's just hope it's controlled to your advantage when you go for a personality test.

Personality Tests

Without doubt, personality is important. It is how you portray yourself to the outside world. It is what you will be judged on when people first meet you, both socially and professionally. When you apply for a job you are very likely to have to fill in a lengthy form of questions designed to show the potential employer what your innermost feelings are on a diverse range of subjects such as money — getting it and spending it — exercise, party-going, pets, companionship, hobbies, family, dreams, desires, and so forth. By the time you've filled out one of these forms you may know more about yourself than you did before, and your potential employer will know as much as you. What all this invasive busy-body "personality testing" is about, so we are told, is to identify management potential and see how you would fit into a team. It may also identify for your potential employer whether you'll tow the company line and not sway the corporate boat by standing up for the workers when a tricky decision has to be made regarding layoffs. "Personality testing" is about making sure you are, in no way, shape, or form, a threat to the company and its profits. No longer are exam passes and other achievements, even hobbies and experience, enough.

Personality testing is carried out in the form of long questionnaires and, also, is assessed through graphology. These methods are employed by companies and other employing organizations, career counselors, and clinical psychologists.

Whether they have any true value is a matter open to question, and in a hundred years time they may laugh at us all, but in the meantime our personality is not our own — it's in the personnel department's files. For that reason, if no other, perhaps it's worth spending a little time considering what our personality is, and whether or not we want to change it.

Personality in Perfumery

It takes years to design a perfume, and millions of dollars to market it. And who knows if anyone will buy it? Perfume houses, then, have had a tremendous interest in trying to establish personality types, so they can more effectively create perfumes that people want, and market them effectively. In marketing research, people will be asked whether a perfume reminds them of a glamorous, cultivated lady, a successful career woman, or a fresh and sensitive young girl, so the perfume houses can have a clearer idea of people's perceptions of the "character" of any particular perfume and can market them accordingly. As part of the drive to know the market, the fragrance house H&R (Haarmann & Reimer), in conjunction with the Research Institute for Applied Esthetics of Freiburg, Germany, have adapted the Luscher color test to identify personality types, which, in turn, can be linked to particular fragrances. According to their system, there are seven groups of female fragrance buyer, classified as A-G: extroverted, introverted, emotionally ambivalent, emotionally ambivalent with extroverted mood trend, emotionally ambivalent with introverted mood trend, emotionally stable with extroverted mood trend, and emotionally stable with introverted mood trend. Each of these personality groups is further defined. For example, the Group D personality is described as "...lively, cheerful, and vivacious, yet easily injured. This group reacts spontaneously to its environment...," and is designated with the "fragrance need" floral, floral-fruity. Group "A" "...quickly impart life to a boring group...." Group B "...would rather stay home than go to a boring party;" Group C "...enjoy dreaming about things that cannot possibly ever come true...." These are of course just glimpses of the much fuller descriptions given to the personality types. They are interesting because they are the links between color preference and fragrance need, as far as this system of classification is concerned.

Classifications are, of course, variable and dependent upon the requirements of particular groups. The fragrance industry needs to be able to tie in its product, which has a particular fragrance, with the marketing approach they need to take to achieve maximum returns on their considerable investment. The Luscher color test is itself used extensively by educational and behavioral psychologists to ascertain personality traits so people can be encouraged to perform better in life. "Color imagers" have another attitude to color — choosing clothes to suit the skin tone and hair color of a particular woman.

"Color therapists" use color light-filters projected onto their patients for healing, while mental color therapists use color projected from their minds to heal — which might sound strange until one considers the fact that all life is vibration, which color is too. The fragrance industry recognize very well that people choose different perfumes for different activities, to complement the moods they may be in at any particular time.

Characterology and Typology

Most of us know our astrological birth sign, and many of us will know whether we are an "earth," "fire," "air," or "water" sign. This is a form of typography, a classification system, that is also about character, or characterology. We talk about someone being "too earthy" or "too fiery," "an airhead," or "wet." When we do this we're continuing a tradition that stretches back in time, for as long as we can see. Classifying people's characters in various ways has been done throughout time and throughout the world. The Sufis have the nine characters of the enneagram; the Chinese have yin/yang and the five elements of water, fire, wood, metal and earth; the Indians have Ayurvedic medicine, which recognizes the three personality and energy types vata, pitta, and kapha; while the Greeks had the four "humors," a concept that was continued in Western medicine until the seventeenth century and beyond. The father of psychology, C.G. Jung, also adapted these four humors of air, fire, water, and earth into the concept of the four aspects of a human being: thinking (air), intuition (fire), feeling (water), and sensation (earth).

We might talk about someone being in good or bad "humor," by which we mean their mood, but this word comes from "humoral," that once described a person's basic physical or mental qualities or disposition. The man who most influenced the course of western medicine, the ancient Greek Galen, used the categories of sanguine (fire) — optimistic and happy; melancholic (earth) — depressed and anxious; choleric (air) — irritable and impulsive; and phlegmatic (water) — listless and not easily moved. The different combinations of the four humors in any one individual constituted their "complexions" or "temperaments" — their physical and mental qualities — and the ideal was to have an equal proportion of all four — balance, in other words. Although the words sanguine, phlegmatic and so on are still used in the English language, they have lost the psycho-physical significance they had in ancient Greece. The choleric person, for example, was not only irritable and short-tempered but yellow-faced, lean, hairy, proud, ambitious, revengeful, and shrewd. These characterizations were the basis for diagnosis for over 1,500 years in the Western tradition, and a person who was innovative and a "born" leader would be described as a fire personality; someone who used their five senses in a practical way would be an "earth" personality; someone who was sensitive and feeling would be a "water" personality; while the thinkers and philosophers were the

"air" type. Medications or treatments would be given taking the personality into account.

Diagnosing people by a combination of physical and mental attributes is still today not the slightest bit unusual. Homeopaths do it every day. Dr. Ronald Livingston, for example, describes the patient who would most benefit from the homeopathic remedy natrum muriaticum: "withdrawn, moody, taciturn, seclusive, sullen, and silent when questioned; while attention and sympathy make him resentful and ungracious to the point of tears."[3] Likewise, a practitioner of Ayurvedic medicine will diagnose you in terms of the three energy forces or doshas — *vata, pitta,* and *kapha,* which he or she will aim to bring into harmony with Ayurvedic medicines, diet, massage, meditation, yoga, or essential oils. *Vata dosha* types are described as enthusiastic and lovers of new experiences but when out of balance they become anxious, exhausted, and depressed. *Pitta dosha* types have a fiery temperament and are ambitious, perhaps overbearing and demanding, but will suffer stress, tension, and anxiety when out of balance. *Kapha dosha* types are calm, strong, and steady but when imbalanced become insecure, lethargic, and lazy. A person might have two dominant personality types and the skill of the practitioner depends on their being able to identify these and bring them into harmony with each other.

Balance is all in the 4,000-year-old Chinese Taoist system, not only between yin and yang, but between the five elements, which are expressions of their interaction — water, fire, wood, metal, and earth — and which are expressed within an individual in terms of their psychological disposition, as well as their physical body. Macrobiotics, a nutritional system developed in the 1880s by Japanese doctor Sagen Ishizuka, aims to balance the yin/yang qualities that exist within us all by the means of foods that are designated either yin or yang. People who are more yin than yang are said to be relaxed, peaceful, calm, sociable, and creative; while those who are more yang than yin are said to be energetic, alert, and precise. Too much yin brings lethargy, loss of concentration, and depression, while too much yang causes irritability and tension. If you went to any person practicing a therapy relating to yin/yang energies, your personality would be assessed to help diagnose where the imbalances are.

Achieving balance is also the aim of the Polynesian Kahunas, medicine men and women of the Huna faith. The whole basis of this system of medicine is the belief that man is a spiritual/intellectual/emotional being and that these three aspects have to be in harmony if disease is not to occur. Indeed, the mind is believed to be the source of all ill-health — even that arising from accidents — because your mind told you to be in the wrong place at the wrong time. The condition of the mind, then, is a crucial aspect of diagnosis, while massage and chanting are aspects of the healing process.

When Dr. Edward Bach devised his Bach flower remedies in the 1930s, he intended psychological and emotional characteristics to be part of the diagnosis, so that a remedy would be chosen depending on the feelings of a person at any given time, and depending on the life-circumstances at the time. Whether chosen by a therapist or by oneself, as well as considering any illness, other things such as relationships or work should be taken into consideration. Sweet chestnut will be recommended for utter dejection, bleak outlook and despair, for example, while red chestnut is more appropriate for someone who is obsessed with care and concern with others. Honeysuckle is for people who are homesick, nostalgic or living in the past, and water violet is for those who are proud, reserved, and aloof. Dr. Bach believed that each person's personality and nature could be matched with a "type remedy," which might be taken for a long period of time, whereas other remedies could be used on a short-term basis to deal with passing problems.

C.G. Jung was very impressed with the old Greek and Medieval idea of the four humors and adapted them into his psychoanalytic theory. The four elements were expanded into eight as follows: *Air* (thinking), *air-fire* (intuitive thinking), *Fire* (intuition), *water-fire* (intuitive feeling), *Water* (feeling), *water-earth* (sensory feeling), *Earth* (sensation), and *air-earth* (empirical thinking). Jung thought that one of these functions was predominant, that the functions to either side were auxiliary, while the function furthermost away from the predominant function (if one sees these classifications as a circle) was subconscious and difficult to express. This view has been criticized, however, because a person can be, for example, both feeling (water) and thinking (air) — a concert pianist, for example.

Another system of personality classification exists in the enneagram — a word which combines ennea, meaning nine, and gram, meaning diagram. This system was made popular by the spiritual teacher Geoge Ivanovich Gurdjieff in the early twentieth century although the enneagram can be traced back in time to the secret brotherhoods of the Sufis in the tenth and eleventh centuries and may go back much further than that. The ancient Egyptians were very seriously into the number nine, believing, for example, that Atum of Heliopolis, as it says in the Pyramid Texts, "came forth from between the thighs of the divine Nine." According to the ennead there are nine personalities: the reformer, the helper, the status seeker, the peacemaker, the artist, the thinker, the loyalist, the generalist, and the leader. These are of course further defined, so, for example, the thinker is not only perceptive and analytic, but paranoid. As with all systems of characterology and typology, each personality type has the potential to be positive or negative.

Webster's Dictionary lists 17,953 different descriptions of personality traits, which shows the immense complexity the human character. Trying to classify these traits into distinct personality types has been, as we have seen, an aspect of human endeavor, and it continues to be so. Today we tend to talk in terms of psychology, so people are defined in the literature as hysterical, obsessional, schizoid, paranoid, depressive, cyclothymic, anxious, or narcissistic. All these sound very negative but in fact it is, as usual, all about potential. So, for example, we are told that the anxious personality can be very competent and decisive.

All the systems of characterology and typology stress that no character is "better" than another and that balance is what it's about. Fire, for example, is enlivening and warming, but it can, if taken to extreme, destroy. Water can be a refreshing stream or a tidal wave that pushes asunder all in its path. It is great to be a thinking "air" personality, but a tornado can rearrange things that were previously well-placed. Earth is a good foundation, but an earth slide destroys all in its wake. Balance and connection with our universal self is, as ever, the ultimate human goal.

———

CHAPTER 13

AROMA-GENERA: THE HUMAN PERSONALITIES OF ESSENTIAL OILS

Introduction

We place people into types all the time. We say, "she is a born worrier," "he won't stand for any nonsense," "she's always apologizing," and so on. Phrases like this are short but they conjure up a whole personality which is a composite of all the other people we've known who are "born worriers," for example. Likewise, when we say "she spends money like water," our mind quickly scans our past experience and comes up with all the other people we've known to spend money like water, giving a category into which we slip this latest entry — "Oh, another one of *that* type."

In a sense this is unfair because we are all individuals and there is no one "type" of person. The person spending money, for example, may be spending it on other people, or on themselves, and

some may be spending money they actually have, while others are spending somebody else's money, or the credit card company's money. Already, this makes five subtypes. There are millions of subtypes and it would be impossible for our minds to keep all the information we have about them if we didn't file them away under some form of "type" classification. Classification helps to keep our mind tidy, even though it may sometimes be unfair and even inaccurate. Personality classification is a trade-off between accuracy and mental overload.

Professional therapists similarly use personality classifications to help us choose from the wide range of options the right combinations of oils for a particular person. It will not be one personality type we refer to, but several layered one upon the other. These factors should be taken into consideration in addition to the therapeutic value of possible essential oils in relation to the physical or emotional problem(s) the client presents. Some of us do this because we have been trained to do so, while others do it subconsciously based on their practical experience, or intuitively. Utilizing this "harmony" with relationship between particular people and particular oils opens up a whole new vista of potential in terms of physical result, but also in terms of emotional and spiritual uplift-ment.

For the practitioner, as a practical aid, personality profile assessment takes no more time than the initial consulta-tion, which should also include questions relating to personality traits such as, "Are you a person who rushes everywhere, or do you take things easy?" "Do you express your anger, or bottle it up?" Questions such as this provide answers that can be as illuminating as knowing where the physical pain is.

This is a book about mind, mood, and emotion — aroma-psychology — and therefore in this context the personalities of the essential oils are extremely impor-tant. The interesting thing is, when you get a harmony between a particular person and a particular oil, the physical problem can clear up more quickly. Not only that, but people who are using this system have seen some almost miraculous recoveries simply by choosing the essential oils only on the basis of their personality typology, not taking the therapeutic values into account at all. And the results are benefi-cial on all levels — body, mind, and spirit. This is true whether the problem being treated is a physical or an emotional one.

During workshops I have given both here and abroad I've noticed a growing awareness of the need to be more easily able to formulate the perfect blend for each individual's psyche. What I am pre-senting here is an introduction to the sub-ject of Aroma-Genera, which will be covered in more detail in a forthcoming publication.

The subject of personality types in relation to essential oils was introduced to me many years ago when I was an appren-tice of clinical herbal medicine in Switzer-land, and working in Germany, Italy, and other European countries. Phytotherapy, as it is known in mainland Europe, uses herbs, essential oils, and naturopathy as an integrated system. It was, and still is, a normal part of diagnosis and treatment to consider the emotional and mental char-acteristics of individual patients. So one might say of an insomniac, for example, "They're angry all the time; we shall use this tea" or "this person changes direction too quickly; we shall use that tea" and so on. Both patients present with insomnia but the diagnosis and treatment will depend on whether valerian tea is used or chamomile. In classical phytotherapy it is taken for granted that a person's mental state will affect their physical body and that, conversely, a treatment using herbs or essential oils could affect the mind. Aro-matherapy also incorporates these ideas — it is only a question of degree and consciousness.

The personality profiles presented in the following chapter have been collected by myself over many years of practical application, through which I have learned to be acutely aware of personality traits. It has become clear to me that there is a system to the use of essential oils vis-à-vis personality, whether or not in conjunction with the treatment of physical ailments. It is this system that I present in this chapter, under the name, Aroma-Genera, which means the different types of personalities, here classified for the first time as *Florals, Fruities, Herbies, Leafies, Resinies, Rooties, Seedies, Spicies* and *Woodies*. These are of course variations on the personality groupings classically accepted in modern-day psychology. Thousands of people have been through my workshops where these classifications have been elucidated. The feedback I have received from these people has been most enthusiastic and I have been asked countless times to provide the material in book form. People's emotional states are expressed through their "personality" and, conversely, personality is a key in the treatment of the emotional state.

Aroma-Genera

The human being is all about potential. We all have good days and bad days. The question is, "How many good or bad days do we have in any given week or year?" The aim of aroma-genera is to maximize the potential so that we more often operate on the positive end of the spectrum of possibility. The nine groupings that follow are arranged as *Abundant Self, Generally,* and *Impoverished Self,* reflecting this potential fluidity. The aim is to become more often abundant, that is positive, and

less often impoverished, or negative.

To choose one's aroma-genera group requires honesty. Read each group carefully and see which most closely reflects your own personality traits. This may be done with a friend or family member, someone who knows you very well but — although other people will know your patterns of behavior — may not know your innermost thoughts. It is then, ultimately, up to each individual to ascertain which group or groups they fall into.

I often find in workshops that, at first, people will choose the aroma-genera class that fits not the person they are but the person they *wish* they were. This is, in a sense, "jumping the gun" because while personality can certainly be encouraged in more positive directions, as we shall later see, the starting point is to establish where one actually is right now.

From a practitioners point of view, one of the most fabulous aspects of aromatherapy is the potential of the blending process. Throughout this book I have referred to synergistic blends — mixtures of several essential oils — and these are the mainstay of our work because blending brings into play the old truism that something can be "more than the sum of the parts." This same dynamic comes into play with aroma-genera. Very few people display the characteristics of one group alone — they are complexes of two, three, or even more groupings. You may then find yourself saying, "I'm a bit of a herbie but also a bit of a leafie." This is fine, and to be expected, and choosing oils and blending them may be based on two, rather than just one, grouping.

One of the challenges of aromatherapy, at least as perceived by the general public, is that there is so much choice. People stand in front of a row of essential oils in the shop and ask themselves, "Which one is for me?" Aroma-genera helps us answer this question. There *are* oils which are better suited to a particular individual and the success of the aromatherapist and layperson alike depends upon being able to make good choices. My aim here is to introduce the possibilities inherent in the confusing diversity of options available, and I present the information with confidence because experience has shown me that it works. When people find the oils that best suit them they can progress in leaps and bounds and become the person they truly wish they were. Another advantage in the system is that it provides a certain amount of lateral thinking and people find themselves considering essential oils they would never have previously thought of using. And, as we shall see, some of the most unusual combinations have a profound impact, not only on the body but on the whole person — mind, body, and spirit.

The Magnificent Nine

Working with the products of nature on a daily basis I have over the years been constantly amazed by the beautiful and effective aromas that can be made when combining particular essential oils. However, sometimes life can be stunningly beautiful in its simplicity. This was the thought that ran through my mind when I discovered the aromas that could be made when blending only those oils that belong to a particular aroma-genera. For example, if you take one drop of every floral essential oil and mix them all together, the effect can be simply divine. A depth of effect is reached that goes well beyond the physical and into the etheric, so that a kind of electrical shudder or wave of energy reaches throughout the whole body. And this extraordinary effect is achieved simply by smelling this combination from the bottle of mixed drops. Something very interesting is happening here, and it happens when you make mixes using essential oils exclusively from each of the other eight aroma-genera groups as well.

What we're talking about here is an effect that is felt on the nonphysical level, as well as the physical. To take a sniff from a bottle and have a shudder run through, not exactly the body, but the space taken up by the body and beyond, which can be felt like a wave is staggering. It is humbling as one realizes that nature has its own simple system, which is expressed in sheer beneficial beauty.

Clearly I have a large collection of essential oils and can make mixes using a large number of *just* floral essential oils or absolutes, or *just* seedie essential oils, or *just* woodie essential oils. But anyone with a fair collection can do the same. Even three essential oils taken from a particular aroma-genera group can give some idea of the potential of this mixing, but the more oils one can use, the better. If you do not have more than one essential oil from a particular group, ask your friends to let you have three drops from their bottles of essential oils that you don't have in your collection. Swap drops with each other, and see how deep and rich the aroma-genera mixes can be.

What is so interesting about this experiment is that you will find yourself mixing oils that, normally, one would never put together simply because you'd think the aromas would be incompatible. In fact, the oils from each aroma-genera group can blend together fabulously. Indeed, the reason I have called this sub-section *The Magnificent Nine* is because people's reaction to the aroma-genera mixes is most usually, "Oh, that is magnificent" — and this is from people who are used to the fabulous aesthetic potential of essential oils. It is not simply that the aroma is splendid, but that the effect is immediately felt as a "rush." Somehow, an extraordinary balance seems to be created when blending in this fashion, a balance that has a deep and powerful effect on the whole person.

I suggest to people that they take nine bottles and label them "floral," "fruitie" and so on, and put in them just three drops of each essential oil you have that falls into that group. Add to the mixes as and when additional essential oils are made available to you, and observe how the aroma gathers depth as more essential oils are added. When you have these nine bottles, which should contain a minimum of three essential oils of that group, they act as an additional means of choosing a person's aroma-genera type, working on the principle that people are attracted to the aromas that will ultimately do them the most good, however emotional that journey may be.

When Is a Fruitie a Fruitie ?

As you can see from the chart at the end of this section, some essential oils fall into two groups. For example, lavender is both a floral and an herb, whereas clove is a fruit and a spice. The reason that an oil can fall into two groups is that two parts of a particular plant may be used in the distillation process. For example, lavender oil is extracted from the flowers, but sometimes also from the rest of the plant and is generally known as an herb in aromatherapy. Clove, on the other hand, is distilled from the buds, which is the fruit of the plant, but it is and has been known to be for centuries a "spice." Clearly, people around the world have different definitions of what is, or is not, a spice, depending upon whether their culture uses the material as condiments in traditional cooking. Resins and roots are exceptions as they are usually only distilled from the part of the plant that defines their category, the resin or the root. The fruities also tend to be categorized under one heading although, for example, cardamom and pimento berry are also classified as spices. Do not let these overlaps bother you — they don't bother nature, which, although simply beautiful, is also beautifully complex.

Moving On

It is not the purpose of aroma-genera to have everyone neatly classified under one group. Indeed, it is possible that the most highly evolved persons carry the abundant self-characteristics of all groups. So, for example, the ideal person might have the enthusiasm of a floral, the good nature of a fruitie, the practical caring skills of an herbie, the vision of a leafie, the wisdom of a resinie, the peace making qualities of a rootie, the spirituality of a seedie, the joy of a spicie and the courage of a woodie. However, none of us are this perfect. All we can do is aim to be as positive as we can, given the real life circumstances we have to deal with.

Only you truly know where your weak points are. You might think you need to get out more and meet people and get more stimulus, or you may feel that you need to be more in touch with your spiritual self. Only you may know how depressed you can get, or how isolated you can feel. The aim of aroma-genera is not only to help you identify these weak areas, but help you adjust your personality so the negatives have less influence and impact on you. We want to replace the negative with the positive, and with essential oils you can literally do that. You can add a drop of joyfulness, or a drop of spirituality, in the form of essential oils that deliver those qualities. Nature *adds* positivity — and it comes in no form more concentrated than in essential oils.

The fact is that people do change for the better. It is not a question of becoming "better" as far as other people are concerned, but "better" as far as *you* are concerned, and that is judged in terms of happiness as well as in terms of good health. These are the natural states, in which we feel most at ease. Aroma-genera helps us attain this ease, this fulfillment, but it cannot be done overnight. Aim first to identify which group(s) you belong to, and aim to become the abundant self of those groups, gradually adding a bit of this, a bit of that, making yourself a fully-rounded individual. This will not be the aim of everyone. Many people will be perfectly happy, and rightly so, being their abundant self within the context of one group. That may be their destiny, and they may have great things to achieve in that aroma-genera group. We are all individuals with individual hopes, expectations, and desires. It is not for us to dictate what makes a person "perfect," but for each individual to establish that for themselves. And, we have the measure — a happy, smiling face.

The following groupings are examples of essential oils and absolutes that fall into the nine aroma-genera groups. Following these are the nine aroma-genera human personality groups.

Florals are defined as those essential oils (and absolutes) that are extracted from the flowers or petals of plants or trees.

FLORALS

Boronia, Cananga, Carnation, Cassia, Chamomile German, Chamomile Roman, Champaca, Genet, Helichrysum,

Hyacinth, Jasmine, Lavender, Lemon Flower, Linden Blossom, Marigold, Melilotus, Mimosa, Narcissus, Neroli, Ormenis Flower, Osmanthus, Rose Maroc, Rose Otto, Tagetes, Tuberose, Ylang Ylang

Fruities are defined as those essential oils that are extracted from the fruit of a plant or tree. For example:

FRUITIES

Bergamot, Black Pepper, Cardamom, Clove, Cubebs, Grapefruit, Hops, Juniper, Lemon, Lime, Litsea Cubeba (May Chang), Mandarin, Orange, Pimento Berry, Schinus Molle, Tangerine, Tonka Bean, Vanilla, Mace

Herbies are defined as those essential oils that are extracted from plants generally thought of as herbs.

HERBIES

Basil, Calamintha, Clary Sage, Geranium, Hyssop, Lovage, Marjoram, Melissa, Peppermint, Spearmint, Oregano, Rosemary, Sage, Thyme Red, Thyme Linalol, Thyme Lemon, Yarrow

Leafies are defined as essential oils that are extracted from leaves of trees or plants.

LEAFIES

Bay, Birch, Buchu, Cajeput, Cinnamon, Cistus, Cypress, Eucalyptus, Eucalyptus Lemon, Eucalyptus Peppermint, Eucalyptus Radiata, Fir, Myrtle, Niaouli, Patchouli, Petitgrain, Pine, Ravensara, Tea Tree, Violet Leaf

Resinies are defined as essential oils that are extracted from the resin or balsam which exudes from trees or shrubs.

RESINIES

Benzoin, Canadian Balsam, Copaiba Balsam, Peru Balsam, Tolu Balsam, Borneol, Elemi, Frankincense, Galbanham, Myrrh, Opopanax, Styrax Levant

Rooties are defined as essential oils that are extracted from the roots of plants.

ROOTIES

Angelica, Galangal, Ginger, Orris, Snakeroot, Spikenard, Tumeric, Valerian, Vetiver

Seedies are defined as essential oils that are extracted from the seeds of plants.

SEEDIES

Ambrette Seed, Angelica Seed, Anise (Star), Aniseed, Caraway, Carrot Seed, Coriander, Cumin, Dill, Fennel (Sweet), Nutmeg, Parsley Seed

Spicies are defined as essential oils that are extracted from various parts of plants or trees commonly known as "spicies."

SPICIES

Anise, Aniseed, Black Pepper, Caraway, Cinnamon, Clove, Coriander, Cubebs, Cumin, Galangal, Ginger, Mace, Nutmeg, Pimento Berry, Turmeric

Woodies are defined as essential oils that are extracted from twigs, wood, chippings or shavings from trees.

WOODIES

Amyris, Cabreuva, Cade, Camphor White, Cascarilla Bark, Cedarwood, Guaiacwood, Linaloe, Pine, Rosewood, Sandalwood, Spruce, Cinnamon

The Nine Personality Groups

Florals

Aspirations: To have status and be admired, to be impressive and stand out from the crowd.

Florals Abundant Self Can Be:

Attractive, enterprising, artistic, well-liked, energetic, dynamic, confident, loving, genuine, flexible, seeking self-improvement, ambitious, enthusiastic, passionate, sensuous, desirable, high ideals, striving for perfection and excellence, inner-directed and aesthetic nature.

The floral type makes the best of themselves physically, are good fun and well-liked. Their lives are filled with enthusiasm, energy, and enterprise — dynamism in other words. They are totally confident and ambitious, not in a nasty way but positive to achieve something in this world and aim to have fun while doing it. Love blossoms from them when in the abundant state and they are passionate, sensuous and very, very desirable. Self-improvement is their aim, which is part of the striving for perfection. The floral type loves perfumes and anything that makes them feel good. Being extremely tactile, they'll choose to wear the best suit they can afford, preferably in the lightest, most flowing wool or silk material. If they wear jeans, they'll have a designer label, or the pair that has the most style credibility at any given time. The house will always be full of flowers and plants, scents, candles, and music. Florals have a very aesthetic nature.

Although they can appear very superficial, florals are very sensitive, soft-hearted individuals, who can pick up on the most subtle mood changes in others and will try their hardest to uplift spirits if they are down. Florals bring a lot of happiness and joy into this gray world and will help other people in any practical way they can — in terms of adding beauty to life. Although very caring, trusting, and naive in many situations, florals are often the object of jealousy, and much misunderstood.

Florals Generally Are:

Flirtatious, romantic, sexual, full of fantasies, seductive, caring, vulnerable, sensitive, concerned with appearance, image and status conscious, pretentious, competitive, conceited, friendly, successful, exhibitionist, self-promoting, self-important, calculating, unrealistic dreamers.

From an early age, about 1 minute old, the floral personality starts to utilize their powers of flirtation — on daddy if it's a girl, and mommy if it's a boy. This will develop later into great powers of seduction — made possible by the fact that they are very sexual. Full of fantasies, the young floral girl will have her head full of princes on white horses and she will have her wedding planned down to the choice of dress and bouquet of flowers. Florals worry about other people and are very inquisitive, especially when discussing other people's romantic liaisons. They never feel guilt — it is simply not in them, or if it is they just blank it out, particularly when it concerns them.

Florals are very much concerned with their appearance, are narcissistic, image and status conscious, and can be totally pretentious. Competition is part of their nature, especially when it comes to love and romance. In a group of teen-agers, a floral goes forward and starts talk-ing to the group of the opposite sex, wanting to get there first and monopolize the most attractive. Florals will use their sexuality for everything. Floral women have no feelings of being inferior to men and will employ every trick in the book to get what they want from them, including short skirts and very high heels. They are not exploited, but exploiting. "Go for it," could be their catch phrase, to which you could add, "And never mind how." Self-assurance marks florals and they get this confidence in themselves because they feel desirable. They are charming and popular and will appear to be very nice people, even though in their minds they may be thinking what an awful dress you're wearing. Florals are very artistic, lovers of dance, art, music — all the good things in life. Generally, florals are very successful, or have attached themselves to someone who is very successful. They feel very self-important and will self-promote without any compunction. Florals are calculating, exhibitionist, and unrealistic dreamers.

Reward is the word that is etched into the mind of the floral type. If they don't have the reward of someone's admiration, life is not worth living. If they don't have a lover who can provide this reward of admiration, they're desperate, half-people, people-in-waiting. They believe them-selves to be outstanding and they need to be shown to be that — the winner who gets all the acclaim and admiration. Their image is extremely important to them. It gives them credibility, so packaging them-selves is a number one priority — so they can get the rewards they cannot live with-out: love, money, success.

Florals Impoverished Self Can Be:

Insensitive, exploitative, manipulative, underhanded, devious, disloyal, envious, power-crazed, vindictive, liars, saboteurs, have difficulty in loving and sharing, have shallow values.

The floral type can be insensitive and exploitative and have very shallow values. They can become manipulative, power-crazed liars, even viscous, malevolent, and underhanded. Impoverished florals can be deceptive and misleading if that suits their purpose. Driven by their need to have the greatest status, florals can be disloyal and betray. Driven by a jealousy of other people's success, they will sabo-tage that person's plans to gain the advan-tage. This can even extend to interfering with other people's lives and relationships because this gives florals a sense of tri-umph and power. When impoverished, the ability to truly love goes, although sex can still be employed as a tool to get what they want. They feel no compunction in marrying for money and then taking on lovers. They can have a problem with inti-macy and commitment (because there is always someone better over the hill), and can be phony.

The floral type cannot help comparing their lives with other people's and are very serious social climbers — opportunistic, calculating, and pragmatic. They have grandiose ideas about themselves — imagining themselves living in huge houses with a big drive (if they don't have it already), impressing people with the huge diamond ring on their hands. Florals will self-pityingly cry for hours if they think that will achieve them something, but they'll be wearing waterproof mascara and looking over their hankie to make sure they are getting the reaction they want. When people don't take floral's advice they can become arrogant and contemptuous. Their exhibitionist nature can lead them into behavior that borders on the decadent.

Fruities

Aspirations: to feel harmony within themselves, have security, respect and approval.

Fruities Abundant Self Can Be:

Appealing, lovable, engaging, faithful, loyal, trustworthy, reliable, dependable, dedicated, cooperative, companionable, bright, joyful, emotionally balanced, independent, self-aware, enthusiastic, nice to be with, passionate, sensuous, inspirational, empathetic, benevolent.

If you are an employer looking for the perfect employee, the fruitie is for you. This personality is hard working, friendly, committed, supportive, and encouraging, plus they take responsibility (both for the task in hand and for themselves) but do not have great ambition and will not be after your job. This personality loves seeing projects to fruition and will enthusiastically put all their energies into something, saying, "Let's make this work." And they can make it happen because they are great organizers.

Fruities are self-aware, emotionally balanced and are usually very nice, happy people. They are liked by almost everyone because of their engaging positivity and friendliness. In fact, fruities are a sheer delight to be around because they're bright, joyful, and playful, and have an altogether benevolent character. This makes them appealing, endearing, and lovable. In addition (their good qualities are many), fruities have empathy with others, and are inspirational. Fruities are faithful and dependable to their friends, as well as to their bosses, and are sensuous and passionate with their lovers.

Fruities Generally Are:

Compliant, dutiful, conventional, organizers, respectful, submissive, jovial, willing to please, supportive, assertive, self-confident, realistic, loving, artistic, emotionally-secure, endearing, responsive, committed, rebellious, dislike authority.

You can't define a fruitie as introvert or extrovert, because they swing between the two in equal proportion. These are the kind of people who keep their friendships from primary school right through life, even to the grave. Although they have many acquaintances, they have few they would call true, deep friends but they offer to all jovial companionship. Fruities are supremely self-confident, which can make them very familiar with other people, not in an unpleasant way but just as an aspect of their warmth, which is rooted in their loving nature. Fruities have a great need to belong, and will make sure that relationships with friends and family are good. This is easy for them to achieve because they are very willing to please, even compliant and dutiful when the rest of us have run. Their respectful nature can turn into a submissive one, although generally fruities are assertive. Bonding is extremely important to fruities, and if their trust is broken, they will be devastated. Fruities can be taken advantage of and when this occurs they become anxious and depressed, quite unlike their usual selves.

Fruities need to express themselves and are very creative in their relationships. They have a very independent nature, great faith in themselves, and tremendous courage. Although fruities are conventional, they do have a rebellious streak and can react against authority if they believe it is behaving unjustly.

Fruities Impoverished Self Can Be:

Contradictory, indecisive, hesitant, cautious, defensive, insecure, clingy, anxious, unreasonable, self-sacrificing, illogical, self-abasing, impatient, oversensitive, disheartened, stagnant, devious, spiteful, sarcastic, immature, masochistic, aggressive, have feelings of inferiority.

It is very sad to see a fruitie impoverished, which can happen if they are taken advantage of, or become world-weary and

depressed. They can become tired and faded, defensive, and indecisive. The fresh, child-like quality that was once so appealing now becomes immaturity and a tendency to cling to other people. They become full of inferiority complexes, untypically insecure. Self-criticism takes over, along with self-sacrifice and servility and, in bad cases, masochistic actions. Disheartened with life and people, the fruitie stagnates and stays at home, becoming more and more impatient, touchy, and oversensitive, and aggressive if people try to help. To protect themselves from prying people, devious methods are subconsciously employed to avoid being used and hurt again. A sharp tongue and spitefulness are sure signs of their impoverishment.

Herbies

Aspirations: To love and be loved unconditionally, to be appreciated and needed.

Herbies Abundant Self Can Be:

Loving, empathetic, charitable, compassionate, unselfish, big-hearted, humanitarian, bounteous, generous, welcoming, caring, supportive, helpful, giving, encouraging.

Herbies are the salt of the earth. They will fix your fence, make sure the old folk down the road are secure when there's been a snowstorm, and collect food parcels for charitable organizations. Not only do they do any little job you ask them to do, they'll see where they can help and do it before you ask. In fact, they are always looking for things to do for people. So, for example, if an herbie is in the garden and sees a plant that would look nice crawling up your fence, they'll take a cutting and give it to you. Herbies are nice, solid, dependable people. If your father is an herbie and you have a crisis, he'll take it on for you, and sort it out so you can get on with your life. Herbies never overcharge on a job. They're steady, reliable, and constant. Herbies want to give service, whether that is in the form of ironing your shirts, taking out the garbage, baking you a cake — anything. They are always helpful, giving, and generous. Thoughtfulness is their middle name. They plan ahead to help people, doing whatever they can or whatever they think people might need. If you've ever wondered who buys birthday calendar books, it's herbies. They never forget a birthday. Herbies are interested in other people and consider it a privilege to be allowed into their lives.

Herbies Generally Are:

Friendly, congenial, sympathetic, neighborly, welcoming, well-intentioned, emotional, demonstrative, motherly/fatherly, self-sacrificing, complacent, enthusiastic, smothering, gushing, nosy, down-to-earth.

This group is sympathetic and have good intentions. They are the stay-at-homers, which is where they really want to be. Herbie females can be made to feel inferior by those feminists who think all women need to be fulfilled in some area outside the home. Herbies need to be at home and are happiest there — preferably with a friend sitting on the sofa having a cup of tea and telling them all the latest drama in their lives. Although male herbies will go down to the bar with his pals, they secretly wish they were in their garage or workshop — which is not an escape to them, but an extension of their home where they can do "man" things. Herbies feel themselves to have been given the saintly role, and they are very charitable and humble and worry about everyone and everything. They're very demonstrative, give a lot of attention and flattery, and can be overenthusiastic. They love to talk about love, and some herbies hug a lot, putting their arms around you and so on.

Herbies can be extremely nosy. They'll exasperatingly ask question after question, never ending. The reason they do this is that they are living vicariously through other people. Although they are happy, herbie's own lives are not usually very exciting so they enjoy listening to other people's exciting experiences. If you've climbed a mountain and tell an herbie about it, they have climbed the mountain too. This is where they get their excitement, and without something to get nosy about they can get miserable. Gossip is as important as food to them, it feeds their imagination. This is the way they balance their stay-at-home lives. This is usually okay for women, who invariably have their pulse on what's going on, but men can get left out so the herbie male will badger his wife until she gives him the latest neighborhood gossip, while the herbie female will badger her male partner to get the office gossip.

Herbies have great empathy and feeling for others. They are caring and sincere, warm-hearted, and encouraging. They genuinely want people to succeed. They will appreciate you if you appreciate them. They see the good in others — which can backfire on them sometimes and they get hurt. But they often disparage themselves, thinking they should be doing more with their lives. They can also feel undeserving. Herbies do their best for other people, often at the expense of themselves, and often they do too much. This is the type that keeps everything and everyone together — that is their role in life, and they know it.

Paula is a typical herbie. The mother of five children, Paula keeps a chart of the children's many activities, which she organizes with military precision, ferrying them all to their various classes and activities. She also manages to find time to make clothes, cakes, jams, and chutneys. Her husband doesn't have to lift a finger and wouldn't even dream of changing a toilet roll. When the demands of a family are not enough, Paula also has her elderly mother to organize and care about, the garden to tend, and the meals she cooks and delivers for the homeless. Non-herbies often wonder how it is physically possible to organize so many people and activities, but it is possible because herbies usually engage in few activities for their personal satisfaction and have very little social life.

Herbies Impoverished Self Can Be:
Resentful, anguished, exploitative, manipulative, domineering, demanding,
self-serving, slovenly, guilt-inflicting, sympathy-seeking, psychosomatically ill, a martyr, a hypochondriac.

Herbies can resent the fact that they seem to do everything for other people and don't usually realize that this is a drive within them. They may feel resentful, but they still can't help themselves taking on everyone's little jobs. The herbie type can become very smothering. They don't like the children to leave home and will not understand why they do this unless it's for a good reason, like getting married or getting a job in another town. "Why are you leaving?," they ask, "I do everything for you, your washing, cooking...." They pretend not to understand the natural desire to break free. When the children leave home, a whole source of information and vicarious living leaves too. Herbies can feel a void in their lives, which they usually fill with long telephone conversations after which, vicariously refreshed with new input, they can enjoy an evening watching soap operas and eating the cake they just made. They may say to themselves, "I'll get a little part time job to occupy myself," although they don't really want to because they're much happier puttering around the house.

One of herbie's failings is to get too intimate — until the person gets so exasperated they cut off all contact. This causes withdrawal symptoms in the herbie, who feels they are entitled to the information. This is when the herbie can become very intrusive and turn nasty — "How dare you not tell me everything." They hover around, wanting to meddle in everything and find out all they can about your business.

When they're impoverished, herbies want a *lot* of thanks — to be over-thanked. Indeed, all the favors have to be repaid. They can also get very possessive and jealous of the people they have helped over the years. Although, in fact, many of the jobs they have done for people were less for those people than for themselves — because they needed something to occupy themselves, just as they need to be involved in other people's lives. In a negative frame of mind, they can exaggerate their usefulness to other people so, for example, if you ask them to go and buy you a carton of milk they will do this but tell other people they had to buy you a week's groceries because you had nothing in the house.

Herbies will complain that they've never done anything for themselves, always for other people, and that nobody appreciates them. Guilt will be inflicted on all those concerned, and will be used as a form of manipulation. Hypochondria and psychosomatic illnesses will develop.

Leafies

Aspirations: To connect with the environment, understand the global perspective and gain wisdom.

Leafies Abundant Self Can Be:

Visionary, knowledgeable, creative, wise, ingenious, perceptive, innovative, intuitive, focused, insightful, cooperative, observant, attentive, understanding, involved, inspirational, enlivening, rejuvenating, contributive.

The leafies are the wise visionaries who know where we have come from and where we're in danger of going. These people's minds are always alert, they take in everything in an instant, shake it down into its component parts and store it away for future reference. Knowledge is their sustenance and they'll spend hours in libraries, getting more of it. They want to understand the world, the universe and everything, and often do. Einstein was probably a leafie, as many brilliant geniuses are. Lateral thinking is a standard procedure for this type of person, as is looking at things holistically. Because they are innovative thinkers, often inventors, they're quite likely to have several original theories kicking around at the same time. The intellectual leeches of this world hang around leafies, hoping to pick up clues, often grasping them and presenting them to others as their own.

The leafie is not only extremely curious and knowledgeable, but also, perceptive, intuitive, focused, insightful, and inspired. Hard work and concentration doesn't frighten leafies and they'll research a subject thoroughly, from top to bottom, so they have all the details to consider. Although they can become very specialized in their particular field, they never lose sight of the whole. These are profoundly creative people, intellectually, and they have an ingenious, original approach. No research lab should be without one.

Leafies Generally Are:

Cerebral, thoughtful, logical, solitary, introspective, idealistic, imaginative, extremist, revolutionary, detached, complicated, non-conformist, invigorating, refreshing, stimulating, vulnerable, melancholic.

Leafies are pacifists and can't abide aggression in any form. If an intellectual rival starts shouting or being rude, leafies wince as if receiving actual blows to the head. Although often categorized as intellectuals, leafies are complicated individuals interested in subjects well outside their usual fields of inquiry, which may have nothing to do with academic pursuits. They are genuinely interested in what people have to say because, with their lateral thinking, they can see relevance to their own interests in many diverse subjects. These are the networkers, who can link facts from ten specialist areas and see a new law of nature.

Because leafies spend so much time thinking, they can forget to experience life and when they do, it can all come as a bit of a shock to the system. They can react to the new input in bizarre ways, trying to incorporate the different levels of experience into one whole. Personally, leafies are thoughtful, introspective, detached, and solitary. Politically, they are idealistic and sometimes extremist. If you were to meet a leafie at a party you'd say to yourself, "Here is an eccentric and nonconformist," and you'd listen in wonder as they expounded on everything under the sun, often coming up with some very original ideas. Esoteric knowledge is, for leafies, just like any other knowledge — there to be researched and understood.

However, leafies can suffer intellectual delusions, almost as if reality were not important. They are also very vulnerable to criticism and can feel threatened by the slightest word. Melancholia can settle over this personality very easily and they can retreat into solitude and refuse to answer the phone.

Leafies Impoverished Can Be:

Compulsive, obsessive, paranoid, cynical, scornful, hostile, hypersensitive, easily intimidated, mean, vulnerable, foolhardy, critical, confused, defeatist, suppressed, prone to insanity.

Although leafies are brilliant, they can be wrong sometimes. When they're impoverished, they refuse to accept it. They'll take great umbrage if people disagree with them. Intellectually, they can reduce a subject so much it doesn't reflect the whole reality, and may make inaccurate conclusions because they can ignore facts that don't fit into their theory. This foolhardiness is not the only danger — they can also become stale.

On a more personal level, the impoverished leafie can become compulsive, ill-humored, scornful, and defeatist. Recluses are often impoverished leafies, who already have a leaning toward secretiveness and isolation. Mental instability is also a danger at this time, starting with melancholy, confusion and suspicion, even paranoia, and going on to delusions and obsessions. Impoverished leafies can become out-of-touch.

Resinies

Aspirations: to have position and purpose.

Resinies Abundant Self Can Be:
*Liberal, charitable, merciful, wise,
nonjudgmental, reasonable, realistic,
balanced, conscientious, moralistic,
ethical, objective, fair-minded, truthful,
spiritual, sagacious, sympathetic,
principled, honest, kind, caring,
benevolent.*

Morality, truth and justice are the forces that drive this personality, often into professions that can utilize these over-riding concerns in a practical way. Right and wrong are the signposts that direct their lives, and purity of thought is their ideal state of mind. Ethical considerations are behind their every move; spirituality is their goal. If all judges were resinies we would have no doubts about the legal system because justice would most certainly prevail. Realism and tolerance temper their advice, which is given honestly and with genuine care. Although they have such high expectations of themselves, resinies have a basic human charity that allows them to relate to others with a nonthreatening, kindly air. These people command respect because their high principles are obvious for all to see. It directs their every move and can be heard in their every word.

Resinies Generally Are:
Perfectionists, efficient, orderly, strong-willed, knowledgeable, balanced, persistent, persuasive, campaigners, workaholics, self-controlled, high-minded, utopian, precise, difficult, responsible, emotionally withdrawn, religious fanatics.

What the resinies are aiming for is a spiritually perfect life, so, if they believe in reincarnation, they will not have to return to this earth again, or if they believe in heaven and hell, they will be going in the right direction. Resinies are very helpful to people, allowing them to off load their spiritual concerns onto them. Resinie's heart is in the right place — each and every day. They know very well their responsibility to the planet and to the human race, even if they don't realize they have a right for a little sustenance and fun too. That may, in fact, be the point of it all. Resinies need to become less the bombastic pulpit-basher and more the laughing, joking Tibetan monk.

Driven as they are by high ideals, the resinie works constantly trying to personally stop the tide of wrong-doing and disharmony in the world. They don't much like parties unless they think there might be someone there who can contribute to their latest altruistic or campaigning project and who, faced with resinie's persuasive arguments and persistence, will usually be persuaded to contribute. Their strong wills carry resinies forward, like explorers across the huge frozen wastes of Antarctica, plodding step by small, painful step toward their goal. Hardship doesn't bother them, they take it all in stride, falling back on their organization and efficiency, which will see them through to the end. Often, people find them difficult because they can be one-dimensional and, frankly, not much fun.

Resinies are not concerned with sensual beauty, preferring spiritual beauty. It's not that they don't *like* sensual beauty or beautiful things, but these things are incidental in their life. Because resinies find it difficult to relax and enjoy themselves, a drop or two of a floral essential oil does them a great deal of good, providing balance. Although generally warm and caring, resinies can also sometimes be emotionally withdrawn, while repressing their sexuality can be resinie's way of denying their human state. Promiscuity holds no interest whatsoever for them.

Resinies Impoverished Self Can Be:

Critical, indignant, angry, unbalanced, abrasive, arrogant, proud, intolerant, menacing, obstinate, dogmatic, unprincipled, judgmental, discouraged, depressed, rash, deprived.

If resinies make a moral mistake they are desolate and find it difficult to forgive themselves. If they are critical, they are most critical of themselves. The constant drive for perfection takes a terrible toll on resinies because they become disappointed with people, themselves and life in general. They can break like a twig under the foot of reality. When they're impoverished, resinies can become self-righteous, dogmatic, abrasive, intolerant, and very, very angry.

If things do not progress forward in a positive manner, and people are a disappointment, discouragement sets in, often leading to nervousness and depression. Resinies feel it is them against the negative forces, so when they're impoverished, there is a strong sense of being threatened. Battle weary, they reproach themselves for their lack of success. Perfectionists as they are, especially in regard to themselves, if they've made a mistake resinies are overcome with shame, guilt, and self-reproach, which is difficult to shake off until they realize that they, too, are human.

Rooties

Aspirations: to have union with everything and traditional values; peacemaker.

Rooties Abundant Self Can Be:

Peaceful, responsive, open-minded, helpful, hopeful, patient, strong-minded, supportive, encouraging, loyal, assured, content, composed, tranquil, unpretentious, kind, caring, good-natured, observant, giving, thoughtful, unselfish, humble, solid, reliable, loyal.

Rooties are very good-natured, easygoing, laid-back and serene. They accept life as it is. The whole world might be in a panic but rootie can dismiss it all, unbothered. Stability is a definite characteristic of this personality as they can accept everything with equanimity, perhaps because they trust themselves and others. Some people might dismiss them as naive because they are simple souls, unpretentious, and gentle, but they also have a capacity to be profound. This is the peacemaker — ever kind and supportive, always making people feel comfortable. If you've had a fight or been made miserable, these are the people to visit because their healing influence will make you feel better simply from being around them. Partly, this reassuring quality is made possible by the fact that they are caring and deeply receptive. Rooties are generally very nice people, always willing to help anyone with their plans, giving encouragement and offering genuine optimism. Rooties are assured in an unpretentious sort of way, composed, solid, and rather more strong-minded than one might at first expect.

Rooties are the ultimate mediators because they are fundamentally harmonizers and healers. Because they are complete in themselves, they can establish profound relationships with all kinds of people, which instills an air of trust when disputes come to be settled. People will take rooties' advice, realizing that peace is their ultimate goal, and because they are impressed by their great dignity. Among their many good qualities are humility, a capacity to give, great powers of observation, reliability, and loyalty.

Rooties Generally Are:

Easygoing, passive, good listeners, down-to-earth, dedicated, try to please, put others first, originality, dislike change, modest, pacifier, controlled, conventional, traditionalists, environmentalists, satisfied.

It's easy to pass the rootie by unnoticed. They don't have the flamboyance of a floral or the obvious drive of a woodie. Some people might call them a plodder,

although they do have original ideas, but they are not sparkling in an obvious sense and so are often misunderstood as dull. Rooties have many very good qualities without which the world would be a less gracious place. They are modest, dedicated, and genuinely aim to please. Composed and controlled, they will step in as the most effective peacemaker.

Rooties could be called conventional traditionalists because they dislike change almost as much as they dislike arguments and disruptions. They'll turn a blind eye to any problem and leave things to sort themselves out. Rooties only see what they want to see and ignore the rest. If the wife or husband is having an affair, rootie will "blank" it out and if their child is being bullied at school, they'll say, "Oh yes dear, you'll sort it out," — or, in other words, don't bring disputes into the house. This stubborn denial of problems, the walking away from conflict, is a form of unresponsiveness and it gets them into serious relationship problems, ironically perhaps. They must decide whether they are really satisfied with their lives, or merely resigned to it.

Rooties ideal life would be to live in the country in a nice cottage, leading a quiet conventional life. Ecology is one of their main concerns. Of all the personality types, rooties are grounded firmly in this earth, which gives them great stability.

Rooties Impoverished Self Can Be:

Neglectful, suppressed, obstinate, disorganized, confused, muddled, easily upset, listless, slack, absent-minded, disinterested, moody, uncaring, down-hearted, sad, low-spirited, sneaky, apathetic, depressed, emotionally weak.

Rooties have to watch out that they do not become too submissive — the doormat type — especially if they are female and are linked to a woodie partner. This tendency stems from their adherence to sexually stereotyped roles, an aspect of their basic conventionality. They can take on too much and, if there's a crisis, collapse into an apathetic heap. Obstinacy is a way they handle conflict, which is of course an anathema to them. The impoverished rootie can be neglectful, disorganized, low-spirited, easily upset, and depressed. Inertia overtakes them and they become emotionally very weak and unstable. If they have been suppressing their opinions (probably in the name of peace), they can become caustic, moody, and sneaky. You can tell whether a rootie is in an impoverished state because they become unfocused and start going on and on endlessly — moaning, muddled, and confused. Disinterest overtakes them as they retreat into themselves. Feeling lost is a classic symptom of an impoverished rootie who needs, at all times, to be grounded.

Seedies

Aspiration: to create beauty and understanding in themselves and others.

Seedies Abundant Self Can Be:

Creative, inspirational, intuitive, knowledgeable, full-of-life, energetic, mindful, observant, considerate, self-aware, honest,

emotionally balanced, harmonious, non-judgmental, sensorial, sensitive, honest, forthright, virtuous, genuine, joyful.

The seedie personality strives to be spiritually rich. Their powers of intuition are so finely tuned they can pick up other people's feelings as if they were radios picking up waves from all the radio transmitters. This intuition is also apparent when it comes to themselves. They know what is and what isn't right for them. They are very much in touch with their feelings. Seedie personalities are sensitive, self-aware, considerate, and insightful.

Seedies have a remarkable ability to go through the same experience over and over again, going to the corner store for example, seeing it and feeling it as a completely new experience each time. It is as if everything is new and exciting, and they notice something new on each trip, marveling at it all. These powers of observation contribute to their considerable creativity, which is occasionally nothing short of inspirational. Not only are they observant — the information goes into their minds and stays there, stored away for future use — seedies are totally alive, aware, sensitive, mindful, and energetic.

Beauty is like spring water to the seedy, it is what uplifts them and makes their lives rich. Romance too is vital to their well being. Seedies have an uncanny ability to avoid bad situations by just sliding away, and, if anyone could do it, the seedie could hitchhike around the world without coming against any trouble because their intuition would sense danger around corners. Another extraordinary capacity is to change like a chameleon, and seedies are constantly reinventing themselves, changing their job or appearance in a flash. One endearing quality is that they don't take themselves too seriously, and another is that they are true to themselves and those around them. Seedies are honest, forthright, virtuous, funny, and joyful. A few are also geniuses.

Seedies Generally Are:

Imaginative, creative, artistic, self-assured, introverted, expressive, caring, giving, spiritual, overly sensitive, deeply feeling, fragile, misunderstood, uncertain, insightful, intuitive, self-sacrificing, amiable, tolerant, even-tempered, self-indulgent, dreamers, harmonized.

Seedies are delicate souls, sometimes overly sensitive, and deeply feeling. This can give them a fragile quality and, indeed, they can be hurt. Florals and seedies make a disastrous combination in a relationship, but a woodie personality can stabilize seedie and bring them down from their dreaming world of beauty and wonders. Generally, they are emotionally balanced with inner harmony, well able to deal with their own feelings but, in certain circumstances, they will withdraw, become shy, and not go outside the front door if they can help it. Indeed, seedies are perfectly happy on their own and can go weeks without seeing anybody, getting on with whatever they are doing, enjoying the chance to grow in their own space, taking time to explore activities that enhance their state of consciousness.

Crowds make seedies feel self-conscious, perhaps because they are so sensitive to everyone's feelings they imagine people can see through them too. They can be very hurt by people, lovers in particular, and are often manipulated, used, or taken advantage of by less-evolved souls. Seedies perhaps give too much of themselves — part of their self-sacrificing, over-tolerant nature. Respect of others is seedie's starting point in relationships, and they will be discreet to a remarkable degree, yet, if you find yourself in conversation with a stranger who suddenly tells you something profoundly revealing and honest about themselves, it's probably a seedie.

Seedies are quite easy to recognize because they are highly individualistic and stand out in a crowd. They are sensual, gentle, and rather too generous for their own good. If they are criticized, they'll swallow it bravely, possibly because they do have self-doubts, but can be hypersensitive, vulnerable, and easily hurt. They are often misunderstood.

Seedies Impoverished Self Can Be:

Self-pitying, melancholy, disillusioned, disrespectful, disdainful, hopeless, self-destructive, emotionally cold, apprehensive, suspicious, aloof, contemptuous, alienated, lost to reality, emotionally burned out.

When seedies become emotionally overwhelmed or mentally exhausted, depression can set in. The negativity is often turned inward so they become insecure with feelings of worthlessness, and have no hope for themselves. The self-indulgent streak, which is usually harmless, becomes, when they are impoverished, an addictive personality — perhaps turning to alcohol or drugs. Emotional burnout causes seedies to become suspicious, undemonstrative and emotionally cold. Self-pity, melancholy, and disillusionment become the order of the day and seedie feels like an outsider, an observer of life, unwilling to join in. Even their creativity disappears, and despite occasional flurries of activity it proves to be unproductive, like the writer who types page after page but is dissatisfied with them all and throws them all in the trash, or the painter who paints over canvases, never getting it right.

Spicies

Aspirations: To have it all — the hedonistic lifestyle.

Spicies Abundant Self Can Be:

Joyous, zealous, animated, exhilarating, appreciative, fascinating, charming, magnanimous, vivacious, sparkling, congenial, warm-hearted, debonair, gracious, loving, seductive, self-assured, practical, dynamic, multifaceted.

The spicie's personality is joyous, exhilarating, and animated. When Londoners were huddled in the tunnels of the underground system during World War II, it would have been spicies who started the singing, "It's a long way to Tipperary, it's a long way to go . . . ," lifting everyone's spirits. Spicies love life and at their best are sparkling, happy, warm-hearted, sponta-

neous, and entertaining. As the ultimate sensation-seekers, they can be very seductive personalities. Spicies can be very intelligent people, multifaceted and multitalented, and are also extremely productive and practical — a combination that can lead to a brilliant career. They are often entrepreneurs, but in any case dynamic, go-getting achievers. Spicies are dynamic and self-assured with a zealous appreciation of life. Their energy and intelligence can make them fascinating people, and at their best they are charming and loving.

Spicies Generally Are:

Extroverted, entrepreneurial, connoisseurs, materialistic, sophisticated, exhibitionists, pleasure-seekers, entertaining, achievers, dynamic, sensationalist, passionate, emotional, power seeking, status seeking, perfectionists, attentive, controlling, arrogant, overconfident, willful.

You can recognize spicies from their over-the-top reactions to everything. If you were looking at Niagara Falls the spicie would be saying, "It's fabulous, just fabulous" in a very loud voice. Nobody reacts as strongly as they do, to everything. If you do something for them, their gratitude and appreciation gushes forth in a torrent. Spicies are extremely excitable and definitely extroverts. They get excited about everything, especially those things that relate to them. Indeed, they can spend so much time thinking and talking about themselves, they can forget that other people have far greater problems or stories they'd like to tell if only they could get a word in edgewise.

I can think of one, a brilliant linguist for whom the authorities had to make a special dispensation so she could go to Cambridge University at age sixteen. One friend went on vacation with her and said she spent so long getting herself made up and dressed (a major preoccupation of spicies) by the time they reached the beach it was too hot and they had to go in again. Exasperating was the word mentioned. Nevertheless, these two remained friends and over the years have had tremendous fun going to zillions of parties and clubs in the spicie's gold Rolls Royce.

Spicies have got to have money, which doesn't interest them from a power point of view, only a spending one, and they can shop till they drop. Their wardrobes will be full of clothes they never wear and their cupboards are full of special gourmet treats they simply couldn't resist buying. If they don't have money they'll go mad with the credit cards or find some way to pretend they have masses of cash, like borrowing friends' most expensive clothes. Spicies are deeply materialistic and will, if necessary, attach themselves to someone who can indulge them. Also, if they have the money themselves, they'll have young men or women playmates to enjoy life with. Spicies do not know how to deny themselves. For them life is there to enjoy.

Spicies are the pleasure-seekers of this world, often connoisseurs of art, antiques and all the beautiful things in life. They are worldly, sophisticated people (or wish to be), and, often, their aim in life is to be a socialite. They can be great trendsetters and, sometimes, shockingly exhibitionistic. Generally, spicies are selfish but fun.

Spicies Impoverished Self Can Be:

Superficial, insensitive, boorish, discourteous, impolite, ill-mannered, impulsive, debauched, compulsive, mean, shabby, loathsome, greedy, self-centered, jealous, demanding, resentful, hysterical, panicky, depressed.

I remember once meeting a Brazilian diplomat who was the classic impoverished spicie. Having had full opportunity over the years to indulge himself in life's pleasures, he sat there totally jaded. Nothing would excite him, even the two young girls bought in for the purpose. He sat there in his silk Givenchy shirt and very expensive suit with a large scotch in his hand, a tray of caviar on the table in front and the two nubile floozies on either side and he looked completely miserable! — the debauchee at the end of the road, with no pleasure left to explore, no new exciting purchase to be made, burned out, and bored.

Spicies can become impoverished both by such burnout and by frustration of their dreams. At their worst, spicies are superficial, impatient, insensitive, boorish, crude, demanding, resentful, self-destructive, mean, and impolite. I say "impolite," but that's being polite because impoverished spicies can actually be extremely rude and ill-mannered, abusive and insulting. They think of everyone as a servant and become very demanding, as if the whole world were designed to feed their need for pleasure. If they want to drive at a hundred miles an hour through a built-up area, they will, and they'll honk their horn as if to say, "Get out of my way, I'm much more important than you." This loathsome behavior can be made worse by their greedy, addictive nature.

To the impoverished spicie, people are there to be used and their needs are completely irrelevant. They might buy you a new outfit, but it'll be one *they* like to see you in, not the one you want. As lovers, they can be jealous and overpowering, and touchy from morning to night. If the typical impoverished spicie cannot find in their wardrobe the pair of shoes that will *exactly* match their outfit, they'll throw a tantrum, scream, shout, throw things around and generally behave like a very spoiled little child. They'll do this regardless of whether they have an audience or are alone. Hysteria, panic attacks, and depression are common. The greatest fear of an impoverished spicie is to be bored, and without a credit card.

Woodies

Aspirations: To be in control and have an impact on the world through self-determination.

Woodies Abundant Self Can Be:
Steadfast, loyal, wise, courageous, eminent, magnanimous, inspiring, supportive, defenders, authoritative, protective, ethical, honest, trustworthy, principled, honorable, strong-minded, decisive, confident, powerful, gallant, champions of causes, visionary, warm-hearted, energetic,
expansive, compassionate.

Woodies are very strong, independent people, bold and forthright. They know what they want and they go for it, striving for their place in the world. Woodies are ruled by intellectual culture, civil rights, civil justice, and wisdom, which they pursue with intelligence, dynamism, and assertion. Because they are very quick thinkers, woodies often talk very fast, backed up by their considerable education.

"Superman" was probably a woodie: bold, powerful, independent, ever able to take the initiative and get a task done. These strong, silent types are real nature lovers and will work tirelessly for the environment, perhaps as a Greenpeace hero, perhaps on the committee to stop road development in their area. Although aggressively ambitious, woodies have a nice disposition, being compassionate at heart, faithful to friends and ideas, honorable in their dealings, and, if a man, gallant with old ladies.

Woodies will do anything they can for a cause they believe in, once they've established the validity of it. "Tell me again," they'll say, questioning your motives about a project. "Tell me again" and "again" and, when they know you are genuine and right-minded, they will climb mountains for you, fight dragons, or do whatever it takes to establish rightness in the world. Having great courage and fortitude, and an endless capacity for hard work, woodies achieve a great deal in their life, both professionally and in terms of social ideals. Woodies are often turned to for help because people recognize that they are ethical, trustworthy, and wise.

When in balance, woodies are intuitive, perceptive, warm-hearted people who will not nag you into the ground about any mistakes you may have made. They seem to be a bit above all that, steadfastly carrying on with their own plans, motivated by an inner moralism, and driven by boundless confidence and persistence.

Woodies Generally Are:

Forceful, intellectual, individualistic, self-reliant, assertive, moral, self-confident, motivated, influential, controlling, content, perceptive, solid, unmovable, enterprising, persistent, earnest, conventional, faithful, steadfast.

Woodies are not puritanical at all so although they may run a youth club, for example, they won't chastise the youngsters for any wrongdoing. They are unhappy in tightly controlled religious groups and, being natural leaders, may start their own less-puritanical and more tolerant breakaway group. Other people can find woodies rather daunting and powerful (because they know what they want), and may feel insecure in their presence but woodies are very fair-minded people and do not treat people unjustly. Although their children may tend to steer clear of their powerful woodie parents, they also know that woodie will give them space to grow and, if they have a problem, woodie will swing into action and sort it out for them. Grandchildren love woodies and are not fearful of them because they appreciate knowing the parameters of expected behavior. Plus this personality has a tremendous amount of patience, especially as they grow older, and are also very caring and generous.

Woodie personalities must be in touch with nature. If they live in town, they belong to a golf club — not for the social aspects, nor for the game itself, but for the joy of walking on grass and looking at nature around them.

Although woodies do like power, and miss it terribly when they retire, for example, they abhor injustice and can genuinely try to see other people's point of view. Their protective nature makes them good union leaders or managers, resistance fighters or politicians, even doctors, reporters, and lawyers. Their principled, strong-minded, decisive nature makes them ideal for high positions of power, in business or politics, to which they can bring an element of vision and inspiration, which could truly change the balance sheet — or the world.

Woodies Impoverished Self Can Be:

Domineering, dictatorial, hostile, threatening, unscrupulous, ruthless, moody, argumentative, expressionless, suffocating, unyielding, harsh, vengeful, egotistical, tyrannical, severe, mean.

The impoverished woodie can easily become a dictatorial tyrant, willful, hostile, ruthless and moody. This is the type of personality we'd all hate to have as a boss. A woodie can become expressionless, under which one senses unexpressed aggression, which can be highly intimidating — an aspect of their power when in an impoverished state.

An elderly city businessman I met once fell into this category. He was dictatorial in all the ways mentioned above, but what really sticks in my mind is the meanness of his attitude not only toward certain members of his family but toward his daffodils. On his kitchen wall he kept a chart recording the performance of the daffodils in his large garden. Each daffodil bulb was followed each year to make sure it was regenerating at maximum potential — i.e., increasing the number of flowers — and if it wasn't, it was simply replaced, no matter how beautiful. Now, that's ruthless.

CHART 13.1
Essential Oils Groups

These are just some of the essential oils which can be included in the following nine groups.

Extraction Methods: Steam distilled — SD; Other — O

FLORALS: This section contains the most absolutes — essential oils that cannot be extracted by steam distillation.

ESSENTIAL OIL	LATIN NAME	CHARACTER	OTHER GROUP	EXTRACTION
Boronia	*Boronia megastigma*	Floral		O
Cananga	*Canaga odorata*	Floral		SD
Carnation	*Dianthus caryophyllus*	Floral		O
Cassie	*Acacia farnesiana*	Floral		O
Chamomile German	*Matricaria recutica*	Floral	Herbie	SD
Chamomile Roman	*Anthemis nobilis*	Floral	Herbie	SD
Champaca	*Michelia champaca*	Floral		O
Genet	*Spartium junceum*	Floral		O
Helichrysum (Immortelle or Italian Everlasting)	*Helichrysum angustifolium*	Floral		SD
Hyacinth	*Hyacinthus orientalis*	Floral		O
Jasmine	*Jasminum officinale*	Floral		O
Lavender	*Lavendula angustifolia*	Floral	Herbie	SD
Lemon Blossom	*Citrus Limon*	Floral		SD
Linden Blossom	*Tilia vulgaris*	Floral		O
Marigold	*Calendula officinalis*	Floral		O
Melilotus	*Melilotus officinalis*	Floral		O
Mimosa	*Acacia dealbata*	Floral		O
Narcissus	*Narcissus poeticus*	Floral		O
Neroli	*Citrus aurantium*	Floral		SD

Ormenis Flower	*Ormenis multicaulis*	Floral	Herbie	SD
Osmanthus	*Osmanthus fragrans*	Floral		O
Rose Maroc	*Rose centifolia*	Floral		O
Rose Otto	*Rose damascena*	Floral		SD
Tagetes	*Tagetes minuta*	Floral		SD
Tuberose	*Polianthes tuberosa*	Floral		O
Ylang Ylang	*Cananga odorata*	Floral		SD

FRUITIES: Although some of the following are not generally thought of as "fruits," they are included here because they are in fact extracted from the fruit.

ESSENTIAL OIL	LATIN NAME	CHARACTER	OTHER GROUP	EXTRACTION
Bergamot	*Citrus bergamia*	Fruite		O
Black Pepper	*Piper nigrum*	Fruitie	Spicie	SD
Cardamom	*Elettaria cardamomum*	Fruitie	Spicie	SD
Clove	*Eugenia caryophyllata*	Fruitie	Spicie	SD
Cubebs	*Piper cubeba*	Fruitie	Spicie	SD
Grapefruit	*Citrus paradisi*	Fruitie		O
Hops	*Humulus lupulus*	Fruitie	Herbie	SD
Juniper	*Juniperus communis*	Fruitie	Woodie	SD
Lemon	*Citrus limon*	Fruitie		O
Lime	*Citrus aurantifolia*	Fruitie		O
Litsea cubeba (May Chang)	*Litsea Cubeba*	Fruitie		SD
Mandarin	*Citrus reticulata*	Fruitie		O
Orange	*Citrus sinensis*	Fruitie		O
Pimento Berry	*Pimenta dioica*	Fruitie	Spicie	SD
Schinus Molle	*Schinus molle*	Fruitie		SD
Tangerine	*Citrus nobilis*	Fruitie		O
Tonka Bean	*Dipteryx odorata*	Fruitie	Seedie	O
Vanilla	*Vanilla planifolia*	Fruitie		O

HERBIES: The majority of herbie essential oils are distilled from the flowering tops or whole plant and are categorized accordingly.

ESSENTIAL OIL	LATIN NAME	CHARACTER	OTHER GROUP	EXTRACTION
Basil	*Ocimum basilicum*	Herbie	Leafie	SD
Calamintha	*Calamintha officinalis*	Herbie	Leafie	SD
Chamomile German	*Matricaria recutica*	Herbie	Floral	SD
Chamomile Roman	*Anthemis nobilis*	Herbie	Floral	SD
Clary Sage	*Salvia sclarea*	Herbie	Floral	SD
Geranium	*Pelargonium graveolens*	Herbie	Leafie	SD

Hyssop	Hyssopus officinalis	Herbie	Leafie	SD
Lavender	Lavendula angustifolia	Herbie	Floral	SD
Lovage	Levisticum officinale	Herbie	Leafie	SD
Marjoram	Origanum marjorana	Herbie	Leafie	SD
Melissa	Melissa officinalis	Herbie	Leafie	SD
Ormenis Flower (Chamomile Maroc)	Ormenis multicaulis	Herbie	Floral	SD
Peppermint	Mentha piperata	Herbie	Leafie	SD
Spearmint	Mentha spicata	Herbie	Leafie	SD
Oregano	Origanum vulgare	Herbie	Leafie	SD
Rosemary	Rosmarinus officinalis	Herbie	Leafie	SD
Sage	Salvia officinalis	Herbie	Leafie	SD
Thyme Red	Thymus vulgaris	Herbie	Leafie	SD
Thyme Linalol	Thymus linalol	Herbie	Leafie	SD
Thyme Lemon	Thymus citriodorus	Herbie	Leafie	SD
Yarrow	Achillea millefolium	Herbie	Floral	SD

LEAFIES: The extraction of leafies sometimes includes the twigs and stems.

ESSENTIAL OIL	LATIN NAME	CHARACTER	OTHER GROUP	EXTRACTION
Bay	Laurus nobilis	Leafie	Woodie	SD
Birch	Betula alba	Leafie	Woodie	SD
Buchu	Agothosma betulina	Leafie		SD
Cajeput	Melaleuca cajeputi	Leafie	Woodie	SD
Cinnamon	Cinnamomum zeylanicum	Leafie	Spicey	SD
Cistus (Rock Rose)	Cistus ladaniferus	Leafie		SD
Cypress	Cupressus sempervirens	Leafie	Woodie	SD
Eucalyptus	Eucalyptus globulus	Leafie	Woodie	SD
Eucalyptus Lemon	Eucalyptus citriodora	Leafie	Woodie	SD
Eucalyptus Peppermint	Eucalyptus dives	Leafie	Woodie	SD
Eucalyptus Radiata	Eucalyptus radiata	Leafie	Woodie	SD
Fir	Abies alba	Leafie	Woodie	SD
Myrtle	Myrtus communis	Leafie		SD
Niaouli	Melaleuca viridiflora	Leafie	Woodie	SD
Patchouli	Pogostemon cablin	Leafie		SD
Petitgrain	Citrus aurantium	Leafie	Woodie	SD
Ravensara	Ravensara aromatica	Leafie	Woodie	SD
Spruce (black)	Picea mariana	Leafie	Woodie	SD
Spruce (white)	Picea glauca	Leafie	Woodie	SD
Tea Tree	Melaleuca alternifolia	Leafie	Woodie	SD
Violet Leaf	Viola odorata	Leafie		O

RESINIES: The oils of Resinies are from the resins or balsam that exudes from trees or shrubs.

ESSENTIAL OIL	LATIN NAME	CHARACTER	OTHER GROUP	EXTRACTION
Benzoin	*Styrax benzoin*	Resinie		SD
Canadian Balsam	*Abies balsamea*	Resinie		SD
Copaiba Balsam	*Copaifera officinalis*	Resinie		SD
Peru Balsam	*Myroxylon balsamum*	Resinie		SD
Tolu Balsam	*Myroxylon balsamum*	Resinie		SD
Borneol	*Dryobalanops aromatica*	Resinie		SD
Elemi	*Carnarium luzonicum*	Resinie		SD
Frankincense	*Boswellia carteri*	Resinie		SD
Galbanham	*Ferula galbanifera*	Resinie		SD
Myrrh	*Commiphora myrrha*	Resinie		SD
Opopanax	*Commiphora erythraea*	Resinie		SD
Styrax Levant	*Liquidambar orientalis*	Resinie		SD

ROOTIES: The extraction of rooties are from the roots of plants.

ESSENTIAL OIL	LATIN NAME	CHARACTER	OTHER GROUP	EXTRACTION
Angelica	*Angelica archangelica*	Rootie	Seedie	SD
Galangal	*Alpinia officinarum*	Rootie		SD
Ginger	*Zingiber officinale*	Rootie	Spicie	SD
Orris	*Iris pallida*	Rootie		SD
Snakeroot	*Asarum canadense*	Rootie		SD
Spikenard	*Nardostachys jatamansi*	Rootie		SD
Tumeric	*Curcuma longa*	Rootie		SD
Valerian	*Valeriana officinalis*	Rootie		SD
Vetiver	*Vetivera zizanoides*	Rootie		SD

SEEDIES: Extracted from the seeds of plants.

ESSENTIAL OIL	LATIN NAME	CHARACTER	OTHER GROUP	EXTRACTION
Ambrette Seed	*Hibiscus abelmoschus*	Seedie		SD
Angelica Seed	*Angelica archangelica*	Seedie		SD
Anise (Star)	*Illicium verum*	Seedie	Spicie	SD
Aniseed	*Pimpinella ansium*	Seedie	Spicie	SD
Caraway	*Carum carvi*	Seedie	Spicie	SD
Carrot Seed	*Daucus carota*	Seedie		SD
Coriander	*Coriandrum sativum*	Seedie	Spicie	SD
Cumin	*Cuminum cyminum*	Seedie	Spicie	SD

Dill	Anethum graveolens	Seedie		SD
Fennel (Sweet)	Foeniculum vulgare	Seedie		SD
Nutmeg	Myristica fragrans	Seedie	Spicie	SD
Parsley Seed	Petroselinum sativum	Seedie		SD

SPICIES: Because the spice oils are mostly taken from seeds and fruits, these oils are also categorized under those groups.

ESSENTIAL OIL	LATIN NAME	CHARACTER	OTHER GROUP	EXTRACTION
Anise (Star)	Illiciuim verum	Spicie	Seedie	SD
Aniseed	Pimpinella ansium	Spicie	Seedie	SD
Black Pepper	Piper nigrum	Spicie	Fruitie	SD
Cardamom	Elettaria cardamomum	Spicie	Fruitie	SD
Caraway	Carum carvi	Spicie	Seedie	SD
Cinnamon	Cinnamomum zeylanicum	Spicie	Leafie	SD
Clove	Eugenia aromatica	Spicie	Fruitie	SD
Coriander	Coriandrum sativum	Spicie	Seedie	SD
Cubebs	Piper cubeba	Spicie	Fruitie	SD
Cumin	Cuminum cyminum	Spicie	Seedie	SD
Galangal	Alpinia officinarum	Spicie	Rootie	SD
Ginger	Zingiber officinale	Spicie	Rootie	SD
Mace	Myristica fragrans	Spicie	Fruitie	SD
Nutmeg	Myristica fragrans	Spicie	Seedie	SD
Pimento Berry	Pimento dioica	Spicie	Fruitie	SD

WOODIES: Extracted from twigs, wood, or shaving from trees.

ESSENTIAL OIL	LATIN NAME	CHARACTER	OTHER GROUP	EXTRACTION
Amyris	Amyris balsamifera	Woodie		SD
Cabreuva	Myrocarpus fastigiatus	Woodie		SD
Cade	Juniperus oxycedrus	Woodie		SD
Camphor White	Cinnamomum camphora	Woodie		SD
Cascarilla Bark	Croton eluteria	Woodie		SD
Cedarwood	Cedrus atlantica	Woodie		SD
Cedarwood	Cedrus virginiana	Woodie		SD
Guaiacwood	Bulnesia sarmienti	Woodie		SD
Linaloe	Bursera glabrifolia	Woodie		SD
Pine	Pinus sylvestris	Woodie	Leafie	SD
Rosewood	Aniba rosaeodora	Woodie		SD
Sandalwood	Santalum album	Woodie		SD
Spruce (black)	Picea mariana	Woodie	Leafie	SD
Spruce (white)	Picea glauca	Woodie	Leafie	SD

CHAPTER 14

INDIVIDUAL PERSONALITY TYPES

In this chapter we shall be looking at the individual personalities of essential oils, that is to say, the human characteristics that each oil displays. People who use oils invariably begin to talk about them as if they were people. Someone might talk about needing geranium, as one might need a dear friend or partner, to offer comfort and solace after a hard day in the concrete jungle. Or another person might talk about frankincense as a source of spiritual uplift — as if they gave the same kind of stimulation and peace as a discussion with a spiritual mentor. Aromatherapists and general users alike seem to come to the same conclusions about oils, the most common generalizations being that lavender is like "the mother," mandarin is "the child within," cypress is strength, while ylang ylang is "the gentle seductress."

Associations such as these have grown and expanded in my mind over the years so that I now have a rather complex image of the personalities of each essential oil, and I've come to know which particular oils could be best suited to each particular person at any given time. Experience has taught me that a certain psyche-matching takes place — the personalities of particular oils match particular personality types of people. To look at it another way, certain essential oils do not match certain people. There doesn't seem to be an affinity.

Of course it is very difficult to explain why such a harmony or disharmony should happen. It is simply one of those things that therapists experience on a daily basis. But it is not a haphazard phenomenon. Certain patterns emerge. Certain types of people have a certain relationship with particular oils, either for good or not for good — which in this case does not mean bad. "Bad," or "not good," in this context simply means that they do not induce the required beneficial effect as quickly as one might expect, and certainly as one might expect with the essential oils that are in harmony with a particular person.

I have included in this introduction oils that are readily available and/or are required study for those undergoing aromatherapy training. The full spectrum of potential extends much further, not only because many essential oils have not been included here, but because each essential oil has chemotypes. What this means is that slight variations on each oil arise because of different growing conditions. For example, lavender that is grown in the valleys is not the same, chemically or in terms of personality, as lavender that is grown high in the mountains. Although the plants may *look* much the same, and are of the same botanical species, the components within them are determined to a degree by the growing conditions, including the type of soil, the other species of plants which are growing nearby, the amount of sun they receive, or rainfall, etc. All these factors contribute to the making of different chemotypes which, in professional aromatherapy, are taken into consideration when treating patients.

Just as a human has a personality and subpersonalities, so do essential oils in the form of chemotypes. Therefore, when we view the spectrum, we have in essential oils a system that can incorporate personality, subpersonality, and multi-personality, and with all the possible combinations of blends can cover all 17,953 states of the human emotional condition noted in Webster's dictionary.

Choosing Your Personality Type

When looking through the individual personality profiles bear in mind that very few people are "classic" types. We may have a "predominant" personality and many other personalities as well. So, for example, if you read Jasmine and find yourself saying, "Yes, that sounds like me but there are some aspects of this character that don't fit," don't worry because you would not expect them all to match exactly. Very few people have all the personality traits outlined under any particular essential oil. No two human beings are the same, we are composites of characters described here.

As you read through the personalities you may recognize people you know or see portions of a particular person's character or personality. We are multifaceted beings and the reason essential oils have such potential is that we can dip into different personalities and create, mix, or formulate an individual blend that includes and reflects the many facets of each individual person.

We all use essential oils each day — in perfumes, toiletries, foods, drinks, etc. — and we're not about to give up these pleasures because the essential oil contained in our favorite soft drink, for example, doesn't happen to fit our own personality type. There are many ways to use essential oils, and by aroma-genera or individual essential oil personality choice, we simply have another dimension to enjoy. With the personality profiles, you may find that there are oils you hadn't really thought of before as having an affinity with you, and now you may be encouraged to use that oil for the first time.

Think of essential oils as drops of positivity, whose purpose is to bring us into harmony with the whole. They are more than fabulous fragrances. They bring well-being, both in terms of physical and emotional health. Use them with positive thought because all life is vibration and thought is vibration too. Essential oils are *positive additions* to life. They can help us move beyond the limitations imposed by circumstance and ego, and make connection with the greater whole, the spiritual dimension, our universal self.

An Introduction to Essential Oils and Absolutes and Their Human Personalities

Although the personalities outlined here are extensions of the larger aroma-genera groups of florals, fruities, herbies, leafies, and so on, either section can be read and practiced as a system in its own right. The essential oils chosen in this and the previous section can be used in all the usual ways.

BASIL   HERBIE/LEAFIE
Ocimum basilicum

CHARACTER
Uplifting, Awakening, Clarifying, Stimulating

USE FOR THESE POSITIVE ATTRIBUTES
Positivity, Purposefulness, Concentration, Assertiveness, Decisiveness, Straightforwardness, Trust, Integrity, Enthusiasm, Clarity, Cheerfulness, Strength

USE TO COUNTERACT THESE NEGATIVE ATTRIBUTES
Indecision, Mental fatigue, Mental exhaustion, Negativity, Lack of direction, Fear, Burnout, Confusion, Intellectual fatigue, Apathy, Bitterness, Resentment, Addiction, Conflict, Fear of intimacy, Shame, Doubts, Melancholy, Sadness

BASIL
Personality Profile

Basil personalities are often the entrepreneurs of the world and, male or female, are able to see what others may not even know exists. For them, opportunities abound. Ambition, flair, drive, and enterprise get them where they want to be and, unless someone bars their way unjustly, they will get there without harming others, and by being honest. Basils have a wisdom far beyond their years, plus a fair amount of luck — often missing ruin by the skin of their teeth, as a brilliant flash of inspiration gets them out of difficult situations. It sometimes seems as if Basils have spiritual intervention in times of crisis — an advantage not a lot of us have.

The Basil personality can be very direct and blunt, particularly if you don't always get their point. They may seem patronizing but they mean no harm and may even feel they're doing you a favor by being blunt. Power holds a great attraction for these personalities and they often become the bosses in commercial organizations, although they can also be found in jobs that involve aspects of law or espionage. They're often the genies of life — the eccentric artists, the mad poets, the sacrificed writers, and perhaps it is their deep wisdom that allows them to glance into unknown realms. Basils will not criticize or think badly of any action, believing that everything has its place, and there is a reason for everything. Perhaps this explains their basic optimism. Basils could be called the protectors of ideas, imagination, and free will.

The sordid or seamier side of life often holds a fascination for Basils, and they could be found indulging in pursuits which the less adventurous would shudder at. It is by walking the fence between what is expected and what is not that gets them into trouble. If they lean too far, they can fall in it — even though their intelligence tells them not to. It is not unusual for Basils to go on to disaster, mental confusion, and madness.

The Basil personality enjoys academic pursuits far more than sporting ones, but although philosophy books may be on the bedside table, so too will be those discussing Tantra, the ancient Indian cult of ecstasy. Basils believe in the communication between mind, body, and spirit and this will extend to their lovemaking. To them, sex is synonymous with spirituality, while marriage is more of a mental commitment — which they'll take very seriously. Generally, Basils are charming and sexy lovers of life, full of bonhomie, despite their calm, sometimes sullen exterior.

Basils are drawn by the mysterious and can be very spiritual, and this interest can take many forms. For example, they may join a sect — possibly rising to become leader; or become very involved with a world religion; they may search through meditation; or explore other, much darker, sides. Basils are certainly fascinated with the paranormal and will apply cool logic to all that is found, describing it with flair and imagination. This fascination can lead to a lifelong exploration of things unknown and can occasionally get them into some very hot water. Basils will also experiment with hallucinogenic mind-altering drugs as they search for the surreal, and spiritual communication.

The eccentric aunt, the intellectual, those who go crazy with passion — all could be Basil personalities, who will fight for the right to be who they are, but are wise enough to let go if they cannot win the battle. The Basil doesn't care because, if need be, there are far more interesting things to pursue.

Norma Gilbert, MIFA, Reg., MIRCST, MBSR, aromatherapist, cranial sacral therapist and tutor:

"Strong, powerful, discerning, and cerebral, like a monarch, basil requires to be treated with dignity and respect and in return will be most trustworthy. Warming and balmy in small quantities, it can bring about a sense of true balance and strength."

BERGAMOT
Citrus bergamia
FRUITIE

CHARACTER
Joyous, Refreshing, Uplifting, Encouraging

USE FOR THESE POSITIVE ATTRIBUTES
Concentration, Confidence, Balance, Strength, Joy, Motivation, Good cheer, Harmony, Completeness

USE TO COUNTERACT THESE NEGATIVE ATTRIBUTES
Depression, Anxiety, Helplessness, Apathy, Bitterness, Burnout, Despondency, Emptiness, Exhaustion, Grief, Hopelessness, Sadness, Loneliness, Stress, Tension, Emotional imbalances

BERGAMOT
Personality Profile

The Bergamot personality is young, fresh, caring, and considerate — everything a grandmother would expect from the younger generation. Being around Bergamot can be as joyful an experience as walking through a field of the sunflowers that inspired van Gogh. Although Bergamot types are not necessarily young in years they will always be young at heart and have a joyful approach to life. While they acknowledge the bad or negative things in life they don't allow them to overcome all the beauty and happiness that can be found. Indeed, they view good and positive things as all-embracing.

This personality is caring, considerate, and full of energy. They're often found in the caring professions or in any job that requires large amounts of energy, skill, and enthusiasm. Being very positive, confident, and outgoing, Bergamots are never afraid to put themselves in line for the best position. They often drift toward the media, in which they enjoy being up-front — maybe as a presenter or spokesperson, a role in which they can display a charismatic personality, a feature too of their personal life. The Bergamot personality is also very good with children as their energy level is very compatible, and they understand the thrill of new adventure. Fun, for a Bergamot, might be climbing up Mount Everest or rowing down white water in a canoe.

This is the outward personality, however. Inwardly, Bergamots may suffer depression and, just as many other personality types can, they can easily plummet quite quickly into the depths of despair when things become too much for them to bear. But Bergamot never really allows anyone to see just how down they can get, or how sad they're feeling. It just isn't in their nature to do so. Because of this, people are inclined to think they haven't a care in the world. Nobody may suspect that behind the mask, Bergamot may be inwardly crying with emotional pain. Only the empathy exhibited toward others who are feeling distressed may give them away.

This might be said of a Bergamot: "You wouldn't think he (or she) would be able to understand how I feel. He is always so cheerful, but he understood, and I felt I could tell him everything. I always feel so much better after I have seen him." Of course this person may be feeling better but poor old Bergamot would have shouldered the distress and, unless they're really on top of things at the time, it could compound the low feelings they already have.

Another phrase applied to someone with Bergamot in their personality profile is, "They'll be all right, they're tough, they can handle it, and they never let anything get them down." If only people knew! Bergamot can certainly get down, but whenever you meet this personality it will be a tonic, and you'll feel the better for it.

Vivienne Lunny MD, MBBS, MDMA, MIFA Reg, MISPA, RQA, aromatherapist and tutor:

"Bergamot comes into the room smiling, bright, happy, and in balance, at ease with the world and is discriminating, loves nature, is tactful, practical, highly imaginative, caring, and productive. Bergamot can see both sides of any issue, which enables him/her to rebalance feelings and emotions."

BLACK PEPPER
Piper nigrum

FRUITIE/SPICIE

CHARACTER
Security, Comforting, Directional, Endurance

USE FOR THESE POSITIVE ATTRIBUTES
Comfort, Stamina, Endurance, Motivation, Changeability

USE TO COUNTERACT THESE NEGATIVE ATTRIBUTES
Emotional blockages, Compulsions, Confusion, Disorientation, Fatigue, Begrudging, Indecision, Irrationality, Anger, Frustration, Emotional coldness, Apathy, Mental exhaustion

BLACK PEPPER Personality Profile

Black Pepper is the older, sterner personality among the essential oils, but having said that, it can also be the livelier types of personality. Black Pepper people often seem old for their age, whether they're the baby who seems to be thirty or the twelve-year-old who acts as if he were forty-two. This type of person will reprimand you for not having behaved correctly at a social gathering — particularly if you are a carefree Melissa type. Indeed, Black Peppers can be very upright and extremely self-righteous (providing it suits them) and, if allowed to be, dictatorial. On the other hand, they can be charming, trustworthy, kind, and very loyal if they wish, and if they like you.

As parents, their children may not understand Black Peppers until they themselves are middle-aged, and although often stern and forbidding to their children, they can instill a sense of security, which can be comforting in that the children know exactly what to expect. Once understood, Black Peppers are very predictable.

In the workplace and at home, Black Peppers can be very stimulating, encouraging everyone to succeed, and tend to take on responsibility for everyone in their family circle. These are more likely to be the financial responsibilities, however, rather than the emotional ones, providing their advice is being taken. If a male Black Pepper has a son, he'll have to compete with the son, and will have to be lord and master. If female, Black Pepper will be the "she who must be obeyed" type. They'll bale their family out of trouble not so much for their family's sake, but for their own reputation, and will have no qualms about cutting a son or daughter out of a will and leaving them penniless.

Black Peppers can be very flirtatious and may boast about their sexual conquests, but this is more to convince themselves that they can be passionate. In truth, they may have an inability to let themselves be free enough to release passion. Although Black Pepper is a hot, warming essential oil, the personality Black Pepper is not warming in love. If they ever recognize true love, it's likely to be discarded for a better social match. Black Peppers go through life having a multitude of lovers, trying to find, once again, the true love they let go — but they'll never admit it of course.

This type will tolerate anyone for the sake of appearances or if they think the other person may be useful to them in some way. Black Peppers do make loyal friends. They're unashamed showoffs and have to be better than anyone else at everything (even if they're not), and they love to show off their knowledge — whether or not it's got something to do with their chosen career or hobby. They're not unknown to adopt a "holier than thou" attitude. Where Black Peppers are welcome is when they help with financial problems, give advice on stocks and shares, or tax returns, procedures in law, etc. They'll know how to get the most out of the welfare state and how, in monetary terms, to exploit the system to their advantage.

Black Peppers can sometimes be exasperating in their lack of empathy toward other people, and their complete lack of lateral thinking. They will lament the number of homeless people, for example, but wonder, "Why do people put themselves in that situation?" Black Peppers will ignore the plight of the majority of the world, as they're only interested in themselves and their families. Yet they often have charismatic power that tricks people into thinking they are leaders of men — which they definitely are not but frequently arrange to be. They just don't have the compassion or understanding needed and will become the dictators if allowed. Also, having a fiery temperament, Black Peppers can often blow their tops with indignation and frustration, usually over the stupidity of others.

Black Peppers are found in all walks of life, to a degree, but prefer jobs that give power and money (which they love), or involve linear thinking (a career in which they do not have to use their imagination or creativity too much). Black Peppers would excel at being lawyers, judges, solicitors, bankers, accountants, financial advisors, or at a life in the military services (army rather than navy or air force), prison services, traffic wardens, and traffic police. They are often found in unsuitable jobs and will never be happy unless they are in charge. The family will take the brunt of Black Pepper's frustration and anger as they take it all out on the family when they get home. Negative Black Peppers will blame everyone else for their emotional state and can be irritable, cold, emotionally stunted, and very emotionally violent. Luckily, it is very rare to find a completely negative Black Pepper personality.

One such character was a retired insurance underwriter from Lloyds of London, who'd made a lot of money from being in the know, and being with the right syndicate. From an extremely modest background, he changed his accent, conveniently forgot his roots, fought, and rose to become a most respected member of the community. When it became apparent that his wife no longer fit the picture, he embarked on a series of affairs, to show off to his friends and colleagues that he was a hit with the ladies, while dragging out his divorce for seven years while he hid his assets so his wife would get the bare minimum. His son, who had been treated as a rival since birth, was dumped with the mother, while the flattering daughter was given all the attention and money. But, to save family face, when the unloved son went wild, the cold Black Pepper father picked up the bill. All his children wanted was for him to say, "I love you," but for Black Peppers, even when they feel love, these are the hardest words to say.

CARDAMOM
Elettaria cardamomum

FRUITIE/SPICIE

CHARACTER
Clarifying, Stimulating, Encouraging, Enthusiastic

USE FOR THESE POSITIVE ATTRIBUTES
Clarity, Concentration, Direction, Motivation, Straightforwardness, Enthusiasm, Confidence, Courage, Fortitude, Purpose

USE TO COUNTERACT THESE NEGATIVE ATTRIBUTES
Mental stress, Apathy, Confusion, Inflexibility, Judgmental, Intolerance, Unreasonableness, Burnout, Suspicion, Sluggishness, Self-pity, Bewilderment, Rigidity

CARDAMOM
Personality Profile

Cardamom is a strong, forthright personality, full of fortitude, stimulating, and straightforward. You know exactly where you are with them — what you see is what you get. There are no hidden motives to their actions and they're direct and encouraging. This personality type gets motivated by good ideas and instills inspiration in others. Their being so enthusiastic could tend to get wearing if Cardamom wasn't also very balancing and able to harmonize everything. This is really their strength — no matter what happens to them, how fraught people may get when they're pushed by Cardamom, in the end harmony will reign. This characteristic of the Cardamom personality makes them very good leaders. They will push and push but in the end others will appreciate the sense of it all. Also, Cardamoms believe in fairness and justice, and that too always comes through.

Cardamoms wear an air of detachment much of the time, as if nothing really worries them, but when they get steamed up they go for the jugular. You don't mess with a Cardamom. If you happen to be confused and in a bad situation, Cardamom will come to the rescue, but not on a white horse bearing gifts. They are much too frugal for that. It couldn't be said that they're mean but they won't squander their hard-earned cash on anyone but themselves. If you go out for dinner together don't expect them to pick up the check. If you don't offer to pay yourself they'll split the bill straight down the middle and if there's one penny left over, they'll suggest you flip for it. Being so financially careful has its advantages — for one thing, Cardamom never gets into any shady deals. And Cardamom does like to have a few pennies tucked away for impulse buys.

The Cardamom personality loves flattery, but they rarely get it, so when a floral comes along full of sweet words, Cardamom will fall for it all. They can be a passionate personality, which may come as a surprise, and they love romance. Indeed, they'll dream up all kinds of crazy, exciting things to do that can seem quite out of character. Who would have thought such a heart beats in them?

Female Cardamoms are perfectly comfortable with their masculine side, which makes them very interesting to men who feel that women don't usually understand them. No Cardamom is dull and all lead interesting lives, making everything seem like an adventure. They will respect the wishes of other people, especially in a love relationship but as parents they can be very strict and expect their children to embrace their high morals. Partners are expected to be individuals, and are respected for it. This isn't always the case with children, who Cardomon expects to be carbon copies of themselves, and enthusiastic and motivated about their schoolwork to boot. They have great difficulty understanding a teenager's need to slump on the sofa listening to loud music.

When a Cardamom gets negative it can be quite alarming. Mostly, they suffer mental stress that can make them apathetic, inflexible, judgmental, or self-pitying. They become suspicious of everyone who tries to help and can become rigid in their outlook and bewildered when anyone with enough courage points it out to them. If the negativity is allowed to carry on for too long, Cardamoms can completely lose interest in life, becoming losers, their sense of fair play and good judgment gone forever.

However, a positive Cardamom is good in leadership roles, providing they learn to delegate, and they make excellent teachers. They aren't overly creative but they have the stamina to carry ideas forward which, in the end, can allow them to achieve more than some creative personalities.

CARNATION   FLORAL
Dianthus caryophyllus

CHARACTER
Secretiveness, Stillness, Originality, Liberating

USE FOR THESE POSITIVE ATTRIBUTES
Self-worth, Communication, Radiating, Creativity, Independence, Tenderness, Nurturing, Encompassing, Cushioning, Openness, Releasing

USE TO COUNTERACT THESE NEGATIVE ATTRIBUTES
Disregard, Neglect, Detachment, Cynicism, Disorientation, Doubt, Mental loneliness, Aloneness, Emotional domination, Emotional solitude, Neglect, Self-criticism

CARNATION
Personality Profile

The Carnation personality will fill your days with love and promise you the earth — and really mean it. Bright ideas and a powerful imagination fill the head of the Carnation personality, who will always have pictures of flowers, trees, or angels in heaven around. They also love all the sensuous things of life — perfume, silks, expensive gourmet snacks, etc. — with which they will pamper themselves. Being the ultimate floral, if they wished, Carnations could become the classic temptresses or Don Juans, but that role is not for them. If the Carnation is female, men will want to take care of her, and if the Carnation is male, women will want to mother him. Everyone can sense Carnation's child-like innocence and trust in people.

Carnations tend to be very gentle people who sometimes cannot quite get a grasp on life events, tending to dream just a little too much, particularly when things aren't going as well for them as they think they should. One characteristic which can cause sadness and depression is their getting too involved with other people's problems, which they take on, but which brings them down, particularly if they feel unable to help.

There is no way a Carnation would hurt a hair on any person's head, and they can be a great comfort to people suffering loss or hardship. With inner wisdom and knowledge, they may be a devotional kind of person, but there is a warmth to this personality that can invite closeness and is, sometimes, unfortunately misinterpreted as sexual advances or social climbing by other people with a more lowly nature.

History in all its forms hold a fascination for this personality and they're quite likely to search for their family's roots or read history books — more likely being interested in the Renaissance than the Tudor period. Carnations also enjoy art tremendously and although they may not take it up as a profession — because they don't have the confidence to promote their work — they'll paint for pleasure, or take up flower arrangement or interior design, anything through which this natural artistic inclination can be expressed.

Carnations are found in all walks of life but they tend to drift toward those jobs that do not push them into the spotlight. Any job that hides them behind a desk that the public comes up to is ideal, such as working in an employment agency, or in a bank, anything that brings them into contact with the public but not in an extroverted way. Carnations tend to be delicate in stature, movements, and mannerisms and their discipline and grace would make them good classical dancers.

Although Carnations don't seem to have much luck themselves — they never win lotteries for example — they do seem to have a magical effect on those around them. If you go to a casino, take a Carnation with you and have them stand next to you at the roulette wheel — luck just might come your way!

Monogamy is the only kind of relationship Carnations want and understand. Infidelity would never even cross their mind. To them, a perfect, faithful marriage is the true joy of life, an essential aspect of being in love. Being monogamous, knowing the partners are for each other only, gives Carnation a special feeling, and repelling advances from outsiders gives Carnation a kick far more exciting than affairs or promiscuity. Carnations need love like a flower needs the sun and, if they don't have it, they'll kid themselves they do, or go looking for a partner. Carnations cannot go through life alone, and if one lover leaves, you can be sure there will be another coming around the corner fairly soon. Without love the Carnation is very down and depressed.

One of the most noticeable traits of Carnations is that they cannot communicate their own sorrows and despairs, which they often have. It seems as if they are always there for everyone else but that nobody is there for them. This is particularly tragic because Carnations find it difficult, at times, to love themselves. The delicate temperament of Carnation leaves them vulnerable to spiteful words and actions and they can bruise very easily and become extremely hurt and sad. As parents, Carnations are very soft and gentle and not very hot on discipline. Consequently, their children take advantage of them and get away with everything.

When they're in a negative frame of mind, Carnations can be self-destructive and depressed, and they cut themselves off from life. They can grieve for years over the death of a parent, for example, or over a love that has been lost. Delicate beings as they are, Carnations can nurse a bruised ego for years, or hide the abused or hurt inner child for a lifetime. It is not unusual, after an episode of being hurt, for a Carnation to go to bed, pull the covers over their heads, and stay there for a week, not emerging even to answer the phone.

Carnations give too much of themselves away. They'll burn themselves out worrying about what they should be doing with their lives instead of simply doing what they enjoy. Partly, this is because they lack the courage of their convictions. When they're on form, however, Carnations are full of laughter, love and care. Indeed, the one thing Carnations always have is copious amounts of love to give to all living things.

Susan Worwood MIFA Reg. aromatherapist and author:

"Carnation is a comforting, yet sensual, personality which makes one feel euphoric, as if sitting in a sanctified place with a sense of inner calm, expectant of the pleasures life has yet to provide."

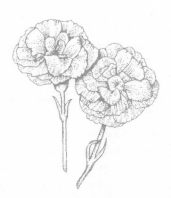

Carnation

CEDARWOOD   WOODIE
Cedrus atlantica

CHARACTER
Grounding, Strengthening, Dignified, Powerful

USE FOR THESE POSITIVE ATTRIBUTES
Focus, Concentration, Strength, Confidence, Balance, Stability, Comfort,
Persistence, Fortitude, Nobility of spirit

USE TO COUNTERACT THESE NEGATIVE ATTRIBUTES
Scattered thoughts, Thoughtlessness, Fixation on past, Anxiety, Obsessions,
Mental strain, Irrationality, Emotional sensitivity, Touchiness, Gloomy thoughts,
Worry, Fear, Too analytical, Paranoia, Selfishness

CEDARWOOD
Personality Profile

The majestic stature of the Cedarwood personality is easy to spot — they seem to glide through life as if they had a royal charter. They may appear haughty and just too grand to be approached about anything mundane, but this would be entirely wrong. Cedarwoods are towers of strength in almost all situations, seemingly in total harmony with the forces of nature, having an ancient air about them, as if they are the repositories of all the world's history. This isn't necessarily the case, even if they make you feel it is. Cedarwoods instill confidence and security in people less able to cope with life's stresses and strains, and can be a great comfort in times of trouble. This ability puts them in the role of family advisor — the person you phone to ask how to deal with your tax

return, or ask how you should approach a financial dispute. You wouldn't ask them to advise you on your choice of friends, or new outfit (or how to get something you don't really deserve) — for that, you'd turn to a Bergamot personality. Cedarwoods appear to be knowledgeable on everything (almost) and will become hurt if a member of the family turns elsewhere for advice. This rarely happens — you wouldn't dare.

However, Cedarwoods are not infallible and are, indeed, frequently wrong because they can be quite dogmatic in their views. The older ones are the worst because they may not even be aware that the world has changed over the last fifty years. If you have this personality for a father or grandfather it can be quite difficult, especially if he holds the family to emotional and financial ransom. This personality excels in the scholarly professions, such as teaching, librarianship, antiques, architecture, and history. They're also inclined towards the sciences and conventional religion although they often have a curiosity about the paranormal too — from a purely scientific point of view, of course.

Unless the Cedarwood is partnered with a balancing type such as a Fruitie, they will dictate the complete running of the household, and all who are in it. They are often amazed that the children will want to leave home and can't really understand why today's young adults want their own lives. Children may not see the loving side of this personality (and may even believe them to be incapable of love), but if trouble strikes, the world had better watch out as Cedarwood will defend their brood to the last. Although Cedarwood is essentially a masculine personality, it's often found in women.

Cedarwoods can become extremely obsessive. They must always have their right seat in their place of worship and their favorite chair at home — and woe betide the visitor who inadvertently sits in the wrong place, who will suffer scowls and dark looks. Cedarwoods always fold their newspapers in the same way and like the cupboards to be organized in a certain fashion. Although their mannerisms lead you to think they would only be at home in a palace, this isn't so, and they're perfectly content in the humblest of places —

even though these characters believe themselves to be truly magnificent.

Cedarwoods of either sex often become confirmed bachelors. It's not that they can't love deeply and affectionately, but it just seems like so much bother. This isn't a passionate personality — not about sex anyway. Excitement is reserved for projects, particularly if they are archaeologists or historians, and Cedarwoods may sacrifice their lives to trying to find the Holy Grail or uncover a particular document, but would never sacrifice themselves to love or abandon themselves to a carefree life.

When negative, Cedarwoods can be hell on earth — demanding, arrogant, selfish, overly controlling, and paranoid. They'll turn every little upset into an international plot against them and may retire to bed with a psychosomatic illness — terminal of course — refusing help from doctors and medicines, and any attempt to make them comfortable — and then say that nobody cares. Subconsciously they seek out partners who are very long-suffering, but loyal.

When they're positive, however, the Cedarwood personality is kind, dignified and very understanding. They can make things seem very precious, even sacred, as they willingly impart their knowledge, often appearing honored to be asked to do so.

CHAMOMILE GERMAN   HERBIE/FLORAL
Matricaria chamomilla

CHARACTER
Strong, Peaceful, Healing, Cooling

USE FOR THESE POSITIVE ATTRIBUTES
Communicative, Relaxed, Understanding, Organized, Soothing, Empathy, Patience, Calm

USE TO COUNTERACT THESE NEGATIVE ATTRIBUTES
Nervousness, Frayed nerves, Anger, Frustration, Emotional dramas, Emotional tension, Irritability, Temper, Tenseness, Overly sensitive, Moodiness, Stormy, Bitterness, Resentment, Indifference, Deep emotional baggage

CHAMOMILE GERMAN
Personality Profile

This deep blue Chamomile is a bountiful type of person, very deep and emotionally strong. They're experts at all activities that require sacrifice and determination. Blues are the father that tucks you in at night, the teacher who helped you with a difficult project, telling you not to worry, and the police officer who helped you home when you were in distress — the type of person you remember as being kind and caring even though you were a stranger to them.

Chamomile Germans have emotional depth and the ability to draw out the best in other people, but seem to keep their own feelings to themselves, preferring to use metaphor to disguise how they feel. The Chamomile German type is liable to be very down to earth, quite up-front, and always appears to be solid in thought — not at all frivolous. They can dramatize things, however, and are often drawn to jobs that involve a certain amount of drama or communication. They may be involved in religion, and feel they have the calling as a priest, for example, but, whatever religion it is they are drawn to, they'll strive to have a deep understanding of it. Philosophy, archaeological digs, ancient monuments, and architecture may be enjoyed by this personality, who is also fascinated by the lives of ancient people and their rulers.

The blue Chamomiles are well suited to a profession in teaching or anything to do with books — publishing, or writing, particularly nonfiction. Being great organizers, they'll organize everything if you let them, including what you have for lunch and who you should invite to your party. If their suggestions aren't taken up, the Blues can get upset, although this doesn't last too long and is soon forgotten. This is a very contented personality, and seems to take everything in its stride.

The negative side of the Chamomile German personality is dark moods and heaviness of heart. In arguments they become irritable as they try to get their point of view across, are confused, tense and easily frustrated, speaking loudly and impatiently — the complete opposite to their normal behavior. When in negative mode they can get easily upset, which disarms people who are used to seeing Chamomile in charge of everything. Often adopting an air of indifference, it leads to break-ups of relationships because it can be difficult for the partner to understand what sparked off Chamomile's bad mood. But this type often lives in the past and some subconscious cue could have reminded them of a past mistake or bad experience. Or it could have been a build-up of things, an explosion (the Blues need to express themselves, not bury it) which gets aimed at the thing or person nearest to them — usually the family or partner.

Of course a strong relationship will ride out the storm, as most of these episodes are short-lived, but while they last Chamomiles have everyone running for cover, including the dog. The deep blue Chamomile Germans are good to have around in an emotional storm, or when grieving, as they provide a strong, solid shoulder to cry on if needed.

CHAMOMILE ROMAN   HERBIE/FLORAL
Anthemis nobilis

CHARACTER
Harmonizing, Peaceful, Soothing, Spiritual

USE FOR THESE POSITIVE ATTRIBUTES
Stillness, Calm, Softness, Gentleness, Relaxed, Serene, Spiritually aware, Emotionally stable, Inner peace, Understanding, Cooperative

USE TO COUNTERACT THESE NEGATIVE ATTRIBUTES
Nervousness, Irritability, Temper, Anger, Depression, Hysteria, Fear, Anxiety, Exhaustion, Worry, Stress, Tension, Grief, Emotional imbalance, Broken heart, Grumpiness, Moroseness, Discontent, Impatience, Short temper, Oversensitivity, Melancholy, Spiritual disconnection

CHAMOMILE ROMAN
Personality Profile

Chamomile Roman is like someone who has been blessed with sunshine and joy, a harmonious disposition and emotional life. They are serene and gentle, and can sometimes seem to be in a dream-like state, as if communicating with unseen angels. Chamomiles often have a strange power over ordinary mortals, on whom they have a calming, almost sedative effect, and people will follow them anywhere, believing implicitly in everything they say.

When a Chamomile Roman commits, they really commit themselves — either to a project or person. Half measures are not for them. They are great company and people will always be eager to visit them, as they are relaxing to be with, have lots of interests, are entertaining, amusing, and charming. In fact they can charm the birds out of the trees, and probably understand the birds' conversations as well. Chamomile Romans do not possess an ego as such and can appear overly humble in certain situations, being embarrassed if lavish praise is heaped upon them, although they may be secretly pleased that someone appreciated their work. This is not false modesty, but just a surprise that anyone would consider what they had done out of the ordinary.

The inner peace that Chamomile Romans appear to have can be misleading because inner conflicts can torment them — mainly on the issue of their living on earth, and not in heaven. They are liable to have changeable moods and emotions, particularly in relationships — and this can cause them (and other people) emotional stress. Chamomile Romans can also become allergic to people — cutting them off, putting notices on the door saying keep away, and being so generally disagreeable that nobody wants to visit. However, this is necessary to enable them to refresh themselves. They pick up on other people's feelings, pain, and distress, and sometimes need time alone to recollect themselves before facing the world again. Romans are not only allergic to people, they can also be allergic to emotional problems or stress — and develop bloating and other intestinal problems, for example. Romans can become very depressed, unable to see anyone's point of view, and get distressed beyond belief if an injustice is done to them.

A negative Chamomile Roman will tend to externalize everything and have what could be called verbal diarrhea. They will tell you every little detail of their day, how mistreated they were, what their work colleagues did to them, and how unjust everyone and everything has been toward them. No details will be left out. This is just Roman's way of discharging distasteful episodes in the day but it can be annoying to the partner because when Roman has finished talking they're emotionally exhausted and drained, and won't want to hear anything a partner might have to say about their day. Anyhow, they will shortly bloom again and will no longer wish to speak about any of it. In fact, to be asked to repeat the events just makes them throw up their hands in horror because, as far as they're concerned, it's now over and done with. This cathartic experience can leave others annoyed to say the least, and can often lead to misunderstandings.

Chamomile Romans are more feminine than their brothers, the deep blue Chamomile Germans, and some human beings carry the characteristics of both.

But above all, Romans are in touch with their spiritual selves. When they're children, this can take the form of seeing fairies or imaginary friends, and it can quite easily carry on into adulthood. Chamomile Roman profiles are gentle and delicate with a serenity many would like to achieve, but which hardly any other personalities do — except perhaps Neroli.

Teddy Fearnhamm IScB France, MRQA, aromatherapist and tutor:

"Chamomile Roman has every quality attributed to caring — it presents a small waterfall of comfort. Think of it — a cascade of Chamomile Roman and you immediately feel loved."

CINNAMON   LEAFIE/SPICIE
Cinnamomum zeylanicum

CHARACTER
Warming, Secular, Fair-minded

USE FOR THESE POSITIVE ATTRIBUTES
Invigorated, Steadfast, Benevolent, Strength, Practical, Energized, Realistic, Direct

USE TO COUNTERACT THESE NEGATIVE ATTRIBUTES
Instability, Severity, Bleakness, Malice, Spitefulness, Coldness, Fear, Nervous exhaustion, Debility, Introversion, Superficiality

CINNAMON
Personality Profile

Cinnamon is the larger-than-life, affable type of person — practical, intelligent, with a strong personality. They can be very conservative in thought and nature, preferring the comfort of the establishment rather than the risk and discomfort of the unknown. This isn't to say they're unadventurous. Far from it, they do enjoy a bit of excitement now and again — providing it doesn't interfere with their well-being.

They are usually large, gregarious types — if not in stature, then in largesse. Both males and females can be aggressive rather than assertive but neither have a sexist frame of mind. They believe everyone has an equal part to play, just so long as it doesn't interfere with their own plans. Although they may appear sexist to others, Cinnamons simply do not think in those terms. To them, people are people. If women want to play football, "Good for them."

Cinnamons take their home life very seriously and will defend everyone in it — partner, children, brothers, sisters, parents, and grandparents. They don't take kindly to anyone criticizing any member of their family. If their children are harmed, either physically or verbally, Cinnamon will instantly be on the warpath and, indeed, may kill anyone who seriously hurt their loved ones.

Male Cinnamons are often admired by their peers as someone who is in control and has everything running smoothly, even if this isn't always the case. Males are often thought, incorrectly, to be having exciting affairs, especially as Cinnamon never denies it, while the Cinnamon woman may very well be hiding a real secret. This personality is often described as strong, or as an "all-round guy" (or gal), and a good companion — if a little vain. Cinnamons enjoy being well-dressed and usually have an expensive car, or at least a respectable one, a nice home and all the material possessions the western world deems necessary for a comfortable life. The home will be full of all manner of electrical gadgetry (even if its never used), and plenty of gardening equipment that looks good leaning against the garden fence. If something wears out, Cinnamons don't bother mending it, they prefer to go out and buy a new one.

Unlike the sacrificing Juniper, who puts everyone else first in line, Cinnamons will first and foremost please themselves. They stand up for their rights and want what is their due — and usually get it. The tax man will be fought with and if the hospital isn't treating Grandma right, the nurses, doctors, and administrators will certainly know about it. Cinnamons expect service and honesty from everyone they deal with, and they never lie or shortchange themselves or others.

Although Cinnamons wouldn't become local vigilantes, they do like law and order, with everything in its place, and no disturbances. They consider themselves fair-minded and despise unlawfulness, lying, or cheating. Direct and forceful, Cinnamons can be too opinionated for their own good sometimes, particularly if an ideal is at stake. Although they try to keep it hidden, they have a strong moralistic streak, which often seems out of character for these street-wise people. Illness seemingly does not affect this character, but Cinnamons are sometimes clumsy and can be accident prone.

Athletics or other sporting activities appeal to their competitive nature. If they're allowed to be, the Cinnamon personality can be manipulating and, because they like to be in charge, overly controlling. They don't use cunning in their manipulation of others, being far too open for that, but will use brute strength of character so people often find it easier just to let them get on with it. It makes life more peaceful. If someone close does argue with Cinnamon, they'll sulk for weeks rather than give in — which is, of course, another way of getting control.

Negative Cinnamons become very superficial, hollow, and conceited. They may start to buy the most ostentatious objects and can become unstable — bullying their partner and friends. Infidelity is an easy temptation for them, mentally if not always physically, but they'll blame their partner for it. If they get found out there will be heated arguments and Cinnamon will become very insecure. Verbal aggression is to be expected at this stage, and Cinnamons can slide into mental stagnation, becoming withdrawn and lacking in motivation. Negativity robs them of the incentive to do anything worthwhile, and despondency can set in. With a little encouragement and praise, however, Cinnamon can soon be back in the game.

Because of their need for material wealth, which Cinnamons believe is necessary for their happiness, they often find themselves in jobs that aren't really suitable for their character. They are better off (mentally if not financially) in jobs such as probation officer, security, social worker, and sports teacher. Although not really entrepreneurial, Cinnamons are happy being self-employed in service businesses that are steady and always in demand, such as plumbing, electronics, carpentry, building and decorating. Being very trustworthy, they instill confidence in their customers and do well financially.

As friends and lovers Cinnamons are steady, lively company and everyone always knows exactly where they are with them. In their positive mode, they hold few surprises, are warmhearted and generally good people to know. They're very approachable and will try to help someone out of trouble if they can, even though they won't consider it their responsibility to do so.

———

CLARY SAGE
Slavia sclarea
HERBIE/FLORAL

CHARACTER
Euphoric, Restoring, Harmonizing, Warming

USE FOR THESE POSITIVE ATTRIBUTES
Calm, Soothed, Confidence, Grounded, Regenerated, Inspired, Tranquil, Revitalized, Uplifted, Balanced, Strength, Relaxed, Restores equilibrium

USE TO COUNTERACT THESE NEGATIVE ATTRIBUTES
Nervousness, Stress, Tension, Changeability, Worried, Anxious, Claustrophobic, Compulsive, Depression, Nightmares, Hostility, Hyperactivity, Lethargy, Obsession, Panic, Mental strain, Fear, Paranoia, Melancholy, Burnout, Delusions, Emotional debility, Absentmindedness, Weepiness, Guilt

CLARY SAGE
Personality Profile

Clary Sage's personality is not that of the wiser and more mature common Sage personality, but is more gentle, melancholy, and thoughtful. Clary will not be rash in their words but will think carefully before they speak, measuring the effect their voice is having on others — making sure it is not offensive. Because Clary Sage has the ability to probe deeply into the psyche of others, they are very aware of the effect they can have on other people. Although they may appear pensive at times they are also playful and don't dwell on things too long, even if they give that impression. If gut feeling or intuition tells them something is finished, they will move on.

The Clary Sage personality has the ability to stir up many long forgotten feelings in people, good or bad, and it can be quite unnerving for some other types — such as the Tea Trees, who do not hide their feelings about anything. Having said that, Clarys are very warm and friendly and enjoy people, along with all their idiosyncrasies. Never judgmental, which is much in their favor, Clarys have the ability to be comforting in times of need, especially during periods of grief.

Clary Sages manage the pressures of daily life well and can handle all kinds of situations. Having an intriguing, fascinating nature, people are drawn to them (although the Clary Sage often cannot figure out why). They are extremely creative and contradictory — being the wise man one minute and the fool the next, and not giving it a second thought.

In work, Clary will not rest until

they're sure a job has been done correctly. Using their psyche as well as their head, they intuitively know when a task is complete. Being so adaptable they can tackle almost any job and shine in creative occupations, such as art, composing, writing, designing, or being involved in advertising, journalism, photography, video, or film.

For most of the time Clary Sages are perfectly balanced between male and female characteristics. If a woman, she may have been called a tomboy when young and if a man, he may have been called a sissy. Both would have been puzzled by this, as they simply don't have this type of sexist attitude. In later life, they can be mistakenly thought to be falsely trying to be one of the boys or one of the girls, but any sarcastic comment on this is met with an answer that will set the ears burning for a week.

Clary Sages are very sexual people and enjoy sensuality in all its forms. When they fall in love, it will be completely — with mind, body, and spirit. Because of the balance between their male and female sides, a relationship with Clary Sage can be a very harmonious experience. However, they are sometimes drawn to the more unconventional type of relationship, if only for the experience. They are deeply romantic and not at all frivolous about their relationships — but can have a lapse of morals where love is concerned. Undoubtedly there is a secret life somewhere, which nobody will suspect. This secret life can be mundane — like going train spotting without telling anyone, or exotic like being a spy.

The female Clary Sage will be very feminine, one of the most feminine of the herbie types, and have lots of aspirations, dreams, and hopes. She's probably waiting for a knight in shining armor to sweep her off her feet. The male Clary Sage will search for the princess with the long shining hair, and the fact that none might exist for him does not dampen the dream. Indeed, Clary Sages will dream the dream until the day they die.

When in negative mode, both male and female Clary Sages can succumb to outside pressures instead of dealing with them and this may happen as a midlife crisis. It can make them hypersensitive and hesitant, and they'll start to find fault in their otherwise exciting relationships, claiming they are dull and uninspiring — being altogether temperamental. It is often when negative moods affect them that Clary Sage will choose the wrong friends and lovers. Negativity cramps their style, and creativity. Clary Sage will become isolated in their feelings, may suffer emotional crises and, by choosing the wrong partner, emotional abuse. They will suffer with nervous and emotional burnout, they'll become compulsive, lethargic and nervous, and may be prone to addiction. The negative Clary Sage can suffer paranoia and fears, and become obsessive. The shift from positive Clary Sage to a negative one can be very dramatic. This is very rare, however, because the Clary Sage personality is more likely to be intelligent, confident, and assured. Generally, they are very courageous and nice people.

Shirley Price MIFA Reg., MISPA, aromatherapy tutor and author:

"Not everyone likes Clary's aroma, but she is one of those people who grows on you — and the more you get to know her, the more you like her and realize how dependable she is. Among her many talents, she is perceptive, recognizing that we like to stay young... Not least, she is a charmer — helping us to succumb to the advances of our partner if we find them inconvenient or demanding when we are tired."

CORIANDER
Coriandrum sativum
SEEDIE/SPICIE

CHARACTER
Enlivening, Motivating, Encouraging

USE FOR THESE POSITIVE ATTRIBUTES
Creativity, Imagination, Good memory, Confidence, Motivation, Optimism, Sincerity, Expressiveness, Enthusiasm

USE TO COUNTERACT THESE NEGATIVE ATTRIBUTES
Emotional tiredness, Weariness, Irritability, Nervousness, Stress, Nervous debility, Doubt, Fear of failure, Sulkiness, Being uncooperative, Vulnerability

CORIANDER Personality Profile

Coriander is a light, sweet, frivolous type of personality — but with hidden depth. They are sincere, imaginative, full of optimism, very warm, and inviting. They're always surrounded by people asking favors and their opinions and, being so accommodating, Coriander never turns anyone away. Corianders enjoy expressing themselves and are masters of body language in getting their point across — throwing their hands in the air to express frustration or giving themselves a gleeful hug if they receive good news. Corianders are people to enjoy.

When they're positive, Corianders are full of imagination and very creative. To say they do their own thing would be a bit of an understatement and whatever they're involved in, it will be different. Take their home, for example. It might be minimalist in the extreme — white and totally empty except for a futon, or they might have a shocking pink dining room with a plastic fish hanging from the ceiling. The heaters might be decorated with sparkles or sequins, or there might be so many objects around the place you have difficulty finding a seat. Coriander definitely does things their own way.

This personality has an extraordinary memory, and they're able to recount an event that happened years ago in precise detail, repeating conversations word for word that you or I would have long forgotten. It can all be very unnerving. They remember not only words, but the expressions people used when they said them and their tone of voice — all of which provides a great store of information for those who become actors and actresses. An animal equivalent to this personality would be the chameleon, and only very close friends will be able to ignore the different characters they take on everyday and see the real person underneath. This is not to say these people have multiple personalities, it's just that they can adopt different looks and behavior patterns at a moment's notice, and discard them just as easily. All this makes them very stimulating people to be with — providing you can keep up the pace. And another thing, Corianders will accept your faults and foibles with perfect, nonjudgmental tolerance.

I once had a secretary who did not fit what might be the stereotype, because she'd sometimes come to work in quite outlandish clothes. This was in the early days of punk and one day she came in with shocking pink hair and Vivian Westwood clothes. A week later she walked in with short black hair and a suit that would look at home in the law courts. She was amazing, there is no other word for it. She laughed a lot and everyone liked her, plus she was good at her job. I was pregnant during this time and she fulfilled my strange dietary requirements without saying a word. If I'd asked her for a coal and cinnamon sandwich, I swear she wouldn't have batted an eyelid. She'd just ask, "With or without mayonnaise?"

Corianders are passionate in whatever they do, even if it just takes a minute, and it can be very confusing (not to say exhausting) to the uninitiated. The person who gets involved with a Coriander will never quite know who they are meeting. As one lover of a Coriander told me, "I'm left breathless but captivated." They eventually drift into jobs where their talent is recognized but may start out in a different field altogether.

When they're negative, Corianders can be very uncooperative, questioning everything. They will sulk and become very vulnerable to criticism, sometimes having a weariness upon them that makes you wonder if they can carry on. They become almost childlike in the sense that they have no confidence or self-esteem. This is particularly noticeable if they're in show business or in any type of job that involves daily contact with the public, such as sales. As they start to doubt their abilities, Corianders become nervous and if they're actors or actresses will develop bad stage fright and lose their memory for lines. This can be a truly terrifying experience for them. Mesmerized into inactivity, it can take the negative Coriander a very long time to recover and, sadly, some performers never do.

If a Coriander falls into negativity, they'll need their family and friends to rally round and slowly coax them back into life. The knocks will show and although they'll be bright and breezy, they'll adopt an air of caution for a while until something new and wonderful happens, which recharges their batteries and they're off again.

Nicole Perez, MIFA Reg., aromatherapist and tutor:

"Coriander begins with a 'C' as in confidence as it often takes confidence and courage to allow the experience of life to move and release our deepest feelings. It's scent pervades, giving a feeling of being slightly drunk and as with alcohol it frees the senses from inhibition and brings our sensuality, but it can also stir our libidinous self."

CYPRESS   LEAFIE/WOODIE
Cupressus sempervirens

CHARACTER
Protective, Righteous, Wise, Direction

USE FOR THESE POSITIVE ATTRIBUTES
Strength, Comfort, Change, Direction, Assertion, Control, Understanding, Balance, Sensitivity, Generosity of spirit, Contentment, Stillness, Confidence, Inner peace, Wisdom, Purity of heart, Stability, Patience, Trust, Incorruptibility, Structured, Softly powerful, Direct, Willpower, Straightforward

USE TO COUNTERACT THESE NEGATIVE ATTRIBUTES
Grief, Sorrow, Self-loathing, Pressurised, Being dominated, Opinionated, Jealous, Lethargic, Weak-willed, Fearful, Timid, Emotional turmoil, Unbalanced, Isolated, Inconsolable, Frustrated, Unable to speak up for oneself, Emotionally tired, Emotionally unstable, Tearful, Loss, Regret, Distracted, Lack of concentration, Absentminded, Uncontrollable passions

CYPRESS
Personality Profile

Cypress represents the strength within. Its character is wisdom, strength, and uprightness. It stands proud, only slightly swaying, always forceful and direct. Cypress is a symbol of eternity that directs itself to the heavens, answering to no one but the great spirit. The human counterpart of cypress is very similar. They tend to be forceful, outspoken, and firm in their views — if perhaps at times a little dogmatic. The air of an authoritarian can often disguise the subtle undercurrent of sensitivity that wells in sympathy to sorrow and loss.

There is never an excuse not to be straightforward with this type. In fact, they demand it, along with your respect in everything, not expecting to be crossed nor, at times, disobeyed. But their wisdom in sorrows of the heart, grieving, and loss, often allows them to give the best advice to people, as does their tendency to see both sides of the story — even if they disapprove of one of them. People will turn to them in times of extreme distress, usually when there is no other path to travel for advice and comfort.

People perceive Cypress to be powerful and able to sort out most problems. If they are not a person's first choice of confidante, it is perhaps because they see them as proud, and even arrogant. This is because of their air of honesty, lawfulness, and their unbending search for truth — even if this isn't always authentic. The Cypress personality doesn't always tread the straight and narrow, and sometimes use their air of credibility to their own advantage. These are clever types, and will have the edge where matters of money or finance are concerned.

Often, Cypress don't see the need for earthly pleasures — including spending money on what could be considered fripperies — considering that there are more lofty pleasures to pursue. They may feel drawn to the role of clergyman, or become active in religious sects, and other very masculine areas such as Masonic orders and so on. Cypress will be the headmaster you dread bumping into when skipping school, but will care enough to ask why you skipped school in the first place. A female Cypress will be in charge of the household and may be considered domineering, although always ready to physically help when someone's world starts to crumble.

Cypresses make great grandparents because children always know the boundaries and feel comfortable in their presence, while Cypress loves the children's free spirits. As the children get older, discipline and respect will be expected, while Cypress will be in the forefront of defending the family. This personality often dwells on spiritual matters, and have no fear of death. Once they have found their pathway, wherever it may lead, Cypress can become unbending in their attitudes and fixed in their ideas, which can be difficult for other, freer minds to bear. Cypress have an air of knowing, but are sympathetic to less structured minds. They help balance the unstable, and patch up the holes.

Jan Kusmirek, MDDH, MED, LLFA, MIFA Reg., LCSP, DM, aromatherapist, medical herbalist and lecturer:

"Cypress... I see it or sense it as reliable, clean, upright yet with the warmth and comfort of masculinity. Not stern or cold like some pines but more solemn or even soothing. It is strangely astringent (personality) so helps to withstand pressure, reduces fear of one's peers, etc. It tightens up and centers."

EUCALYPTUS   LEAFIE/WOODIE
Eucalyptus radiata/globulus

CHARACTER
Energy, Stimulation, Balance, Sheltering

USE FOR THESE POSITIVE ATTRIBUTES
Emotional balancer, Energy balancer, Concentration, Logical thought, Centering, Rationality, Cooling, Predictability

USE TO COUNTERACT THESE NEGATIVE ATTRIBUTES
Exhaustion, Heated emotions, Mood swings, Lack of concentration, Cluttered thoughts, Temper tantrums, Irrational thoughts, Explosive nature, Argumentative

EUCALYPTUS
Personality Profile

Just as there are many species of eucalyptus tree, so there are many variations on the Eucalyptus personality. Here, we are talking about the Eucalyptus globulas personality, which I shall simply refer to as "Eucalyptus." For the most part Eucalyptus' are very calm, rational people. They don't have any special abilities and wouldn't stick out in a crowd. Everyone seems to know one. Eucalyptus remains calm in a storm and, when they're in positive mode, try not to make a fuss, preferring to sort things out for themselves. They don't gossip and can keep a secret.

In general, the Eucalyptus personality is content and well-balanced. Some people might call them dull but they're a refreshing change from some of the more dynamic personalities. They do have an adventurous spirit, which takes the form of planning a project and quietly getting on with it. They don't make plans just for the sake of it; they are into action. This side of their personality can be surprising as they suddenly announce that they're off on an adventure vacation trekking across swampy marshes. They won't divulge too much of their plans to anyone — being highly suspicious people — but will just tell you what you need to know. For them, that is sufficient. After all, they reckon, it's their business, not yours. You could say they're too secretive but they just don't think anyone should be interested in what is a private matter. This can be very annoying to the more outward types such as Fennels, who will share their every thought. Generally, Eucalyptus is a stable personality, able to diffuse an argument simply by being in the room. They have the coolness not to argue back, unless in negative mode — but that's another matter. Eucalyptus appears cool, logical and, at times, calculating. It seems as if everything must have an explanation or be proven before they'll consider it. Although this personality is very laid-back, they can have an exhilarating effect on others, instilling enthusiasm and confidence. They do this by logical reasoning, which gives the more imaginative personalities a good basis from which to launch their ideas and creativity.

Eucalyptus types go in for the sciences and are often found in the medical professions — such as doctors, nurses, and pharmacists — but they're also quite likely to be accountants, bankers, and solicitors. They are good in those professions that don't require much creative thought and that have strict guidelines

that must be adhered to. They will never make any earth-shattering discoveries, even as scientists, unless they have a fair proportion of a more imaginative personality within them. Basically, they're happy knowing that $2+2 = 4$ and $4+4 = 8$.

In their private life, Eucalyptus is very similar — choosing carefully where they live and who they have as their partner. Sometimes, but not often, you find they choose a floral partner, but this is not a good match for them as their cooling nature tends to put out the flames of the passionate florals and it all ends in tears. Eucalyptus is very predictable in love. They'll make a list of the potential partners' good and bad points and go for the one who compliments them in some way or other, and who won't rock the boat too much. As a partner, Eucalyptus is entertaining and can make one laugh.

A negative Eucalyptus is another matter. They can store up resentments and slights, hoarding them until one day they snap! They'll become explosive, which can be very surprising to others, as they never let on to anyone that they've been feeling hurt and disillusioned. So when the explosion comes it can be very heated — and you'd better run for cover. They'll shout and yell as years of pent-up resentment comes flying out in a barrage of verbal abuse. Others may stare in surprise, unable to believe that Eucalyptus could go so obviously over the edge. However, it's all over as quickly as it started and they'll apologize with, "Sorry about that, I don't know what came over me," embarrassed that anyone had seen them with their guard down.

It's not good for anyone to keep things bottled up and if Eucalyptus doesn't find some regular means of release it can lead to nervous exhaustion, temper tantrums and, eventually, burnout. If this happens it can take a long time to get them back on their feet because they feel they were indulgent to release their emotions in that way and to sink into such a state. They are easily addicted to anything that relieves their emotional discomfort and it can be difficult for them to be weaned off.

Eucalyptuses are good, solid characters, who are often shy, believe in reasonable behavior. They can be very willing to help others, not expecting thanks or praise. Indeed, they'll probably be embarrassed if it's offered.

EUCALYPTUS CITRIODORA (Lemon) LEAFIE/WOODIE
Eucalyptus citriodora

CHARACTER
Soundness, Trust, Vitality, Harmonious

USE FOR THESE POSITIVE ATTRIBUTES
Stimulant, Concentration, Enthusiastic, Uplifting, Vitality, Understanding, Creativity, Regeneration, Optimism, Letting go, Encouraging, Empathy, Positive change, Freedom, Expressiveness, Comforting

USE TO COUNTERACT THESE NEGATIVE ATTRIBUTES
Sluggishness, Emotional crisis, Emptiness, Confusion, Disillusionment, Restlessness, Fear, Despondency, Emptiness, Loneliness

EUCALYPTUS CITRIODORA (Lemon) Personality Profile

This personality is fresh, alive, and loves freedom. Eucalyptus Citriodora are like the youngest member of the Eucalyptus family, constantly expressing new ideas and full of vitality and laughter. Indeed, expressiveness and enjoying life to the fullest is what this personality is about. What excites them is new things and new ideas and anything that catches their imagination and is inventive. Citriodoras will be the whiz kids on the latest computer games, and they'll invent a gadget if they find it's needed — a capacity made possible by their tremendous imagination. When you're around a Citriodora, you feel as if you're on the edge of making a new discovery — which you very possibly are.

The one thing Citriodora cannot stand is being tied down or feeling hemmed in. They love, and indeed *need* freedom — freedom to express themselves, freedom to move wherever it pleases them to go, and freedom to be who they really are. This can be quite disconcerting if you're in a relationship with a Citriodora because they'll only want to see you (and be really happy to do so) when they want to. Although they may agree to compromise, this on-off quality can make having a relationship with them seem rather like having a relationship with a roller coaster, especially if you're a home-loving Marjoram.

Citriodoras have a freshness and exuberance that they bring to everything they do, whether this is in a relationship, at home, or at work. In the workplace they are a veritable dynamo, very dynamic and go-getting, yet they're also very sound and trustworthy. They abhor disharmony and will often try, through humor to bring about balance. Secrets are very safe with this personality and you can have absolute faith they will not exploit any weakness they may discover in you or anyone else. If you're going through an emotional crisis, Citriodora will be a tower of strength, listening attentively, never criticizing or judging, or even remarking on any aspect of your behavior that others would call pathetic. For all their love of freedom, Citriodoras are very sound people.

When Citriodoras get down-hearted, it's usually because there is just too much to do, too many ideas to process, too many places to visit, and too many people to see.

Will Citriodora ever be able to do it all in one lifetime? This question bothers them and they are often drawn to the idea of reincarnation, if only because it gives them the opportunity to get more done. People disillusion Citriodora, rather than events, and they can feel empty and lonely if they somehow forget (in the rush) to include love and romance on their agenda. Instead, they leave it all to fate. Overall, Citriodoras are fun people, creative, and enthusiastic and, if you can handle friends who knock on the door at 2 o'clock in the morning for a cup of coffee after not seeing them for two years, great friends.

Judy is a typical Citriodora in that she is bright, funny, encourages and comforts everyone. Whenever she sees her friends she boosts them up so they can forge ahead or take that vital risk that moves them closer to their goal. This is one of the reasons why Citriodoras are so well loved. When there are steps to be taken into the unknown, Judy is always willing to hold her friend's hands — when she's around. And there's the rub, because, like any Citriodora, Judy begins to feel uneasy and trapped after a while, and must put on her wings and fly. Her friends would get a postcard from India or Australia once in a while and then, knock, knock, she'd be on the doorstep again — as if four years hadn't even passed. However, she started to feel lonely, as if she'd missed out on meeting Mr. Right by being constantly on the move. Eventually, so I'm told, Judy married an Orange type personality on top of the Andes mountains, and they are now living happily in Brazil.

FENNEL, SWEET
Foeniculum vulgare dulce

SEEDIE

CHARACTER
Clearing, Resolute, Enlightened

USE FOR THESE POSITIVE ATTRIBUTES
Enlivened, Motivated, Fortitude, Clarity, Forceful, Perseverance, Courageous, Reliable, Confident, Assertive

USE TO COUNTERACT THESE NEGATIVE ATTRIBUTES
Mental blockages, Emotional blockages, Boredom, Unable to adjust, Fear of failure, Hostile, Overburdened, Lack of creativity

FENNEL
Personality Profile

The highly active Fennel personality will take brisk walks, exercise regularly, and be a member of a sports club. At school they will love athletics, be on a sports team, and they may even receive a sports scholarship. Fennels are constantly active and always on the move. They don't walk — they hurry along — leaping up the stairs rather than waiting for an elevator. Fennels buy exercise tapes to use at home, they belong to swimming clubs and probably play racquetball on the weekend. They excel at any type of competition — at work as well as at play.

Fennel is a very assertive personality, invigorating, and determined. They'll decorate the house while everyone else is only thinking about it, redesign the garden over a weekend, and change the furniture around on a whim — and still find time to visit friends. They're very kind people, and will help their neighbors or friends if they can't find anything else to do at home. As children, they'll willingly walk the dog, run errands and generally be helpful, getting bored easily and preferring to do anything rather than sit still.

Emotionally too, Fennels are very active, moving from one emotion to another — crying one minute and laughing the next. It's very easy for Fennels to build a brick wall to hide their emotional pain, and it can take forever to knock it down and get to know them deeply. They'll talk for hours and hours about themselves and then you realize they actually told you nothing. Nothing important, anyway. Not that these are superficial people, although at times it may seem that way. Although apparently easy going, they're actually shifting gears constantly, so you can't really catch who they are. They're not big on profound relationships, thinking they may hold them back in life, and often end up alone if they can't find someone who can fit into their plans. Fennels can be very tiresome because you never get a straight answer, even to a simple question like, "Which day shall we go to the movies?" This personality is just too frightened of commitment. Although sometimes exasperating, Fennels are never dull.

Fennels are very intelligent people, quick-witted and creative and needing a lot of mental stimulation. The partner should be an equal, rather than one who simply complements their personality. Providing you don't need to understand how they tick, and don't want to dig too deeply into their motives for doing things, Fennels make terrific friends. Being intellectually sharp, Fennels are often ahead of the game — as if they have insider knowledge.

This personality makes good stockbrokers and financiers because they love the risk element in making a deal that might make them, or lose them, ten million dollars. Money is very important, and they enjoy making it, so also make good entrepreneurs — whether male or female. Fennels are assertive and know what they want and go for it, but not at the expense of others — unless it really can't be avoided.

When they're being negative, it's a complete reversal — Fennels will become what can only be described as a slob, and slump in a chair, not bothering to see friends. Activities fly out the window as Fennel loses their competitive edge, not really bothering about anything — which can be a disaster if they have a job that involves quick thinking. The only race they think about will be the one on TV. The more negative they become, the sharper their tongue becomes and anybody who passes them on the success ladder will be ridiculed and become the subject of sarcasm.

Unless something snaps them out of this negative mode, Fennel will get more guilt ridden. For their family and friends it'll be like watching the Titanic go down, a horrifying loss of potential. It takes a brave person to attempt to budge them, and the best thing is flattery. Once they're roused, it will be painful to watch them try to repair the damage to their health and business contacts. The Fennel, meanwhile, will be completely perplexed as to how they allowed all this to happen.

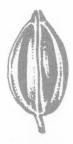

Fennel

FRANKINCENSE
Boswellia carteri

RESINIE

CHARACTER
Elevating, Spiritual, Meditative, Wisdom

USE FOR THESE POSITIVE ATTRIBUTES
Comfort, Healing, Emotional stability, Enlightenment, Protective, Introspection, Courage, Resolution, Fortitude, Acceptance, Inspiration

USE TO COUNTERACT THESE NEGATIVE ATTRIBUTES
Fears, Grief, Blockages, Over-attachment, Burnout, Exhaustion, Insincerity, Panic, Anxiety, Disconnection, Repression, Resistance, Self-destruction, Apprehension, Despair

FRANKINCENSE
Personality Profile

Frankincense people are compassionate and interesting and something of an enigma in that they often display an air of mystery and secretiveness, even hinting at an understanding of the nature of the universe. There is a driving forcefulness about this personality, a strength and fortitude supported by maturity, conscientiousness, confidence, and efficiency. At the same time, Frankincense can be impetuous, compulsive, and generous.

Frankincense personalities are often geniuses and may well have invented practical contraptions for use around the home and at work. They don't rely on others to do things for them, preferring to use their own initiative, and are sometimes called eccentric. Frankincense will drive fast on dangerous mountain roads, ski down runs nobody else would dare, and swim in shark-infested waters without batting an eye. It's not that they're reckless but they believe they are protected in ways that the rest of us are not.

The Frankincense personality has what one might call parapsychological tendencies. They're very sensitive to atmospheres, sensing unhappiness or evil in a room or house, although this wouldn't necessarily be mentioned if they didn't think you would understand. Although no particular personality has more psychic experiences than another, some *notice* them more than others, and Frankincense notices the most. They also sense the intentions of other people, which is a very useful tool.

Frankincenses are very steady, upright citizens and are often found in jobs that command respect and even honor. In business, their ability to sense accurately whether a deal will turn out well or be a waste of time is a very useful tool for them to have. Although this profile may make them seem rather cold, Frankincenses are very kind, warmhearted personalities with a knack of making people feel both confident and secure. They would make good counselors as their advice is often very down-to-earth and practical, not impossible for mere mortals to carry out.

The Frankincense person may not think of themselves as religious and may avoid places of worship, but they carry a profound love of God in their hearts. Frankincense question things in terms of good and evil and have a love of all things spiritual, which gives them a deep wisdom. They are often excellent speakers, clear and eloquent, but are inclined to be somewhat blunt.

If they're negative, the Frankincense personality can be destructive and bitter, full of skepticism and cynicism, inclined to become guilt-ridden, insecure and uncertain, liable to suffer anxiety attacks and stress, also becoming short-tempered and agitated. This is such an enlightened personality, however, they soon realize what's going on and make a concerted effort to change direction — into positivity. Frankincense is a well-balanced personality and remarkably gifted. They are terrific communicators and are friendly, warm, and loving.

Maureen Farrell, MRPharmS, FRSH, MIFA Reg., MISPA, aromatherapist and tutor:

"Frankincense — the traveler, the pilgrim on the Way of Life — a steadfast companion in a journey through grief and in letting go of fear or suppressed emotions. For me, the resins and resinoids most frequently used in aromatherapy come into the category of Wounded Healer."

GERANIUM
Pelargonium graveolens

FLORAL/HERBIE

CHARACTER
Balancing, Healing, Uplifting, Comforting

USE FOR THESE POSITIVE ATTRIBUTES
Consoling, Cushioning, Solace, Adjustment, Elevating, Regenerating, Humour, Friendliness, Stimulant, Balancing, Soothing, Security, Assuring, Shielding, Mothering, Stability, Tranquillity, Steadiness

USE TO COUNTERACT THESE NEGATIVE ATTRIBUTES
Anxiety, Depression, Acute fear, Extreme moods, Confusion, Rigidity, Instability, Abuse, Moodiness, Lack of self-esteem, Insecurity, Sensitivity, Tension, Stress, Hurt, Overly emotional, Crisis, Apprehension, Aggression, Irrationality, Discontent, Worry, Heartache

---

GERANIUM
Personality Profile

The Geranium personality is friendly and comforting, not in any way extroverted or overly talkative. This is one of the mothering types of personalities, always taking care of someone or something. Geraniums just get on with things. They allow everyone freedom to have their own thoughts, never interfering unless you want them to — which can be infuriating if you don't have the courage to ask for help (as Grapefruits will). Geraniums seem to be able to create a feeling of security and stability wherever they go. This doesn't mean they're boring, far from it, but they just seem to have the knack of making everything all right again. Say for example, you

feel frustrated and hurt about something and need to make a phone call to sort it out, Geranium will make you a cup of coffee, settle you in a chair and make the call for you. Your tension is relieved because you don't have to make the unpleasant call and you feel cared for (and about three years old).

Geraniums never look for thanks or appreciation but usually take it for granted. They have the ability to wash away your tension and stress just by being there, and caring, and they do care a great deal for their family and friends — which are very valuable to Geraniums. They tend to take on too much, however, and don't leave enough space for themselves and unfortunately those who are helped may not even notice that help may be needed in return sometimes.

Geraniums are seldom eccentric, outlandish characters prone to great strokes of genius. They are just steady and stable, but often do have the most bizarre friends and companions, flamboyant, and colorful — the complete opposite to themselves. This feature makes the even more popular and they have the most interesting dinner parties, the most interesting house guests, and their homes are always full of people. This isn't because they are not sensational cooks — they tend to serve good home cooking — nor because they are sparkling conversationalists. What attracts people to them is their marvelous ability to make people feel worthy and wanted.

Geraniums may be surrounded by fascinating people but fascinating people are often too full of their own self importance to think about lending a hand. Geranium will set the table, cook the meal, clean up, wash the dishes and glasses and if someone asks, "Oh, do you want a hand?" they'll do it knowing that, more often than not, Geranium will say, "No, you carry on with your conversation, I'll do it" (unlike the Lavender, who'll leave the cleaning for someone else to do).

Within the family, this generosity of nature can really be exploited. This personality will continue to do their children's laundry twenty years after they're left home, mind the grandchildren, and take on the chore of washing and repairing the entire football team's uniforms. Unless they occasionally shout, Stop! very loudly, they can easily become the gofer. Geranium is the ultimate personality for being taken for granted, never really getting their due. They often come into their own in middle age, and may surprise everyone by suddenly packing a bag and going in search of personal happiness. They can get very anxious and depressed if they're not appreciated, and may find they are suffering from more than one kind of broken heart.

Negative Geraniums have mastered the art of inflicting guilt on their families and use it at every opportunity. They can also be prone to imaginary illnesses as a way of getting (much-deserved) attention. Unfortunately, this often has the opposite effect, and drives people away. Not all Geraniums are meek, but they can be very meek — bordering on the doormat type. These personalities may have suffered emotional abuse as a child and feel they somehow have to make up for what they perceive to be their fault.

Geraniums are a much undervalued personality. They have generously comforted those who suffer, those with broken hearts, the grieving and the stressed out, often without praise. Whether male or female, Geranium is a warm, kind, and generous personality who deserves to be appreciated for the very special person they are.

GINGER
Zingiberaceae officinale

ROOTIE/SPICIE

CHARACTER
Warming, Strengthening, Encouraging

USE FOR THESE POSITIVE ATTRIBUTES
Confidence, Warmth, Fortitude, Empathy, Courage

USE TO COUNTERACT THESE NEGATIVE ATTRIBUTES
Sexual anxieties, Lack of direction, Purposelessness, Unfocused, Apathy, Burnout, Confusion, Fatigue, Loneliness, Sadness, Resignation

---

GINGER
Personality Profile

The Ginger personality is often called the strong, silent type because with them, actions speak louder than words. If you think of a large, gentle giant, you'll get the picture. This doesn't mean Ginger types will be either large or gentle but explains the largesse and warmth this personality exudes. Ginger types couldn't be described as being sedative — they are stimulating and lively company with a very wicked sense of humor, definitely everyone's favorite uncle.

This personality can be very masculine, forceful, and profound; able to sort out their problems philosophically without relying on anybody else. The personal space of people around is respected and Gingers never crowd you or become possessive. That's something the Tuberose personality finds hard to take, whether a member of the family or in another type of relationship with Ginger but, in fact, these two match quite well, balancing each other out. Ginger's lack of possessiveness is part of their charm and they don't expect to have interdependence. Gingers expect you to do your own thing, just as they expect you to leave them alone to do theirs.

Ginger personalities make good listeners but bad conversationalists and prefer jobs that don't entail much conversation. As their caring nature often needs expression, they're good in one of the caring professions that involves listening — counseling, psychology, probation officers, social workers, and so on. They also seem to do well as farmers dealing with animals and will be more inclined toward natural farming methods. Animals respect the quiet strength of Gingers, making them good vets and veterinary nurses, partly because they have the ability to comfort the owners. An ideal job for this independent soul would be looking after the animals in an African game park.

Although Gingers don't invite people into their home very often — they like their privacy too much — they will be welcoming when people come by. Although they believe their door is always open, others can sense that Gingers actually want to be left alone.

In love, Gingers will dedicate their lives to the loved one, even though they don't often say the magic words, "I love you." Because they allow their partner their own freedom, this is often misunderstood. But don't think freedom means infidelity; it doesn't. Ginger expects fidelity along with respect from partners, parents, children, friends, and business partners — and if they don't get it, their Ginger temper really becomes apparent. Don't cross a Ginger, or you'll be sorry. They'll hunt you down and their temper, once roused, will make sure you pay for any wrongs against them or their loved ones — and beware, grudges can be held for years and years.

Gingers have a very sexual nature, love making love, and will choose a mate who shares their enthusiasm. This is one way that Gingers can express themselves perfectly. They exude a powerful sexuality rather than sensuality, which can be unnerving to more timid profiles, but it explains why florals are often drawn to them.

Negative Gingers are just awful. They withdraw into a silent world of sulking, and appear confused, apathetic, and with no memory of who they formerly were. They will not get depressed as such, but can lose their purpose and joy in life, becoming directionless as if resigned to whatever fate has in store for them. Great bouts of loneliness can engulf them, no matter how many people are around.

After knowing the warm, positive Ginger, this drop into sadness seems profound indeed. They're liable to be unstable at times, particularly if unemployed or passed over for promotion. It's not that they seek power, they do not, it's already built into them, but they'll be upset that they haven't been treated with the respect they deserve, whether for work or some other achievement. They don't like "losing face," as the Chinese say.

Gingers may suffer in silence from emotional burnout — a quite common trait of this personality that often results in their sex drive diminishing, which is devastating to a Ginger. Luckily, the Ginger personality has remarkable powers of recovery and although these negative bouts may come often, they can go away very quickly too. Ginger is a great friend or relative to have around you because they'll always listen to your problems with patience, sincerity, and kindness. Just don't forget to sometimes ask them about theirs.

GRAPEFRUIT   FRUITIE
Citrus paradisi

CHARACTER
Radiating, Cheering, Joyful, Liberating, Boosting,

USE FOR THESE POSITIVE ATTRIBUTES
Joyful, Positive, Confident, Clarity, Balanced, Attuned, Alert, Inspired, generous, Uplifted, Emotionally purified, Spontaneous, Cooperative

USE TO COUNTERACT THESE NEGATIVE ATTRIBUTES
Depression, Dependency, Sadness, Grief, Apathy, Mental pressure, Mental exhaustion, Emotional Violence, Self-doubt, Self-criticism, Aggravated, Frustration

---

GRAPEFRUIT
Personality Profile

The Grapefruit personality is about freshness and newness. These are happy, warm people who are usually bursting with energy (even when they're sitting down), a wonderful radiation of pure energy that gives light to everything they do. Even in the poorest countries, where you might think everyone is weighed down with daily problems of survival, the Grapefruit personality can be found with a big smile on their face, cheerfully helping a neighbor.

The Grapefruit personality has a very deep concern for humanity, and the direction the world is taking. They can't really understand why we allow people with no consciousness or consideration for their fellow man to take over the controls, and why we do nothing about it. Grapefruits

are not particularly concerned about money, although they're not blind to its importance in allowing us to get through life. Being "comfortable," to them, doesn't mean having lots of money, instead "comfort" means being contented.

Grapefruits love people and they dislike seeing someone not fulfilling their potential. They become great motivators, the "get up and go" people, although not overbearing, not saying, "Do something worthwhile with your life," rather, they give out subtle, discreet suggestions, which the recipient doesn't realize were intended to give them confidence or motivation.

Infused with happy joyfulness, Grapefruits sing and laugh the loudest and are not in the least self-conscious. They might have difficulty toning all this down, however. Having no fear of other people, no matter how illustrious they may be, Grapefruits are able to clearly see unspoken intentions and innermost thoughts. Other people are often unaware of this ability of Grapefruit, seeing only the superficial, jolly exterior.

Grapefruits are very clear thinkers. They make wonderful healers because, if nothing else works, the placebo effect of their infectious enthusiasm creates well-being because Grapefruits are attuned to their spiritual selves, and have an affinity with the unseen realms. Because they have a global perspective and care very strongly for the future of the planet, Grapefruits are very good in jobs concerned with the environment. It's almost as if they've been put on this earth as guides of light and happiness for the rest of us, and would make very good leaders, if goodness was a prerequisite for leadership. It's a pity they are often ignored in favor of the more ambitious personalities. As group leaders they can instill enthusiasm on a grand scale, but may tend to overdo it.

Grapefruits make thoughtful, caring partners and lovers, and very good parents, but they may mentally (never emotionally) neglect their own children as they spend so much time trying to save the children of the world. This can lead to resentment and discord. It's fairly easy for a Grapefruit to become bogged down with work or other responsibilities, or to get emotionally overloaded with the problems of this planet, weighed down with the inhumanities human beings can commit against each other. It all becomes too much. Tired and irritable with those nearest and dearest, an overwhelming sadness can rest on their shoulders like a mantle.

Happily, Grapefruit's light is not easily extinguished and it's always there, ready to be rekindled. When they're right, Grapefruits are warm, generous and very cleansing, mentally. Grapefruit is tempted by the prospect of being able to make a clean sweep, and helps many people to do just that.

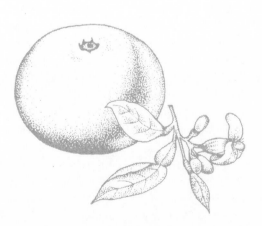

Grapefruit

HELICHRYSUM
FLORAL
(Immortelle or Italian Everlasting)
Helichrysum angustifolium, H italicum, H orientale

CHARACTER
Gentleness, Harmonizing, Caring, Warming, Meditative

USE FOR THESE POSITIVE ATTRIBUTES
Calm, Accepting of change, Buffered, Dreams, Energy, Patience, Idealism, Understanding, Perserverence, Inner strength, Acceptance, Awareness, Positive inner child

USE TO COUNTERACT THESE NEGATIVE ATTRIBUTES
Abuse, Stress, Tension, Emotional crisis, Depression, Lethargy, Mental exhaustion, Emotional exhaustion, Tiredness, Emotional blockages, Disorientation, Overwork, Loneliness, Insecurity, Hypersensitivity, Grief, Addiction, Negative inner child

HELICHRYSUM/ IMMORTELLE
Personality Profile

The Immortelle profile is one of quietness, introversion, and youth, with a quiet knowing that comes from being sure of the spirituality of all things, and the understanding that there are greater things in heaven and earth than we can see. Fragile innocents in a harsh world, Immortelles are frequently called naive because of their compassionate nature and understanding of the frailties of others. This type can easily accept changes of any sort as they're not fixed in their ideas or thoughts.

The Immortelle person is spiritually highly evolved and often seem almost fairy-like, having a high consciousness and mental agility. If wronged, they can forgive quickly, and do not bear grudges, but will not encourage the company of anyone who does commit a wrong against them. This cold shoulder can be difficult for the persons concerned, who often don't realize what it is they have done wrong.

This personality has a dry, cheeky, kooky sense of humor and is great fun to be with. Friendship is very precious to Immortelle who, with an inner strength and genuine love, is always encouraging and helpful. Immortelles are always able to see other people's points of view — even if they don't agree with them — and accept other people's way of doing things. Immortelles always try to at least understand other ways of thinking and doing.

Because of their inner strength and open heart, Immortelle is willing to see new points of view. They love exploring new ideas, walking new pathways, and heading in new directions. They can easily leave people and problems behind, and don't worry about the past. Having a strong sense of what is right and wrong, Immortelles have a willingness to develop and can learn life's lessons very quickly, developing ideas as they go along, learning from everyone and everything, from mistakes as well as successes.

This personality may have suffered abuse as a child — either emotional, verbal, or physical. The sensitivity felt by Immortelle is partly due to their caring, in a corner of their heart, for a child hurt a long time ago. The neglect as a child may have taken the form of lack of love or emotional warmth in the home, and Immortelle may have had difficulty understanding why they were feeling hurt. Rejection is a very powerful emotion that can be carried throughout life — whether that rejection comes from parents, peers, teachers, or siblings. They carry the emotional wounds very deeply (as does a Chamomile Roman type, but in a slightly different way). Immortelle may always be searching for the comfort needed to assure them that everything is all right. The Immortelle personality often appears guarded, as if protecting themselves emotionally, but this is an inaccurate judgment because it's just that they feel no need to externalize and express their emotions to everyone. Sometimes a crisis of identity will occur if Immortelle did not receive enough nurturing love as a child or young

person. They have no difficulty in acknowledging the child within themselves, just as they can acknowledge unseen forces, such as guardian angels or God. They just don't always tell you.

Young at heart and youthful in appearance, Immortelles will have the air of eternal youth about them, even in the last stages of their journey on earth. They're very emotional and will cry like a baby at sad movies, being able to identify with the dramatized sorrow as if it were their own. Immortelles are often very shy but if they could overcome that shyness, would become the world's greatest actors and actresses because they've got such good empathy with other people, or exemplary speakers of truth, outspoken and direct — representative of people, animals, and plant life.

Immortelles can get very apathetic and tired — both emotionally and mentally — often in middle age. When depressed, they cannot be consoled and will often be irrational and irritable, preferring to shut themselves off from the world, just hiding in bed or lying on the sofa, refusing to accept help. They can also become disoriented and confused and lose their valued friendships through simple things like never phoning, missing meetings, being late, and standing people up — and through a host of other annoying but not life-threatening faults.

Despite all this, the Immortelle personality is a floral who loves beauty, delicacy, and joy — all qualities they carry within their beautiful open heart. These are sensitive, caring, and loving people and their idiosyncrasies should easily be forgiven.

HYACINTH
Hyacinthus orientalis

FLORAL

CHARACTER
Gentle, Trusting, Soothing, Enlightening

USE FOR THESE POSITIVE ATTRIBUTES
Calming, Forgiving, High self-esteem, Perseverance, Equilibrium, Trust, Faith, Courage

USE TO COUNTERACT THESE NEGATIVE ATTRIBUTES
Instability, Stress, Repression, Apathy, Lovesick, Dejection, Distress, Grieving, Sorrow, Powerlessness, Regret, Unforgiving, Naiveté, Dependency, Apprehension

HYACINTH
Personality Profile

The Hyacinth personality is forgiving and trusting, and this personality's gentleness and good nature are apparent in everything they touch. They love beauty and beautiful things and can decorate a room exquisitely simply by using their ingenuity and artistry and a few pots of paint, taking immense trouble over every little detail. When you come for lunch the table will look fabulous with little pretty touches to catch the eye. Of course, there will be flowers — that goes without saying. Indeed, Hyacinths are happiest when they are tending gardens and plants and taking care of animals (who don't talk back).

Having an unshakable belief in people, Hyacinths think that good will always triumph over evil. Needless to say, they are often disappointed. Their faith in the human race is a virtue that is easily taken advantage of, particularly by those with no scruples. Time after time, sweet Hyacinth will be drawn into plans they don't really want to be involved with and schemes that are detrimental to their well-being. Relationships are just the same, and Hyacinth is just the personality to choose the wrong man or woman to be their life partner — one who will strip them of all their emotions, and their money. They try to make the best of it because that's how they are.

Hyacinths are very mindful of other people's feelings and love to be privy to their secrets. They don't mean to pass them on, but do, sometimes thinking other people won't repeat what they say. Hyacinth never seems to understand that some people live vicariously through others and need interesting tidbits of information to keep their lives exciting. Hyacinth likes talking too. So, innocently,

Hyacinth inadvertently passes on secrets, not realizing that they may be the subject of discussion at a dozen social events before running out of steam.

Hyacinths never have any trouble talking about their own problems, usually concerning the opposite sex. No matter how naive, gentle, and caring they are, they can drive the more assertive types, like Bergamot, to distraction. Hyacinths can take on almost any job provided that the circumstances are right. For example, they make good salespeople as long as they have faith in the product; they make good secretaries and assistants as long as the boss is honest with them and the job doesn't entail any underhand dealings. They'd be marvelous at animal breeding and any job involving flowers and plants. Although they love music, dance, and theater, these professions are much too cut-throat for Hyacinth, even on the administrative side.

Negative Hyacinths often emphasize their fragile, delicate nature to get sympathy if all else fails, creating the illusion of a tragic personality, and can act out this role to the fullest, particularly if they find it working to their advantage. However, tension, stress, and stress-related disorders are invariably genuine, common to this personality type.

Hyacinths make Good Samaritans — listening to people in trouble and, being basically very charitable — and would be happy working in any capacity in the charity field. Being very intuitive and known as "sensitives," these are nice, gentle, soft people who need space to breathe and be who they are — without any interference.

JASMINE   FLORAL
Jasminum officinale, J. grandiflorum, J. sambac

CHARACTER
Euphoric, Sensuality, Welcoming, Intuitive, Soothing,

USE FOR THESE POSITIVE ATTRIBUTES
Uplifted, Confident, Sexual, Assertive, Relaxed, Optimistic, Open, Sensitive, Harmonized, Aware, Profound, Inspired, Joyful

USE TO COUNTERACT THESE NEGATIVE ATTRIBUTES
Depression, Anxiety, Pessimism, Tension, Indifference, Repression, Bitterness, Jealousy, Low self-esteem, Guilt, Emotional frigidity, Emotional abuse, Emotional violence

JASMINE
Personality Profile

From the top of their head to the tip of their toes, the Jasmine personality is pure femininity. We're talking womanhood in full bloom. Jasmine is a no-holds-barred personality, the passionate seductress, gentle and charismatic, bewitching all who come into her presence. Before all the men reading this go rushing out to find one, let me say that ultimate femininity can dwell in the heart of most women but only the true Jasmine has the courage to expose it to the world.

Jasmines are beautiful from within, whether they're a model on the cover of a magazine, or a tribeswoman in the Amazon. Their beauty has the ability to transcend the daily battles of existence; it's a glimpse of the archetypal female, Mother Earth — giver of all life. Jasmines are the mermaids that touch the hearts of man, the petal that drifts gently by on the breeze. No wonder that this personality, like the perfume, has enchanted the world since time began.

Jasmines are joyful, happy people, comfortable with who they are. They have no wish to stop enjoying the sensuality of their surroundings or fabulous objects, and have no wish to become part of an androgynous society. They enjoy all the things that are generally considered, in the Western world, to be essentially feminine — delicate silk underwear, perfume, the touch of cashmere against their skin, or the sweet smell of a newborn babe. If they can afford it, they'll dine on strawberries and champagne and, whatever their financial status, will enjoy the sight and aroma of flowers. Jasmines have no intention of forsaking these pleasures for anyone.

Jasmines won't stand for sexual harassment and anyone bold enough to attempt it with them will receive a barrage of abuse powerful enough to blast them onto another planet, but are flattered when someone suggests they are looking nice, and enjoy old-fashioned courtesies and thoughtfulness — which they also give to others. Whether they're brunette, blond, black, or red-headed, whether they're nine hours old or ninety years old, whether they're pretty or ugly by conventional standards, Jasmines will have people lining up just for a smile. They have a wonderful ability to really listen and the time and attention given to others instills confidence in them. Past lovers will remember Jasmine with a smile, and Jasmine will remember every lover and friend they ever had. Usually independent, these are intelligent, assertive, confident people.

Having a great sense of humor, Jasmines are great fun to have as friends — imaginative and alive. There will be no dull moments with them. They're the kind of friend you can call at midnight after a dreadful day, without worrying whether they'll be upset that you bothered them so late. Jasmines are passionate lovers and understand the spirituality of sex, enjoying it without guilt or hang-ups. It doesn't matter to them whether the soulmate is rich or poor, just as long as they're right for each other.

Jenny is a Jasmine personality, a social worker, who fights for her clients in court, not missing a trick as she presents an argument, then sending the sweetest smile across the room to the judges. She wears perfume and exquisite fabrics and somehow manages to get her way every time, without realizing how she's done it. The charm of the Jasmine personality is inborn, and subconscious most of the time. This is what is so attractive to other people.

The male Jasmine personality is charming, charismatic, and at ease with his femininity. He is devastatingly attractive to the opposite sex, as Jasmine females are to men. He'll be able to hold his peers spellbound as he recounts tales about his latest passion over lunch. The male Jasmine uses his sensuality to get what he wants more consciously than the female, and can flirt with both sexes. Jasmines can be very unnerving if you're not used to them — particularly at work. After a heated debate they may storm out of the room but, disconcertingly, almost surreally, will find time to touch the petal of a particularly beautiful flower as they pass. This personality is found in every kind of job although they're happiest in those in which they can use their instinctive intellect and behavior. They'll be unhappy as an accountant, but will enjoy the challenge of physics. They also make good designers, artists, and gardeners.

Jasmines can become depressed at the discord in today's life, and self-destructive.

Indeed, negative Jasmines can be lethal to themselves. Passionate jealousy can become a serious problem and, as they turn their passion inward, can become addicted and obsessive. Of course, this affects everyone around them, which makes things worse, and Jasmine can become paranoid, miserable and prone to emotional illness. The depths of emotion that Jasmine are able to reach can only be truly understood by another floral, also delicately balanced between the conscious and subconscious. In negative mode, Jasmines can make everyone's life hell on earth, and can easily destroy their own careers and relationships. It takes a long time for them to pull themselves out of the mire, and they require a lot of help. Fortunately, nearly always, they have generated many friendships and, in these times of stress, the chaff is separated from the wheat. After they recover from a negative phase, Jasmines will carry an air of fragility and melancholy. This doesn't affect their passion, however, and it even makes them more desirable to some.

This joyful personality is often attacked by those who don't understand just how fragile they may be feeling, and this can lead to all kinds of problems. However, if you want warmth and gentleness, with passionate benevolence, there is no other personality quite like the true Jasmine.

Nicole Perez, MIFA Reg., aromatherapist and tutor:

"The character of Jasmine is represented by the two J's — as in Jasmine for Joy. This, to me, is the true character of Jasmine. Jasmine has the most uplifting and beautifying effect on people. It elevates us to higher spheres, it is also renowned for increasing sensuality as well as personal charisma."

JUNIPER   FRUITIE/WOODIE
Juniperus communis

CHARACTER
Cleansing, Purifying, Sacredness, Visionary

USE FOR THESE POSITIVE ATTRIBUTES
Self-worth, Spiritually supported, Peace, Inner vision, Uplifted, Strength, Vitality, Cleansed, Meditative, Conviction, Sincerity, Enlightened, Wisdom, Humility

USE TO COUNTERACT THESE NEGATIVE ATTRIBUTES
Nervous exhaustion, Emotional exhaustion, Guilt, Lack of self-worth, Dissatisfaction, Anxiety, Abused, Listlessness, Weakness, Transience, Emptiness, Conflict, Defensive

JUNIPER
Personality Profile

The Juniper personality is radical in that they have no concern for human authority, preferring to be directed by their intuition or religious belief. They have a reverence for anything sacred and will inevitably take a spiritual path through life — whatever form that may take. As children, they may be drawn to church or other spiritual places, without knowing why, even if their parents never go to them. One young man I had as a patient always had the desire to go to church but was never taken by his parents so joined the local church youth center held in the church hall and would pop in to the evening service every day on his way home from college — and his parents never knew a thing about it. The Juniper personality doesn't consciously seek out spiritual places, but just seems drawn to them. The Juniper personality has a profound spiritual ease that is obvious to all who come into contact with them. This doesn't mean they are religious fanatics, in fact they may never tell you how they feel about spiritual matters; apparently this feeling is a private matter between them and God. This spiritual thread runs through everything Juniper does through life.

Juniper is also a personality of spring — of things fresh and new. To others, it sometimes appears that Junipers are immature because they take such delight in new experiences and knowledge. This is a misjudgment, however, because Junipers are simply not afraid to enjoy themselves in a way that expresses their delight. They rejoice in simple pleasures like meeting new people, taking a trip to the country, having a drink with friends or lunch with the family. Although these things would have been experienced many times before, each time is like the first to them, fresh and new. This is actually a very endearing quality because it shows Juniper's appreciation of the uniqueness of each occasion and the fleetingness of the moment, and their ability to live in the present. Junipers always have time for other people. They'll invite you along to whatever activity they may be going to, not out of obligation, but because genuine pleasure is taken in sharing your company.

When they're negative, Junipers appear very vulnerable, as if their very soul is being attacked. They become uneasy among other people and disquieted by all manner of things. Anyone used to their usual easygoing nature may sense the disquiet being generated. During these bouts of doubt and anxiety Junipers can become very weak-spirited, depressed, and exhausted — as if they've fought an enormous battle. Their faith never falters though, which is a great strength. No matter what life throws at them Juniper will always pull through and once again laugh and believe in themselves and others.

Junipers are best suited to professions that allow them freedom of thought and speech. They don't take kindly to authority or to being the underdog, and are best suited to jobs in which they can be left on their own to carry out the work in their own way, although they can have a wishful nature, approaching things in ways that are not always practical or efficient. This type of person has difficulty choosing romantic partners because they need someone who understands why they need to withdraw into themselves for inner reflection, without feeling excluded. There are many personalities Juniper is not compatible with and they often wrongly feel that they will never find their soulmate or true love.

Teddy Fearnhamm IScB France, MRQA, aromatherapist and tutor:

"Definitive personality; Peter Pan/Juvenescence. Clears and detoxes the mind as well as the body — promising a fresh vitality and promoting the desire to live up to our expectations and the dreams we had when we were very young."

LAVENDER   FLORAL/HERBIE
Lavendula officinalis, L. angustifolia

CHARACTER
Harmonious, Calming, Healing, Caring, Compassionate, Embracing

USE FOR THESE POSITIVE ATTRIBUTES
Secure, Gentle, Compassionate, Balanced, Reconciled, Vital, Clarity, Comforted, Acceptance, Inner peace, Relaxed and alert, Rested, Aware, Emotionally balanced, Spiritual Growth, Meditative, Visualization, Rejuvenated

USE TO COUNTERACT THESE NEGATIVE ATTRIBUTES
Anxiety, Irritability, Stress, Tension, Mental exhaustion, Panic, Hysteria, Shock, Apprehension, Fears, Nightmares, Insecurity, Lost inner child, Restlessness, Moodiness, Distracted, Addiction, Obsessional behavior, Trauma, Conflict, Emotional violence, Agitation, Jitteryness, Depression, Psychosomatic illness, Nervousness, Worry, Over-excitedness, Burnout

LAVENDER
Personality Profile

Lavender could be called the mother, or grandmother of essential oils, able to care for a multitude of physical and psychological problems and, like a mother, accomplishing several jobs at the same time. Lavender is the most useful essential oil and is usually the first that any student of aromatherapy learns about. It is the preferred essential oil of the nursing professions, who use it more for its calming and sedative properties rather than for its anti-infectious ones. Lavender is the most commonly used essential oil in aromatherapy treatments and aroma-psychology research. There are several species of lavender that are distilled to make essential oil, and there are subtle personality variations between them, but here we are looking at the personality of *lavendula officinalis* or *angustifolia,* the most commonly used species.

Lavender is the perfect balance between the masculine and feminine traits that are within us all, and that all *grande dames* exhibit boldly. Lavender is completely mothering in its personality — electric, formidable, yet gentle and kind, and the perfect embodiment of Mother Earth. Embracing Lavender is direct, pure of thought, brave, and humble. It makes men gentle, and women strong.

Even in times of hardship a Lavender personality bravely continues overcoming obstacles that are placed in their way, having the ability to give generously of themselves — caring for others, often with gentleness and sacrifice. This type will be the first to offer to hold the baby to lull it to sleep, and the first to come to the rescue in times of trouble when help is needed. Lavenders seem to have an inexhaustible amount of energy to call upon, which their own calm exterior belies. They are the ones who will sit and talk to your plants or feed your cats when you go away, who will do the shopping for sick neighbors, and who are always ready to listen.

The Lavender personality loves the earth, the flowers, and trees, and will fill their homes with living things if they can. True Lavenders have a built-in correctness and spirituality. Nurses, buddies, and foster parents are just some of the roles taken on by people who have a fair proportion of Lavender in their makeup. They're also often found fighting for a cause, but one usually nearer home to than the rain forests — such as for facilities for nursing mothers, or the physically disadvantaged. Whatever they put their campaigning energies into, it will be for a home issue, in one form or another. Lavender types are often subject to flights of fancy and are happy to search for the elusive solution to life's problems — an aspect of mothering to a certain extent. A male Lavender is often drawn to the Gaia principle and New Ageism, and will go looking for the goddess within himself, or may go into farming where the mothering instinct can have expression in the care of animals and crops. Whether male or female, Lavenders are very versatile, and if stuck in a city job they'll be drawn to volunteer jobs such as helping the homeless and otherwise disadvantaged.

A negative Lavender will be highly strung, wound up, and absorbing energies off everyone, never discharging them. They won't disclose their problems or troubles to anyone as they believe they must always care for others, overdoing it, never resting or sleeping properly. Unexplained headaches and migraines are conditions that afflict this personality, along with aches and pains — which go away as soon as everything returns to normal.

Lavenders are gentle men and women. These intelligent people often become teachers, but whatever they do, they will be kind-hearted, benevolent, humane, worthy, and valuable.

LEMON
Citrus limomum, C. medica

FRUITIE

CHARACTER
Purifying, Stimulating, Directional, Versatile

USE FOR THESE POSITIVE ATTRIBUTES
Joy, Emotional clarity, Direction, Awareness, Calm, Concentration, Lively, Conscious, Strength, Clarity of thought, Memory, Emotionally invigorated

USE TO COUNTERACT THESE NEGATIVE ATTRIBUTES
Resentful, Depressed, Bitter, Touchy, Apathetic, Lethargic, Humorless, Indecisive, Bad attitudes, Distrust, Mental Blocks, Stress, Mental fatigue, Turmoil, Irrationality, Fear

---

LEMON
Personality Profile

The sweet lemon is like a breath of fresh air on a summer's day, positively wonderful to have around. Lemon types are lively and casual — unbothered by the struggles and strains of living, able to take it all quite calmly, dealing with each problem as it comes along. They have a sense of energy about them and are very active people. Lemon types sparkle, full of life, with a very positive approach, in the form of an unshakable confidence in everything they do. Even if this personality has never attempted a particular job before, they categorically believe it can be done with success. This "never doubt yourself" attitude can rub off on other people which is a blessing for personalities who have difficulty starting or finishing projects.

Lemon's enthusiasm seems to rub off onto those around, with subtle and permanent effect.

The lemon personality type can be sweet, sour, or confusingly balanced between the two. Even sweet Lemons can be sharp and inclined to be rather critical, not understanding why everyone doesn't strive for perfection as they do. Work colleagues often come in for harsh words, and the mistakes of Lemon's children are not easily tolerated.

Although lemons have no difficulty in concentrating or being engrossed in a job, it has to be one they like otherwise they won't be interested. It's no good trying to get a Lemon involved in a business deal, no matter how much money it could make, if the project isn't interesting. As Lemons often reach the top of their chosen profession, they are much sought after on the work front, but do better owning their own business, where it is easier to set the pace of the work and where Lemon's originality and intuition can be put to good use. Lemons are workaholics who, if they enjoy their work, will let it dominate their lives — but always with a casual air about it. If a business deal is lost, Lemon will not fret but go out for a nice lunch with someone whose company they enjoy.

In relationships, Lemons can be wonderful as they always have an answer for all life's problems. As lovers, Lemons can be thoughtful, original, and very energetic — as they are in most things when in positive mode. Positive Lemons never seem to have any illnesses, and germs just seem to pass them by — a fact that often makes other people wonder what their secret is. They are athletic people who love sport and competition, often playing amateur or professional sports or becoming sports teachers or trainers; while those who make their living in commerce or industry usually take up sport in their spare time. Whatever the sport, Lemons often become the captain of the team.

Lemons do not usually bear grudges unless in negative mode, and then you had better watch out. That carefree manner can become scornful, sarcastic, and sharp-tongued. A negative Lemon can be scattered, selfish, arrogant, uncompromising, and a bully. Lemons can turn to negative mode if they're unable to express themselves either in the workplace or during outside activities. Burnout and overwork are other situations that can propel them into negative mode, although these can quickly be readjusted with a vacation in the sun, under clear blue skies.

Lemons who are oscillating between positive and negative can be very confusing as they smile one minute and scowl the next. As Lemons are workaholics, they're inevitably under stress and when the crunch comes, everyone is in their firing line. Their mood swings come very fast, confusing those around them, as positivity turns to deceit.

———

LINDEN BLOSSOM   FLORAL
Tilia vulgaris

CHARACTER
Consoling, Serenity, Security, Patience

USE FOR THESE POSITIVE ATTRIBUTES
Relaxed, Calm, Soothed, Self-confident, Secure, Balanced, Structured, Stable

USE TO COUNTERACT THESE NEGATIVE ATTRIBUTES
Nervousness, Anxiety, Nervous Tension, Emotional debility, Hysteria, Over
excitement, Insecurity, Emotional blockages, Possessiveness, Jealousy, Anger,
Stress, Irritability, Mood swings, Guilt, Lovelorn, Oversensitivity, Indecision

LINDEN BLOSSOM
Personality Profile

The sweet perfume of Linden Blossom gives a clue to the character of this profile — sweet, calm, gentle, and very feminine — whether the person is male or female. If male, he will be in touch with his feminine side, appearing to understand women — a "new man," one might say. If female, she will be "womanly." This profile has a calmness about them that affects other people deeply. Usually these types have very rounded personalities. They stand no nonsense from anyone and are happy and content with themselves. Confident with who they are from an early age, Lindens will be determined to follow the path they have set for themselves, carrying on regardless of any opposition to their plans. These are open and up-front people, helpful when the mood takes them. They're a very interesting personality as they can

change and wear many guises.

Lindens are perfectly happy to reside in the shadow of their partner or family, nurturing their growth and encouraging their ambitions, perhaps hoping to win a large amount of cash so they will never have to work again — or leave the home domain. When arriving back from a vacation, Lindens say, "It's good to be home, I don't know why I bothered to go away."

Lindens love nothing better than being at home with their family, if possible, and often have large families. This personality can cook up a meal out of practically nothing in a minute, get the grass stains out of your clothes, and could write a book full of useful hints about running a home efficiently and taking good care of a family. Guests are welcome but will not get preferential treatment over Linden's own family, who always come first. In return, Lindens expect their family to adore them.

Due to lack of ambition, Lindens are

often found in jobs that do not suit their temperament. They tell themselves this is a temporary situation but once in a familiar routine, will be reluctant to change, enjoying the train route, or the people they work with, or the way in which the company is run. These are people who will stay in a job forever, providing it pays them sufficiently, the work is moderately satisfactory, and they're not expected to sacrifice too much. Workmates like Lindens because they're calming in a panic — when a deadline has to be reached, for example. (Just don't expect them to stay late). Lindens are by no means timid, however, and will not suffer fools gladly.

A Linden woman can flirt outrageously just because it's fun, and with no ulterior motive — like trying to catch somebody else's man. She flirts like a three-year old on her father's knee, all fluttering eyelashes and coy expressions with the milkman and the office clerk, yet rarely suffering sexual harassment, perhaps because of a child-like innocence. Linden males also flirt and will be quite surprised when it's taken for anything other than a little bit of fun. In fact, they don't know they're doing it and it can quite often lead to trouble — particularly when they try it on a Tuberose personality.

Many Lindens find that their idealized perfect partner simply doesn't exist so they end up with people who are inevitably less than perfect in their eyes. Although drawn to people similar to themselves, this is a disastrous partnership decision for them. They aim to partner successful people, and this can take many forms, not necessarily financial. Indeed,

money is not the Linden's measure of success. Once in a relationship, infidelity never crosses their minds, and they would be hurt if anyone thought otherwise.

In love, Lindens can act more like a parent than a lover and will want to be in touch every moment of the day, just to make sure their loved one is all right. Being incurable romantics, in the first stages of romance Lindens will send poems, love letters, flowers, chocolates, and all the traditional lover's gifts. This phase does wear off and then they'll wonder why there's no romance in their lives. In fact, this lack of romance is often due to a poor choice of partner and Lindens often turn to daydreaming.

If not satisfied with their life, at some stage in life Lindens will look back on the past with regret and this can turn into recrimination, aimed at whomever they're with at this stage. This is when other activities start to take an interest, particularly as the children start to leave the nest. Lindens never get nervous or excited and are unlikely to shout in temper or anger. Instead, they sulk — which is not always good for their psyche.

In negative mode, Lindens are possessive of their partner or children, always reminding everyone of what could go wrong. They become the worriers, the "what if?" type — "What if the world blows up?" "What if you have an accident, or there is no work, or I get fired?" Negative Lindens half expect to get mugged on the way home. If anyone is more than half an hour late, they'll wait by the phone getting more anxious by the moment. Lindens can easily end up having anxiety attacks over things they cannot possibly control, while their families are caused to have tremendous guilt and their children may find it difficult to cut the ties that bind them.

Lindens hoard papers, books, old toys, clothes, and furniture until the house is full of junk. Negative Lindens can easily start to envy the possessions of others, blaming everyone around them for their lack of money, success, and recognition. They use the "Nobody cares if I live or die"

speech to get sympathy. If all this becomes a regular occurrence, Lindens can drive friends away, children out of the home, and their partner insane. "I gave up everything for you," will be heard, along with "You never really loved me." Selfishness will rule supreme. Luckily, before this happens, a bit of praise (a lot actually), coupled with reassurances and continual expressions of love, will put Lindens back on their feet.

MANDARIN   FRUITIE
Citrus reticulata, C. nobilis

CHARACTER
Gentle, Peaceful, Revitalizing, Sympathetic

USE FOR THESE POSITIVE ATTRIBUTES
Calm, Uplifted, Refreshed, Inspired, Soothed, Sprightly, Integrity, Tranquil

USE TO COUNTERACT THESE NEGATIVE ATTRIBUTES
Anxiety, Depression, Grief, Inner child, Abuse, Dejection, Emptiness, Dwelling on the past, Overexcitable, Desolate, Emotional trauma

---

MANDARIN
Personality Profile

The Mandarin personality is sweet, gentle, kind, and loving — one of the softest personalities. Their kindness is extended to all living, breathing things including plants, fish, animals, humans, as well as to inanimate objects like the teddy bear that

was precious to them as a child, and still is. They'll have boxes full of letters from old friends, photos, dried flowers, and champagne corks kept from rendezvous long ago. Everything is lovingly protected. Gentle in everything, the Mandarin personality has a meek manner but this doesn't mean their spirit is meek — which is a mistake many people make.

Mandarin personalities are child-like

in that they need love and protection. Unconsciously, they draw out protectiveness in others with an air of needing to be looked after, even if they don't actually need it. Women want to "mother" male Mandarins, knitting them sweaters and cooking them dinner, while men find themselves carrying the grocery bags for the female Mandarin, helping with chores and protecting them from the wicked world. Mandarins don't complain about all this attention, and rather like it, but to be constantly spoiled in this way can get on the nerves of even the gentlest, sweetest person and Mandarin will feel at some point the need to break free. This they will eventually do, after some diplomatic scheming. The last thing a Mandarin would do is hurt somebody's feelings or bruise their ego.

Mandarins are very uplifting and, as the saying goes, can "gladden the old man's heart." They often take care of the older generation, who appreciate their courtesies. The fact that the Mandarin personality can spend much of their life caring for other people shows they are quite tough, despite their child-like qualities. This toughness becomes apparent when they're left entirely on their own to fend for themselves. They manage better than most of us — proving what a paradoxical and complex character they are. With careful nourishing, they bloom and outlive everyone, still carrying on when stronger types have fallen by the wayside. Perhaps nature looks more kindly on the docile and cautious.

Actually, Mandarin might have drifted into this personality just for the sake of

peace and that becomes a problem when their true selves break free of whatever restrictions have been built up. Friends and family can't believe what's happening, as Mandarin shed their meek personality like a snake skin. The Mandarin personality is sometimes adopted as a result of childhood trauma, in one of its many forms — from actual physical abuse to unkind words overheard and taken into the subconscious. The child decides it's better to be meek, gentle, and caring as a protective mechanism, so they might avoid getting more of the same.

Mandarins love children and will protect them fiercely, ever watchful and mindful of what dangers could befall them. This constant awareness of potential dangers can make Mandarins reluctant to have children but when they do, the children complain of lack of freedom. Hopefully, they won't choose a partner who repeats the patterns they suffered as a child. They need someone who won't take advantage of their good-naturedness and kindness, and who helps them become more assertive and carefree.

A negative Mandarin can become hysterical at the slightest thing, and compulsive — usually about cleanliness, both personal and domestic. They have nightmares and experience fear out of all proportion — afraid to meet people, afraid of life — and will be nervous, jumpy and full of unnecessary grief. When their emotional sanity is shot to pieces, they can become quite uncontrollable, like creatures much too fragile to walk this earth.

One typical Mandarin personality who came to me as a patient was Jennifer, who had reached the age of sixty without ever having thought of doing anything for herself. She came from a household that forbade any extroverted behavior, with a very authoritarian father. She escaped at the age of seventeen into a loveless marriage to a man ten years older, who needed someone to care for him, rather than a loving relationship. For over forty years she cooked and cleaned, doing everything for him and their children, constantly at everyone's beck and call. She went to work as a school cook and handed her wages over to her husband at the end of the week. Everyone thought she was contented, driving the kids back and forth to their activities, and her husband to his rotary club or for a night out with the boys. Only her best friend, another meek

Mandarin type, knew how boring she found it all.

When her husband died suddenly as a result of an accident, Jennifer realized she didn't even know where her husband banked their money. She got furious with herself, with her parents, and especially her husband for leaving her like this. Jennifer has to become assertive, enjoying her new independence. She sold the house and eventually moved to France where she fell in love for the first time, and started a new life. Finally, she said, she had found herself. Of course the children said, "What about us?" and the rest of the family thought she'd gone completely mad, but Jennifer was happy at last — with someone who realized how precious her kindness and gentleness was; a true partner.

MARJORAM, SWEET
HERBIE/LEAFIE
Origanum marjorana

CHARACTER
Comforting, Soothing, Warming, Strengthening

USE FOR THESE POSITIVE ATTRIBUTES
Calm, Balanced, Direct, Self-assured, Integrity, Courage, Confidence, Focus, Perseverance, Restored, Sincere

USE TO COUNTERACT THESE NEGATIVE ATTRIBUTES
Anxiety, Hysteria, Hostility, Withdrawn, Mental strain, Tantrums, Anger, Irritability, Overactivity, Weak will

MARJORAM, SWEET
Personality Profile

The marjoram personality is warm and friendly, always ready to offer comfort and solace under their wing. These people make really good friends and are solid, calm, steady, organized, potentially strong, and straightforward. Although they generally prefer to watch events from the sidelines, they can be outspoken if necessary. It's quite difficult to gauge their feelings because emotions are rarely shown, and are certainly never overdramatized. Generally, Marjorams keep to themselves and will not intrude upon another person's privacy unless asked to. The steadying influence of Marjoram is often mistaken for dullness or lack of imagination, but this is a mistake soon recognized once you get to know them. They do enjoy life, but choose to show it in caring.

Marjorams are great animal lovers. They'll take in any stray cat or dog and look after the neighbor's hamster when they go on vacation. Marjorams often feel more in tune with animals than with people and are often found in jobs relating to animals, such as vets, vetinery nurses, animal rescue teams, animal wardens, and the like. Although not active campaigners, they are quite likely to be found working in the offices of organizations concerned with saving whales and dolphins or, if they have the money, will send donations to help the cause.

Marjorams don't hang onto money for long, not because they spend it on themselves, but because it goes to family or friends. It'll be the Marjoram who lends the Jasmine personality the money to buy a new outfit for a hot date, and the Marjoram will stock up the refrigerator with goodies to please the Cardamom. These things are done out of the kindness of Marjoram's heart, with no thought of reward. But, because Marjoram is so generous, they are often taken advantage of. Sadly, because Marjorams don't expect any rewards, they often don't even receive a courteous "thank you." This can actually make Marjoram very depressed, because all they really want is for people to appreciate their kindness and when they realize they're being taken advantage of they can become irritable, withdrawn, and often emotionally cold.

Marjorams find that people drop into their houses as if it were their natural right, which is all very well except that people often forget to invite Marjoram around to their place in return. Relationships can be very one-way. Often, Marjorams don't get invited to parties, not because they weren't intended to come, but because they were simply forgotten. They're like the toothbrush you use several times a day but forget all about when you're not using it — an essential but invisible part of life. If Marjorams are romantically teamed up with a floral you can expect sexual disharmony. Although Marjorams are gentle, kind people, they aren't very sexy, much preferring to curl up with a good book in front of the fire, than share a candlelight bath with their partner.

Marjorams can quite happily live in a house that is tumbling down around their heads, with a threadbare carpet and doors that don't shut properly, because they're just not bothered. The same goes for appearance. Old, comfortable clothes are preferred and Marjorams will stick with the style adopted in their thirties right through to old age, never changing. They cannot see the need to buy anything new, thinking that if you already possess something, why throw it out? They actually take pleasure in making things last for as long as possible. This attitude can cause problems with the family, who are also expected to make do with what they've got.

Marjorams are good people, not necessarily the "go-getter," but needed to stabilize and ground the more flamboyant types. They are sincere, having great courage, stamina, and perseverance.

MELISSA
Melissa officinalis   HERBIE/LEAFIE

CHARACTER
Calming, Supportive, Sensitive, Fostering

USE FOR THESE POSITIVE ATTRIBUTES
Strength, Revitalized, Happy, Gentle, Spiritual growth, Relaxed, Peaceful, Positive, Progressive, Cheerful

USE TO COUNTERACT THESE NEGATIVE ATTRIBUTES
Nervous tension, Stress, Anxiety, Irritability, Overexcitement, Restlessness, Melancholy, Sadness, Grieving, Sorrow, Emotional crisis, Depression, Mental exhaustion, Lethargy, Negativity

MELISSA
Personality Profile

The Melissa personality is bubbly, fizzy, full of energy, and usually delightful, with a multitude of interests and activities. This personality finds time to go to yoga class, attend interesting talks, and will know about all the events worth seeing, listening to, or being part of. Not only that, they find time to do it all as well as hold down a full-time job and, possibly, take care of a family. Melissas never forget to phone home, feed the cat, walk the dog, or make sure the essential groceries are in the house. How do they do it? The fact is that Melissa is not only highly organized, like the Grapefruit personality for example, but they have such a love of life that even one second is, to them, too precious to waste. Melissa doesn't waste time thinking, *"Shall* I do it?" but just muddles through without giving it much thought, just doing things because they *want* to.

Melissa has a youthfulness, and a revitalizing effect on just about everyone they meet, so are very much in demand. You can find many imitations of the Melissa personality but a true Melissa is unmistakable. Their house is full of things, but this is not collecting for collecting sake; they gather things around them that they need for some reason, that are relevant to them at a particular time. For example, they might purchase an Indian art object without any particular purpose but then discover in it something they feel a connection with, and go on to collect many Indian art pieces. When they no longer feel connected to whatever it was that appealed to their soul, Melissa will dispose of the collection, going on to something else.

When Melissas come to look after their health they throw themselves into a quest of knowledge as if it were their vocation. No stone will be left unturned. Melissa will read everything available on the subject, and discuss it with everyone, gleaning more information all the time. However, this knowledge will not be used on themselves. It's almost as if by absorbing all the information about a particular disorder, the actual treatment is no longer required.

Melissas are very enthusiastic and like to try new and exciting things. Some people might accuse them of being "over the top," but this is unfair — there's noth-

ing wrong with having an open mind and being positive about things. Some people find them frivolous and perhaps not serious enough. Again this is unfair because Melissas are actually very serious people and are usually born with a good sense of judgment, sometimes bordering on that of a sage.

Because they bubble with so much enthusiasm, Melissas are not usually thought of as candidates for meditation or other solitary practices, but they do indeed excel at receiving insight and truths that are lost to others who are not so open to all that life has to offer. Melissas live very much in the here and now, although they have respect for the past and thought for the future.

Partners who cannot let go of the past are very bad for Melissas, dragging them into the negative vortex. The soft-hearted Melissa cannot absorb this fundamentally opposing view. Melissa wants to get on with life and anyone harping on about the past prevents them doing that. Indeed, Melissa cannot take the weight of unnecessary guilt or emotional baggage and if forced to take it on, will crack and become negative. They can become anxious and lose interest in life, stop their many activities and just sit in front of the TV, never going out and seeing friends. The wrong partner can turn these bright effervescent people into zombies, and the sad thing is that Melissa may not even notice this process happening, until it's too late. The shocking thing is that their partner and friends may welcome this change because it means there is more time for them. At least if Melissa is at home on the sofa, one knows where to find them. Parents are usually the first to recognize what's going on and, sadly, can welcome the change with, "Good, they've slowed down, more time for me to visit and get attention."

Melissas attract jealousy, spitefulness, and unadventurous souls who feed off their vivacious, outgoing nature, and admire their control of life. The trouble is, these people want to *tame* Melissa and make her (or him) more like themselves. Throughout it all, however, Melissa will always try to find the good side in people. Melissa is a very sweet-natured personality and, despite the attempts of negative people to make them otherwise, essentially independent.

Elizabeth Jones, OBE, MCSP, DRE, MIFA Reg., MISPA, physiotherapist and aromatherapy tutor:

"Uplifting, joyous, quickens the spirit, having a subtle, piquant character, unlike the more direct citrus note of sage lemon. A 'happy' oil."

NARCISSUS
Narcissus poeticus

FLORAL

CHARACTER
Hypnotic, Empowering, Mesmerizing, Sagacious

USE FOR THESE POSITIVE ATTRIBUTES
Inspired, Creative, Stillness, Meditative, Inner vision, Aspirations, Idealistic, Sensuous, Visionary, Discovery, Truthful

USE TO COUNTERACT THESE NEGATIVE ATTRIBUTES
Hysteria, Nervousness, Irritability, Tension, Grief, Addictions, Withdrawal, Loneliness, Illusions, Disillusionment, Longings, Hopelessness, Obsessions, Trauma, Emotional wounding, Misery, Anguish, Emotional analgesia

NARCISSUS
Personality Profile

Before saying anything about the Narcissus personality, I must first dispel any preconceived associations that may be made with the personality trait "narcissism." This word comes to us from the ancient Greek tale of a young man, Narcissus, who fell in love with his own reflection and eventually was turned into a narcissus flower. Narcissism thus means to have a morbid self-love or self-admiration. In fact, by strange coincidence, the very next word in my dictionary is "narcosis," meaning "the production of a narcotic state" and it is this that more accurately reflects the quality of narcissus, the flower and essential oil, the aroma of which can achieve mystical effects on the emotions and mind. Indeed, it was probably the hypnotic effect of the plant narcissus which induced the person Narcissus, so long ago, to transport into another, unreal world — a world in which he could so detach from himself, he thought he was someone else. So, while the fragrance of narcissus is most certainly a hypnotic, it would be quite wrong to think that the Narcissus personality suffers from self-admiration and love.

The Narcissus personality is one of closeness, of clandestine moments, poised between the conscious and subconscious. This is the personality of the seeker of truth — no matter how deep or painful that journey may be. Because Narcissus is deep and thoughtful, people often refer to them as old souls that have been reincarnated. There is nothing carefree about them, although being masters of camouflage they're very often able to give the opposite impression. Narcissus is found at the trendiest parties, laughing and joking, and at the art event or reception of the year, pursuing someone who may give them a contract. They enjoy being involved in the most "happening" events — and this can lead to the impression of superficiality. In fact, they are quietly weighing the objectives of everyone and subtly rooting out dark secrets, while sensing the place of everything, as well as everyone, in the room.

Because the Narcissus personality is ever changing, it's not easy to get to know them intimately. They change the color and cut of their hair, their clothing style, their friends, lovers, houses and even the country in which they live. Like many other free, creative people, Narcissus is often misunderstood. It is wrong to accuse Narcissus of not having any passion, or for not being understanding, but the accusation of delving into things too deeply may sometimes be justified.

Narcissus points out other people's mistakes and notices potential dangers at work or play — and 98.9% of the time they're correct. It is precisely this ability to see what's ahead, their precognitive faculty, that infuriates others and leads them to mistrust Narcissus. But, through it all, Narcissus has complete trust in their own judgment, which is excellent. Being a friend of Narcissus is an experience in itself — once they feel comfortable with you you'll see that they can be hilariously funny, with a wicked, dry sense of humor.

This personality type is always

impeccably dressed, with clean, pressed clothes and mended, polished shoes. Loving fine things that have been crafted with sweat and tears, Narcissus will fondle a piece of carved wood as if actually identifying with the pain and sacrifice of the tree from which it came. Not only that, they can tune in to the feelings of the man or woman who carved the wood and even imagine the chips of wood that fell to the ground in the process. Everything is experienced in the round, totally beyond three dimension.

The presence of Narcissus is inspiring — a mystical transference of self-confidence and assurance. They're very kind in their words, even if they are not always genuine, saying "it does no harm to be graceful," and are invariably found in jobs that match their abilities — anything that requires creativity, inspirational actions, and intuitive behavior. They make great composers, writers, painters, architects, and scientists and are often black-balled for ideas that seem to be "off-the-wall" but which will, in time, become accepted theory.

Narcissus personalities have freedom of mind and consciousness and there are no ties which can bind them down or hold them back. This is irritating for others, even their family. But they make great parents, never questioning their offspring's motives for doing anything, just accepting them for who they are — independent beings. This, in turn, gets Narcissus in trouble because people accuse them of having no interest in anyone other than themselves, of being arrogant and too involved in their own affairs to worry about their children (or anyone else). But of course they worry about other people. They've probably had premonitions and think about them more than anyone could ever guess.

Narcissus personalities are what one might call "relaxed passionates." In love they'll be both tender and passionate and love both physically and spiritually, seeing no point to love unless a spiritual bond can be forged with the partner. If they become negative, however, their love can turn inward and, preferring their own company and thoughts, all overtures of love will be rejected. Being distant and withdrawn is used as a protection from more hurt and thoughtlessness. Those who have the capacity of loving unconditionally, like Narcissus, need to withdraw sometimes as a self-protection mechanism. If, they were subjected to emotional trauma as a child, Narcissus could retreat into a shell never to emerge unless coaxed out by gentleness and love, such as can be given by the Rose Otto type of personality. Any early trauma will be carried over into adulthood, ready to resurface at times of stress.

It seems that the Narcissus personality needs acclaim, kudos, and even exaltation, when in negative mode. This is when their egos become very fragile and Narcissus becomes self-effacing, self-limiting, and doubting of the intuition they previously trusted. No longer listening to their inner dialog, Narcissus can turn to new ways to seek truth — such as using drugs.

Generally, however, Narcissus type people are gentle souls, much misunderstood. They seem to have brought knowledge forward from past lives, knowledge that gives them both anguish and pleasure. But only Narcissus will

know the extent of all this because they will never tell anyone the whole story.

Vivian Lunny MD, MBBS, MDMA, MIFA Reg., MISPA, RQA, aromatherapist and tutor:

"Narcissus has a spiritual quality and a flair for dissolving different boundaries, breaking through mental and spiritual blockages. This personality can be very persuasive, seductive and broad-minded. It despises pettiness, while loving freedom, joy, laughter, and fun. It clears away low self-esteem."

NEROLI (Orange Blossom)   FLORAL
Citrus aurantium, C. brigaradia, C. vulgaris

CHARACTER
Spiritual, Pure, Loving, Peaceful

USE FOR THESE POSITIVE ATTRIBUTES
Lightness, Lifting of sorrows, Spiritual, Connected, Completeness, Joy, Understanding, Guided, Calm, Stable, Regenerated, Peaceful

USE TO COUNTERACT THESE NEGATIVE ATTRIBUTES
Anxiety, Stress, Tension, Shock, Emotional crisis, Sadness, Longing, Panic, Grief, Inner child, Abused as child, Abused as adult, Depression, Hopelessness, Fear

---

NEROLI
Personality Profile

Neroli, also known as Orange Blossom, is one of the most spiritual personalities — another angel, like Chamomile Roman. Whatever their age, there is a built-in wisdom that extends far beyond that of worldly knowledge. Neroli is another personality that seems to have found a way to be ageless, forever young in a spring-like way. This is not the rashness of youth, but the fresh enjoyment of everything from the smallest flower to the tallest tree.

The Neroli personality is not a cynic,

and will always be able to find happiness in something, acknowledging imperfections in people but easily bypassing them to find the good. This is not a blind judgment. This personality is fully aware of the evil that exists in the world, just as the Frankincense personality is, and will be quite open about it, possibly recognizing it in people before others do, but in charity will say, "Something has to make a person like that." If nasty gossip is heard about someone they will be the first to point out the person's good points, reminding the scandal-mongers of things of merit that the person may have done.

In today's aggressive world Neroli's good intentions may seem misplaced, and they get mistaken for being daft or stupid, easily taken in by people. But Nerolis like to give their fellow man every possible chance, within reason. This personality has high morals — and will not lie, cheat, steal, murder, or harm anyone or anything. Apart from that, anything goes. Being a floral, they can understand overwhelming passion but will not condone extramarital affairs — yet will not condemn them either. Always giving credit where credit is due, Nerolis are altogether good people.

If you have a lover of friend who fits this personality, they will never crowd you, sensing when you need to be alone and ready to have fun when you are. Unfortunately, Nerolis can easily be taken advantage of by people they love. Friends and family get so used to being put first, it often leads to Neroli types having their own needs go unrecognized. Yet they do not bear grudges or resentments.

Neroli strongly believes that no one on this planet has any right to dictate how they should think, feel, and act. This can sometimes get them into hot water. They respect authority as necessary for an orderly life but all other matters are between god and themselves — so you'd better not interfere. This basic respect of authority can mutate into a strong sense of injustice as this sensitive personality battles with the understanding that some people in power are not as honest as they portray themselves to be. Neroli can have a hard time grappling with the fact that not all people on this planet realize that you can't take it with you when you go, so why be greedy now?

Neroli types are happiest when searching the mysteries of life as a hobby. Saddened by the lack of understanding in the world today, they can turn to being supersensitive souls. This can be tricky if you work for a Neroli or have one as a partner because, half the time, you won't understand what it is you did wrong.

Nerolis can be very deep emotionally, and if in a negative frame of mind, are easily angered, usually with the "you just do not understand" kind of line. They can stray from reality, and be unaware of it, and may be inclined to dismiss many of the facts of living today, just because the ideas don't fit into their philosophy. It is at this point they may become withdrawn and timid, and refuse to enter into the physical world, deciding it's just too bad out there — prone to dark, deep depressions, feeling that the world is against them. These types may say they are communing with angels, have visions, and so on, and who can say they are not? But they can get drawn in by tricksters during these negative periods and start to mistrust their own inner feelings and knowledge.

Nerolis are good in jobs that do not have to deal with any of the things they abhor, particularly deviousness, so won't do well in politics or law, nor will they want to take jobs that deal exclusively with money. They are good in professions that are fairly straightforward, such as crafts, carpentry, electronics, engineering, conservation, and teaching. They are very good with children and make great play-leaders or, because of their empathy, care-givers for the physically and mentally challenged. Many Nerolis are found to be florists or gardeners, and may choose to become spiritual counselors of one kind or another, playing an active role in their chosen religion or belief. They're clear-sighted and calm, with a peaceful air, seemingly quite balanced emotionally — and between their male and female sides, believers in great love for all.

ORANGE
Citrus sinensis, C. aurantium

FRUITIE

CHARACTER
Warming, Happy, Resolute, Energizing

USE FOR THESE POSITIVE ATTRIBUTES
Joy, Uplifted, Sunny, Balanced, Light-hearted, Regenerated, Strong, Creative, Positive, Self-confident, Sympathetic, Courageous

USE TO COUNTERACT THESE NEGATIVE ATTRIBUTES
Depression, Hopelessness, Sadness, Apathy, Resignation, Withdrawn, Self-con-sciousness, Anxiety, Emotional violence, Emotional abuse, Worry, Selfishness, Obsessions, Addiction, Burnout

ORANGE Personality Profile

Very few people dislike the smell and taste of the orange fruit, and there are very few people who wouldn't fall under the spell of the cheerful, optimistic Orange person-ality. These sunny people are a joy to be with. They're open-hearted, witty, funny, honest, and embrace ideas and sugges-tions as easily as they embrace people. The Orange personality is never shy and loves to touch, giving a quick cuddle if you need it. Luckily, their personality doesn't lead people to think they have ulterior motives, which is a good thing because they're inclined to touch a lot — children, adults, family, friends, work associates, and strangers.

What people notice first about the Orange personality type is their great sense of humor. They have an easy, friendly smile, an amused look in their eyes, and openness and understanding seems to exude from every pore in their body. What a pity there aren't more Orange personalities in the world. They're quite often found mixed with elements of the Neroli or Petitgrain personalities, complicating the matter of recognition. The Orange type is warm, sweet, and sensuous, and has a positive effect on everything and everyone — not in an overbearing way, but in a gentle, harmonizing effort to make everything all right.

Oranges are found in all walks of life and are very adaptable, although particularly in any sort of job that needs kindness and an empathetic approach. They enjoy working in areas which utilize their natural flamboyance, such as show business and, if successful, will devote time to charity work. They make good supervisors and administrators, being good organizers who won't stand for any nonsense. Any job close to negativity or human suffering affects their sensitivity, and disillusionment and burnout will eventually result.

Negative Oranges become despondent and emotionally distorted. They're liable to be the receivers of emotional abuse and violence, particularly if the wrong partner is chosen. Because of their deep faith in the human race, Orange can become victimized if they're not careful, or are unbalanced, and can quite often resort to obsessive behavior such as continually washing their hands, checking that they've locked up over and over again, and so forth. They tend to put their feelings of unhappiness aside and do not recognize the harm they are doing to themselves. This is further aggravated by the fact that other people don't see the sadness and hopelessness and when they do, it may be too late.

When you're so used to seeing someone always in positive mode, happy and optimistic, you'd think it would be easy for people to recognize depression when it comes along. Not so. Orange's family and friends are likely to say, "What's wrong with you?" or "Cheer up, it's not like you to be this down." But, replying, "I'm fine" with a smile, poor Orange may be sinking further down each day. Not only does Orange refuse to recognize that they need help, other people get so used to Orange being cheerful and helpful, they just don't see that Orange can have problems too.

Oranges make marvelous parents and are popular with all children, including their own. They are like the mothers in situation comedies who keep the family together through endless dramas, work themselves to the bone, and are sunny and funny while they do it. Oranges can be loud, overconfident and, because of the amount of energy they have, exhausting. An inner radiance gives them incredible beauty, and their vitality makes them very thoughtful, considerate, fun lovers, and, when single, they'll have prospective partners lining up to take them out.

ORMENIS FLOWER (Chamomile Maroc)
Ormenis multicaulis

HERBIE/FLORAL

CHARACTER
Unhurried, Composed, Mindful, Mystic

USE FOR THESE POSITIVE ATTRIBUTES
Calm, Empathetic, Courageous, Earthed, Relaxed, Mindful, Able to let go, Attentive, Meditative, Consoled, Soothing

USE TO COUNTERACT THESE NEGATIVE ATTRIBUTES
Stress, Tension, Anxiety, Dread, Overactive mind, Highly strung, Impulsive, Indecisive, Confused, Bad temper, Emotionally controlling, Emotional blockages, Abused, Fearful

ORMENIS FLOWER Personality Profile

Ormenis Flower has long been mistaken for and used as chamomile when it cannot be said to be anything like it, nor have the chemical constituents of chamomile — although it does come from the same botanical family. It's use in aromatherapy derives from the fact that it has long been sold as chamomile, and is far cheaper. Over the years, the qualities of Ormenis have been hidden behind this misnaming but its true personality is easy to smell. Ormenis is rich and balsamic with hidden depths that are unmistakenly alive and very vibrant.

The Ormenis profile is of the secret person, one who always likes to keep their true selves hidden. They are masters of disguise in everything they do, and very efficiently hide their emotions and true intentions. Ormenis is a slow, dilatory type of person, who takes everything at their own pace, with no hurrying, rushing, or rashness in their movements. Everything will have a motive, and every step will be a deliberate one. Although they may have been planning something for weeks, Ormenis can make it seem unplanned and fateful, but in fact, this type never leaves anything to fate. Everything is carefully planned and calculated.

Ormenis personalities may talk for hours and hours about a project they intend to start, but it may never get off the ground. "Why hurry?" they'll ask. "There is plenty of time to sit, think, and talk about it." Laid back isn't the word for it and to Grapefruit personalities, for example, Ormenis types can be infuriating. Fortunately, some projects do actually make it off the drawing board.

Ormenis people like to be in charge and like to be thought of as thinkers — wise men or women not in the medicinal sense, but in metaphysical *knowing*. Secrets are safe with them so don't tell an Ormenis if you want a rumor spread, but take them for an ally. You can unload your problems onto this personality but be prepared for a long speech advising and counseling you, and you'll be expected to carry it all out. They tend to have an answer for everything, and if they haven't, they know a man who does. Ormenis types are full of wonderful and exotic stories and experiences and make wonderful storytellers. As a family member, and with friends, Ormenis is always able to calm explosive situations.

It's difficult to see when Ormenis is in negative mode because most of the time they appear to be in control, although paradoxically passive, and being in control is what their negativity is about. Negative Ormenis types can be very controlling, expecting to be obeyed no matter what, immediately and without question. They can cut you dead in the street, or be abusive, and may stop talking to you one day and never speak to you again. This type do not listen to reason easily (except their own), and may be very patronizing and condescending toward others when in this negative mode. They seem to have a coldness of emotion completely in contrast to their normal warm selves. Ormenis types appear more male in character than female, although this personality is very much attuned to the earth's ways. Ormenis seems to be an adaptogen between the male and female parts of us. It brings a warmth that the chamomiles can never bring, and is the personality of the wise person who values the earth and all its treasures.

PATCHOULI   LEAFIE
Pogostemon cablin

CHARACTER
Grounding, Soothing, Unruffled, Assured

USE FOR THESE POSITIVE ATTRIBUTES
Invigorated, Restored, Reasonable, Lucid, Astute, Stimulating, Persistent

USE TO COUNTERACT THESE NEGATIVE ATTRIBUTES
Depression, Anxiety, Indecision, Lethargy, Sluggishness, Egotistical, Tension, Stress, Mood-swings, Touchiness

PATCHOULI
Personality Profile

Patchouli is well balanced between the earth and the sky, grounded yet able to lift up and reach for the unattainable. As this type is grounded, often having an effect on people around them, giving the impression that they are slow or sluggish — which couldn't be further from the truth. There is an elderly quality about Patchouli, ancient, and steady, no matter how old they may be. Patchoulis are born age forty.

As a child, Patchouli may seem dull compared to their hyperactive siblings, and parents may worry that they never seem to want to play with the other children, being perfectly happy on their own. But by the time Patchoulis reach their teens, they'll be further advanced than their peers — both emotionally and intellectually, which may find them having older friends. Patchouli will convince the family that they have ambition, strength, and courage to attain their dreams, even if they don't have the talent for it, but because they have the determination. It is Patchoulis' ability to stick to things, and be tenacious, and in most cases will allow them to succeed. Once a course has been determined, Patchouli will strive hard to reach the highest positions.

This personality is very astute, never missing a trick, always ready when a good opportunity presents itself. Not that Patchoulis are opportunistic, they just happen to be in the right place at the right time, so why let the chance go to some-body else? Patchoulis stand their ground and when at school will be a strong member of the debating society.

Activities that might be considered slightly oddball will appeal to Patchouli, who may very well end up being an intrepid explorer. They also enjoy delving into the psyche and, with their gift of being able to draw people out of their shell, make good psychologists. Patchoulis are intensely interested in all sorts of obscure subjects that other people may find boring and irrelevant to life (like how long it takes a snail to cross a road compared to a worm). Once they get hooked on a subject, they'll keep exploring, over and over again, until completely satisfied that they have an answer to their questions. This personality gets indignant and outraged by all sorts of things in society and are inclined to send letters to newspapers or television companies, not for publicity, but as a way of protesting and exercising their right to do so. Patchoulis do not have a lot of friends, nor do they encourage their family to invade their personal territory — whether their space is one room or a mansion — being perfectly happy on their own and quite capable of seeking out the company of others when desired.

The Patchouli personality can do well in science or related professions where their powers of reason can be put to good use. As Patchouli has the power to convey a complicated message in a more easily accessible form, they make good commentators and would do well in journalism, particularly of the investigative kind, or as a documentary filmmaker. These people will do well in any job that requires reasoning and is intellectually stimulating, from librarianship to cabinetmaking.

Patchoulis are not boring people and can be found burning the candle at both ends — until they burn themselves out. Being so grounded, it never occurs to them that they are just as fragile as other personalities and need to watch their health. When they do become ill, Patchouli becomes immobilized — unable to function or even think clearly — touchy, and trying. Depression often follows illness until they can get back on their feet again.

In relationships, Patchouli likes to be in charge and will seek a partner who is able to take a passive role. The same goes for friendships. As the years go on, Patchouli seems to go into reverse, appearing younger in spirit and more adventurous, seeking out new experiences and relationships. Patchouli is a mysterious personality and you can never be quite sure how their lives will develop. Warmhearted, but slightly overbearing at times, they tend to hang onto people as if afraid to let them go, yet still want to be alone.

Anna Marie Joyeux, MIFA Reg., aromatherapist:

"I see Patchouli as a link between the spiritual and the physical level. It is grounding, but at the same time can awaken the spiritual side of a person or balance it if they are feeling confused on the spiritual level."

PEPPERMINT   HERBIE/LEAFIE
Mentha piperita

CHARACTER
Clarifying, Awakening, Stimulating, Penetrating

USE FOR THESE POSITIVE ATTRIBUTES
Regenerating, Emotionally refreshed, Self-acceptance, Concentration, Vitality, Vibrancy

USE TO COUNTERACT THESE NEGATIVE ATTRIBUTES
Mental fatigue, Shock, Helplessness, Overwork, Sluggishness, Lethargy, Apathy

PEPPERMINT
Personality Profile

The Peppermint personality is difficult to forget once you have met one as they cause an immediate reaction: either you like them or you can't stand them. Some timid souls find them brash and overpowering, but they are never dull. Peppermint has an almost fearless spirit and this spills over into their relationships with people and animals. Unusual things will surround Peppermints, who are drawn to bright colors, loud clothes, and even louder friends. They are very quick thinkers — the salesmen of life — alert to opportunities, and excellent speakers with a quick intellect. On a good day Peppermint can remember the names of a whole gang of people they haven't met for years.

Peppermint's swiftness and quick thinking, combined with a good sense of humor, makes them witty, and they'd certainly make good stand-up comedians. Whatever they choose to do for work, they are usually dynamic. If working for someone else, they will charm them with wit, agility, and adaptability. Jobs that are totally involving, both physically and mentally, suit this personality well. It might be flying a plane, sailing a ship, or a stressful driving job. Whatever it is, it must combine mental agility and physical stamina to truly satisfy this type.

Peppermints are friendly people and quite concerned about the fate of others, even though they do like to be the center of attention. They are not always thought of as honorable, but they are, and they can be quite old-fashioned about it — particularly if out to impress members of the opposite sex, who flock around them. This personality type enjoys mixed company over their own gender. As friend or lover, be prepared to take a back seat to Peppermint's life.

Peppermints will be very loyal in relationships — no matter how stormy — but confusion often arises because the partner doesn't always know what the game-plan is. The younger males are inclined to brag because they're sure to get an audience that way. As an older person, Peppermint becomes the parent who always plays the clown at the PTA school play — "a jolly good person," you hear people say about them.

A negative Peppermint is inclined to struggle between highs and lows, sadness and happiness. These swings can be quite severe, and if they continue, Peppermint will start to get sluggish, dull, and lethargic, forget about everything and become intolerant and frustrated. At this point the refrigerator might become the focus of comfort. Peppermints can put on weight, get depressed and, eventually, become mentally incapacitated.

Positive Peppermints are often found as healers because they have an empathy and sympathetic approach to life and are able to stay calm and still enough for the healing to flow. They are popular in this profession because they can charm the client and make them feel at ease. These are sparky people who often act as a catalyst, inspiring others to get up and go.

PETITGRAIN   LEAFIE/WOODIE
Citrus aurantium, C. brigaradier

CHARACTER
Revitalizing, Balancing, Restoring, Clarifying

USE FOR THESE POSITIVE ATTRIBUTES
Harmonized, Uplifted, Joyful, Relaxed, Inner vision, Strength, Self-confidence, Stability, Optimism, Expressiveness

USE TO COUNTERACT THESE NEGATIVE ATTRIBUTES
Disharmony, Confusion, Difficulties, Depression, Mental fatigue, Nervous exhaustion, Insomnia, Sadness, Disappointment, Rigidity, Betrayal, Anger, Irrationality, Introversion, Pessimism

PETITGRAIN
Personality Profile

Petitgrain, the orange leaf person, is often closely associated with the Neroli and, to a lesser extent, Orange personalities. This isn't surprising as all three essential oils are distilled from different parts of the orange tree. One person might have elements of all three personalities, which can make them difficult to categorize or recognize. At first, the Petitgrain personality may seem somewhat subdued or overshadowed by the more flamboyant Orange, or the more spiritual Neroli, but in fact Petitgrain feeds the ego of Orange and balances the spirituality of Neroli. Petitgrain is like the firstborn in a family, often carrying responsibility for the siblings, but not overloaded by them, because Petitgrain has copious amounts of energy that can be equally distributed between various activities, apparently in tune with the rhythm of life. A link between sun and earth, Petitgrain personalities are the providers of comfort and emotional nourishment.

This personality appears to be in control, capable, and never fazed, but are often underestimated and their qualities are not always given the recognition they deserve. Petitgrain may serve on a committee for years, gently guiding and counseling, doing all the work while others take the credit. They are respected at work and deemed responsible and steady.

Petitgrains are by no means dull and can make stimulating company if given the chance, being good conversationalists and interested in other people's opinions — at least they give that impression, being too polite to do otherwise. Petitgrains will be totally taken with anyone who is "less than responsible" and one often wonders if they wouldn't secretly be happier if they "let go" a little bit themselves. This isn't to say that Petitgrains aren't happy. They always appear contented and they'd never admit to being otherwise — it would be, to them, "terribly bad form."

Petitgrains are the keepers of the small niceties that stop this world from going out of control. They're the maiden aunt who insists on tea at 4 o'clock or the middle-aged father who wants to give his children a sense of decency. Petitgrain parents will take the time and effort to point out both the good and bad and try to present as many sides to a story as possible. They often feel that the world is toppling off its axis and that things need to be balanced and harmonized, but remain basically optimistic and can stimulate others into change.

Being optimistic doesn't stop Petitgrain from being the provider and making sure there's money in the bank for a rainy day and a roof over their head. This personality isn't usually very well off, however, because promotions at work are given to whiz kids instead — not because Petitgrains aren't capable but because they are the anchors of the workplace and are just too valuable to move upward. Jobs that involve something other than making money for the shareholders interest these people (although if able to afford them, they'll have a few shares themselves), such as governmental office or a profession associated with care, hospital administration, and the like. Petitgrain may dream of being an adventurer or film star but wouldn't even try to pursue something so ambitious.

In a relationship, Petitgrain will only be as attentive as necessary and may have difficulty expressing how deeply they feel about a person. But when they fall in love they fall very hard and very deep. This can be a disaster for them if the relationship doesn't continue because their trust (more so than their heart) will have been broken. As lovers, Petitgrains wouldn't set the world on fire and although they have a warm nature it is not fiery or passionate. Because Petitgrains don't like to take risks, and may not feel they've met the right person, long-lasting romantic relationships often elude them.

When they're negative, Petitgrains get very disillusioned with the general lack of concern for human life expressed in this world and often try to alleviate these feelings by doing something positive themselves, no matter how small. Although often mistaken for being snobbish and cold, they are far from this. But they aren't gushing or sentimental either, which seems to them somewhat intrusive. Negativity makes Petitgrains irritable and their energy level drops so they may appear ill, and become very fixed in their ideas. This is especially the case when they want advancement but find their way blocked. If this happens Petitgrains can become quite eccentric, preferring their own company to anyone else's and cutting themselves off from human beings in general. You can still find them sitting in the sun, feeling the earth beneath them, and talking to the flowers or admiring the architecture, but they'll have no time for people. They'll become impatient, ill mannered, and rude in an effort to get people out of their life. But this only happens when they've been deeply hurt. Petitgrains becomes impossible when negative, particularly for their partners. They become snappy and find fault in everything, their nurturing instincts gone and despair in its place. Confusion, pessimism, and rigidity can set it.

Generally, however, Petitgrains are stimulating and can harmonize the most fraught situation. They have a calm that transposes people, giving them the confidence to go out and do things for themselves. These are complex characters with profound spirituality and wisdom. They will not, however, belong to any particular religious group because their conception of a deity is completely universal.

PINE
Pinus sylvestris
WOODIE/LEAFIE

CHARACTER
Acceptance, Understanding, Patience, Self-forgiveness

USE FOR THESE POSITIVE ATTRIBUTES
Humility, Simplicity, Assured, Buffered, Forgiving, Perserverence, Sharing, Mindful, Trusting, Directness, Direction, Acceptance of love, Tenacity, Confident, Exhilarated

USE TO COUNTERACT THESE NEGATIVE ATTRIBUTES
Regrets, Guilt, Self-blame, Dissatisfaction, Self-critical, Worried, Overly responsible, Nonconfrontational, Self-reproach, Unworthiness, Exhaustion, Masochistic, Shameful, Feeling rejected, Unsympathetic, Miserable, Feeling inadequate

PINE
Personality Profile

Although one would think that, like the Cypress, the Pine personality would be upright, direct, and sometimes self-righteous, it is not, being like no other in that it is the child betrayed. Pine persons are the soft, gentle types who often go through life afraid to make a sound, or a mistake, and

when they do will always say it was their fault. This personality can be self-critical, full of guilt, and constantly apologizing for everything and everyone. Never mind that it isn't their fault. The Pine type is invariably "wrung out" — you cannot carry the world on your shoulders and not feel exhausted.

Pine people are never satisfied with themselves, their work, or play, and then blame themselves for not having tried harder. Pines are often the workaholic who has forgotten that it's okay to play sometimes — the sky won't fall in on them if work stops for five minutes.

Pines do not accept that anything can change, and may not wish it to, thus perpetuating the negative aspects of their life. However, there is a lighter side to Pine, who is capable of giving love in enormous quantities, and they're fearfully protective of their family and any causes that have caught their imagination. Pines can have large amounts of energy and are often able to help people in a similar situation to themselves without realizing it, becoming a home from the storm for troubled souls. Pines can help you see through the mists, and become clearer and calmer.

Because the Pine personality can be rather masochistic, it is important that they recognize this tendency so that any guilty feelings can be transformed into a positive look at what is really happening, and in this way Pine learns to accept love instead of just giving it. They need to learn to understand their needs and desires, accept that it's okay to have them, and to reach out to obtain them; it's okay to want to receive love — and you don't have to be passive about it. Using Pine essential oil can help put back the clear-sightedness needed to take a good, hard look at what you need, and it helps you to slowly put into practice the art of striving for it without setting unrealistic goals for happiness and life. Like a good walk in an alpine forest, Pine can help you make important decisions calmly and confidently.

Molly is typical of those who fall into the trap Pine personalities set for themselves. She got engaged on her sixteenth birthday, left school and became an apprentice hairdresser. By eighteen she had been talked into marriage and felt obliged to help her young husband build up his career as an electrician, spending every evening after work placing advertisements, doing the books, washing his overalls, and tidying up the electrical equipment he left all over the living room floor. She gave up her dream of owning her own salon, and concentrated on her husband's needs, and her growing family of four children. After all, she said, he was trying to make a good life for them all and she shouldn't complain.

When the husband started to buy second-hand equipment that too ended up all over the house, Molly would patiently clear it up, making a little space for herself, apologizing every time she moved something. Although it irritated her like mad, and she grew to hate her home, and avoided it whenever possible, she still carried on telling herself that it would all be okay one day. After all, she said, they needed the money. The children had to be fitted in around the wires, plugs, soldering irons, and various boxes of tiny screws — a difficult thing with small children, who kept moving things about, for which she got the blame.

Gradually the strain became too much and Molly snapped. She had a breakdown which, of course, she thought was her fault. Wherever she went, others would burden her further with their own horror stories and tales of abuse but somehow, listening to others locked out her own problems. When she was released from the hospital, with the help of various therapists, she started to look at what she wanted. It was a long, slow process during which her husband left her — taking his mess with him. Molly learned to take walks in the countryside, enjoy her children, and that it was okay for her to say what she felt, and that she was a lovable human being.

ROSEMARY
Rosemarinus officinalis

HERBIE/LEAFIE

CHARACTER
Vigorous, Strengthening, Restorative, Centering

USE FOR THESE POSITIVE ATTRIBUTES
Energy, Upliftment, Confidence, Creativity, Clarity, Structured, Concentration, Stabilized, Fortified, Sincere, Purified, Aware

USE TO COUNTERACT THESE NEGATIVE ATTRIBUTES
Loss of memory, Learning difficulties, Lethargy, Disorientation, Fatigue, Indecision, Nervous exhaustion, Overburdened, Overworked, Strain, Emotional exhaustion, Sluggishness

---

ROSEMARY
Personality Profile

Rosemaries are young at heart and seem to have found the elixir of youth. These are imaginative, happy, sensitive people, quite determined at times, but quite gentle souls, who are free of mental restrictions. They can be very creative and have quite a refreshing approach to the eternal problems of love and happiness.

Rosemary enjoys security and will aim to be in a secure position in love and in life because it's within a secure environment that they can express themselves fully. Nevertheless, juggling things around is a feature of this personality, who can easily balance two jobs, four hobbies, and many friends. With a knack of putting things in order and well able to manage time and negotiate with people, Rosemary can achieve a great deal and will never do so by intentionally manipulating others.

Rosemary has a spirit that vibrates at an astonishing level, and some other types may find it difficult keeping up the pace. This vibrancy extends to their mental states, and to their ability to organize and concentrate on the many tasks they set themselves. Rosemarys have high ideals and like to think of themselves as slightly above the cut. They are not consciously arrogant, it's just their way. Challenges and new activities are welcomed, especially if they involve traveling. Their lighthearted approach can get them into trouble because others can take offense. Rosemary judges things by the head, rather than the heart, and in general are open and trustworthy and make great mates. However, be prepared to be dragged out on cold, wet mornings to join in with the latest enthusiasm.

Rosemarys are usually very environmentally conscious, and vegetarian — or at least trying to be, believing in animal rights. They don't want to be leaders but will be found going on marches or lobbying, or in jobs concerned with ecology, conservation, or gardening, and would suit politics, trade unionism, and teaching.

If they find themselves in jobs to which they are unsuited, Rosemaries will develop their negative traits. A lack of sincerity shows first, then they become surly, withdrawn, and temperamental. In a relationship that is not altogether alive, they tend to become reproachful and have unaccountable traumas and dramas.

They become, as they sink further into reproachfullness, very sharp-tongued and quite unlikable.

Rosemarys like beauty and their eyes may tell them to choose a gorgeous, "drop-dead-for" type — usually a floral — and this might be fine while flirting and playing games, but no good when it moves to the bedroom. Rosemaries are not the greatest lovers, being much more interested in *why* humans have a sex drive, than in sex itself. It can be difficult to be intimate with a Rosemary, although you would never believe it at first. Either male or female, they can also be abusive — turning their sexuality into anger. As young people they'll have lots of affairs, trying to find out just exactly what it is that interests everybody so much, but as they get older, will look for a secure relationship that doesn't ask too much of them in terms of romance — a good buddy rather than a lover.

Rosemarys remain happy into old age, and even when injustices befall them, they feel invincible, protected by the gods. You can call on Rosemarys to help clear out old ghosts and memories from your cupboard, and clean the dark secrets out of your life.

Palmarosa

ROSE MAROC
Rosa centifolia

FLORAL

CHARACTER
Passionate, Harmonious, Reassuring, Comforting

USE FOR THESE POSITIVE ATTRIBUTES
Motivated, Inner vitality, Revived, Confident, Passionate, Cooperative, Sense of freedom, Fulfilled, Forgiving, Sensual

USE TO COUNTERACT THESE NEGATIVE ATTRIBUTES
Grief, Bitterness, Fear of letting go, Fear of love, Fear of sexuality, Jealousy, Resignation, Passivity, Deception, Lack of ambition/motivation, Self-destruction, Vengefulness

ROSE MAROC
Personality Profile

Just as Rose Otto represents the gentleness of spirit, Rose Maroc represents passion of the spirit. This is the passionate Rose, with a deep, hypnotic personality — vivacious and alive. The Maroc personality is deeply erotic in nature, and their lives are full of excitement and emotion.

The Rose Maroc is alive in every sense of the word. They love dramas — other people's, because Roses have no room in their own life for such time wasting. Life is too short for that. Everything this personality does is done with great fervor, delighting friends with sensuality and appreciation of life's pleasures. Imagine a flamenco dancer — that is Rose Maroc: very erotic, fully aware of their sexuality, and of the effect it can have on others. Many of the traits of Rose Otto are in the

Rose Maroc personality too, the difference is that Rose Otto does everything with gentleness, while Maroc is soft but purposeful. This spiritual personality appreciates all life's sensual pleasures, so long their enjoyment does not cause detriment to others.

Rose Marocs can comfort the deeper emotions and affect the souls of others. These Roses often become artists, poets, composers, musicians, singers, dancers, cooks, body workers, or become involved in film, photography, journalism, or design. They tend to wilt in any profession that does not allow them free reign of expression, yet, like many people, may not have the choice.

When in a negative mode, Rose Marocs can be overbearing and deceptive. They often unwittingly become involved in power struggles. If truly wronged and hurt, these are the Rose personalities that could become jealous and vengeful —

particularly if someone hurts a member of their own circle. For themselves, they never worry and just accept the hurt and pain.

If the more spiritual side is neglected, Rose Maroc can become controlling and impatient, and when driven to succeed, can even become self-destructive. Although they get accused of bullying and always knowing best, nothing is done out of malice but out of concern for the individual. They'll seek out the truth in all things, and won't tolerate lying or cheating, prud-ery or puritanical morality.

Marocs are often the power behind the throne of great men and women (and the not so great — which is why they need Rose Maroc). Parents can be charmed just as much as lovers and friends, and Roses give unconditionally to everyone if deserving of their attention. Growing older, Roses can become eccentric and, if totally negative, impossibly cantankerous. But the younger generations love older Rose Marocs because of their wild stories and charming tolerance.

ROSE OTTO — FLORAL
Rosa damascena

CHARACTER
Loving, Harmonizing, Comforting, Happy, Caring, Euphoric, Gentle, Peaceful

USE FOR THESE POSITIVE ATTRIBUTES
Comforted, Contentment, Devoted, Motivated, Inner vision, Revival, Joy, Happiness, Inner freedom, Acceptance, Completeness, Wisdom, Spirituality, Patience, Love, Sensuality, Purity

USE TO COUNTERACT THESE NEGATIVE ATTRIBUTES
Depression, Sadness, Grief, Anger, Anxiety, Bitterness, Emptiness, Fear of loving, Fear of not being loved, Broken heart, Guilt, Shyness, Jealousy, Touchiness, Emotional crisis, Resignation, Inexpression, Hopelessness, Despair, Abused, Emotional violence, Hurt inner child

ROSE OTTO
Personality Profile

The Rose epitomizes the floral characteristics of the truly feminine personality — both the positive and negative sides. Although all Roses come under the same banner, there are subtle differences between the Rose Otto from Bulgaria, Turkey, France, or India, and as more species are distilled and become available, such as the Rose di Mai, so other slight variations will be noted. However, generalization does suit the Rose personality as all Rose types are only a slight variation on a theme — except for the absolute of the Rose Maroc.

The Rose Otto personality is one of gentleness and apparent perfection. Although thought of as mainly feminine, the Rose is also the feminine in the male. Some males carry more of this type than others, and surprisingly perhaps the negative Rose personality is often detected in males. Bulgarian Otto of Rose is more suited to the feminine while Turkish Otto of Rose is more masculine.

Whatever the species, Rose is perfection personified. It's the ultimate female — one who can give unconditional love. This, and spirituality, is what the Rose personality strives for in themselves and others. The Rose is charming and lovely, an exquisite person. They will be well-mannered, ever-mindful of any hurtful phrases, caring, gentle, and joyful. Roses are able to laugh at themselves, admit their silly actions and wrong deeds with no self-recrimination, or ego, always accepting full responsibility for their actions. Roses have the wisdom to know that there are far greater things in the universe than them, and that humans do make mistakes. Indeed, their presence and understanding is so peaceful, you'd think they were angels.

The pure-hearted generosity that Rose extends to other people is often misunderstood, but Rose seems to understand this as their fate and just continues anyway. Others are drawn to them, perhaps in the hope that some of their spirituality and inner vision might rub off. Bewitchingly lovely, Rose's words will be well-chosen, often soothing and peaceful.

As much as the Rose personality might seem like the ultimate spiritual human being, however, they live in the real world and are real people, fighters who won't tolerate anyone undermining their efforts at work or at play. Full of confidence, they tend to play a lot, and are another floral who uses their sensuality to get what they want — although this is often subconscious, just part of their sensual selves. Empowered, Roses can be the ultimate lovers — full of sexual confidence, sensual, aware of their partner's needs, and fully understanding of the spiritual elements in love and sex. People with a Rose profile enjoy life as it is, but you can't shackle this type if you try, in marriage for example; they'll be gone. However, this type never seem to bear grudges and will always consider themselves your friend.

The Rose personality loves cooperation, and uncooperative people shatter their rose-colored world. They may find it difficult to understand why everyone doesn't operate on the same level as they do. Self-indulgence is enjoyed without guilt, whether this is reading a book when they should be at work, or playing in the park with a child when the car needs washing. Serving humanity is a trait of the Rose, providing it doesn't interfere with the pleasures and pathways of life —their life. If you get in the way, you could be on your way. Roses can be very blunt at times, and hate to lie, seeing no point in it. If a

Rose tells you to pack your bags, that doesn't mean they don't love you anymore, just that they have to move on.

The Rose personality is found in jobs where the appreciation of fine, sensual things can be utilized. They are the silk merchants and art dealers, the models in fine gowns, the filmmakers and photographers, the artists and sculptors, composers and musicians, the writers, philosophers, and spiritual counselors. Places of spiritual worship hold a fascination for this personality, who may experience déjà vu, prophetic dreams, insight, and the all-important *knowing*.

When Rose is in a negative mood everything becomes fate. Interest disappears and complete apathy takes over, along with moodiness, feelings of abandonment and resignation to their situation. They seem to barely exist in this world, all life drained out of them, as if stuck for eternity in a slow whirlpool of emotions with no exit. Only their sensuality remains.

Rose will blame outside influences for how they feel — not another person, but illness or job failure. It isn't always easy to see this side of Rose because to the outside world they appear much the same — concerned with others, caring and considerate. But the spark will be gone and eventually Rose will become boring company. People will leave them, and it becomes self-perpetuating. You hear, "I wonder why nobody visits me any more?" When ambition is thwarted, it becomes worse. The more sensitive Rose can just give up on life altogether. They will still love their friends, and give love, but they'll shut themselves off from receiving love — and a Rose without love shrivels up and dies.

If a loved one dies before Rose they'll be inconsolable, often dying of a broken heart. The Rose type doesn't grieve a little; they will grieve through to their very soul, for a very long time. As Rose's love touches the spiritual in the loved ones, the loss will be profound. Even if a brave face is shown to the world, the grief will still be there, deep inside.

———

SANDALWOOD   WOODIE
Santalum album

CHARACTER
Enlightenment, Meditative, Balancing, Connecting

USE FOR THESE POSITIVE ATTRIBUTES
Warm, Comforted, Sensitive, Serene, Trusting, Harmonized, Peaceful, Wise, Sensual, Expressive, Good self-esteem, Open, Insightful, Unity

USE TO COUNTERACT THESE NEGATIVE ATTRIBUTES
Anxiety, Nervous tension, Possessiveness, Manipulating, Unforgiving, Obsessive, Lonely, Accepting, Cynical, Insecurity, Recurrent nightmares, Selfishness, Distressed, Uneasy, Hasty, Aggressive, Irritable, Dwelling on the past

SANDALWOOD
Personality Profile

The Sandalwood personality is serene and in charge of their emotions, fully aware of their direction in life, even anticipating the rocky sections ahead. Their inner calm is like that of an old soul, and Sandalwoods are certainly familiar with the concept of reincarnation. Their laid-back, philosophical attitude mistakenly leads to them being accused of detachment. Sandalwoods are very still people who listen more than they talk, sizing you up — which they are very good at. This personality never consciously strives to be ahead of anyone else in their thinking or deeds, but usually are, so invoke a lot of jealousy.

The Sandalwood personality has a direct line with the universal telephone exchange and instinctively knows when something is missing or not quite right.

They leave no stone unturned in the search for truth and are sometimes mistaken for being terribly serious, which they can be, *but* they're also able to laugh at themselves and other people without any malicious intent. The Sandalwood personality is supportive of people trying to pick up the pieces of their lives. But having a difficult time finding solutions for their own problems, they ignore them, and hand out solutions to everyone else. Sandalwoods can be quite tactile people, in a gentle sort of way, depending on the mores of the culture in which they live. At times, they may long for the answer to life, appealing to the heavens to reveal just a little bit more. Understanding humanity so well, Sandalwoods make good healers.

Sandalwoods are very sensuous and sex is important to them. They may even have studied the secrets of Tantra, the ancient Indian cult of ecstasy, and will be amused by the antics in the Kama Sutra.

These people are not afraid of their sexuality and will view it as one of the precious gifts we've been given here on earth to help us through this lifetime. Sex is never simply thought of as a means of procreation, or used for any ulterior motives — like making contacts or getting money. The Sandalwood personality is easy-going and comfortable, making them self-assured, calming people to be with, at ease with both genders.

On the negative side, Sandalwoods can be possessive of their knowledge, manipulating, bossy, controlling, and unable to admit mistakes. They may be prone to fits of anguish about their plight, and unforgiving. It has also been known for Sandalwoods to cut people out of their lives completely — as if they never existed. If negativity strikes, Sandalwood can be prone to sleepless nights because of stressful dreams, and become irritable, uncooperative, and dissatisfied.

As partners, Sandalwoods expect an equal relationship and continual support. If they don't get it, the partner will be changed. When Sandalwoods fall desperately in love they can become intolerant of any company other than the loved one. The Sandalwood personality makes a good parent and their children's friends will usually spend more time at their house than their own, particularly as teenagers, when Sandalwood is ready to answer questions about life, love, and sex.

Sandalwoods are good in any job that needs direct communication and ingenuity. Otherwise they'll become easily bored. They make good artists, writers, theologians, psychologists, counselors, and buyers for companies, but also seem to have leanings towards botany and archaeology, and make good members of management teams. In fact, they'll make a serious effort in most professions, as long as it engages their intellect.

Elizabeth Jones, OBE, MCSP, DRE, MIFA Reg., MISPA, physiotherapist and tutor:

"Infinitely soothing qualities. Deep, woody, subtle, in no way overpowering. Has a timeless, soporific character."

THYME LINALOL
Thymus vulgaris, sp linalol

HERBIE/LEAFIE

CHARACTER
Gently Empowering, Invigorating, Assisting

USE FOR THESE POSITIVE ATTRIBUTES
Fortified, Balanced, Tolerant, Courageous, Supportive, Decisive, Alert, Focused, Concentration, Warming

USE TO COUNTERACT THESE NEGATIVE ATTRIBUTES
Lack of direction, Intellectual or physical exhaustion, Weakness, Overreactive, Nervous debility, Blockages

THYME LINALOL
Personality Profile

These charming, intelligent, proud people pride themselves on being honest and straightforward and in having command over their actions and deeds. Thyme Linalols have an exuberance and freshness about them that transfers to almost everything they do. They are always full of new ideas and projects. This isn't always apparent at first because they like to hold back a little until they know a person well. The Thyme Linalol personality is able to command attention although they don't ask for it. They're considerate, thoughtful, and discreet.

Thyme Linalols have a built-in genius which allows them to look at things in fresh and unique ways, bringing life to any project they become involved in. Forging forward in everything they do, leaving others behind, Thymes have a vivacious spirit, inner strength, and fortitude that far outweighs any weakness they may have. This isn't brute strength but gentle persuasion, and Thymes can be very supportive. The great affinity Thymes have with children is probably due to the fact that children feel confident with them, going to them with troubles and worries. This protectiveness extends to members of their family, who can always rely on Thyme's assistance and support. This personality falls in love easily, partly perhaps because they spend so much time alone, so when they do fall, it's hook line and sinker, becoming prone to bouts of love-sickness and emotional trauma.

Thyme Linalols are the strong, silent type but when in negative mode, are quick to anger. They're prone to nervous problems, and if they push themselves too hard they may suffer nervous exhaustion, even nervous breakdown. This personality can become hypersensitive and may occasionally retreat from the world. As children,

Thymes often seek solitude, perhaps playing with an imaginary friend, even if they have brothers and sisters. As an adult, Thymes are at ease with their own company, sometimes preferring the chance to be peaceful and reflective.

Thyme Linalols often have a revolutionary outlook and are colorful characters. They're honest, open people who ultimately believe that the world is a good place. Because they go where angels fear to tread, they make good, easygoing travelers and their unique ways of looking at old problems gives them an inventive streak,which is helpful in science. Because of their ability to understand difficult moral situations and their capacity to relate to events happening to other people, this personality can do well in personnel, counseling, or spiritual leadership.

TUBEROSE — FLORAL
Polianthes tuberosa

CHARACTER
Transformative, Spontaneous, Extroverted, Centering

USE FOR THESE POSITIVE ATTRIBUTES
Motivated, Enthusiastic, Encouraged, Expansive, Sensuous, Sensitive, Spontaneous, Expressive, Frank

USE TO COUNTERACT THESE NEGATIVE ATTRIBUTES
Stress, Irritability, Emotional conflict, Oversensitivity, Jealousy, Bitterness, Anger, Confusion, Disorientation, Hostility, Insincerity, Resentment, Selfishness, Falsity

TUBEROSE Personality Profile

The Tuberose personality is daring, attractive, hypnotic, charming, and good company. They love gossip, but beware, if you do tell them your deepest, darkest secrets, they are not above blackmail. This inclination is further compounded by the fact that the Tuberose personality loves danger and will take huge risks for the sake of excitement. Tuberoses have an obsessive nature — whether they lament losing a lover or the fact that they didn't have the opportunity to spend their usual ten minutes chanting under a tree. Their addictive nature often gets them into hot water.

The Tuberose personality will use all their skills of seduction to get exactly what they want. Their physical appearance is extremely important to them and they'll always be nicely dressed, with manicured nails and well-groomed hair. If female, she wouldn't contemplate opening the door to let the cat out unless she was fully made up or wearing dark glasses. Looking good and being desired are Tuberose's number one priorities, important because physical attraction can be used to gain power — sexual, economic, and political. Tuberose loves power of any kind, and they'll use lovers to gain money, fame, or prestige. The age of their lover is immaterial to them. Older lovers are taken for the prestige they can confer, while younger lovers are taken for their prowess. An older Tuberose personality will go through younger lovers like a bag of toffees — discarding the wrappers without a care.

The male Tuberose is often overly fussy in his dress — to the point of obsession. If he doesn't have the money to buy his own designer suits, he'll borrow a friend's. He's a born flirt and will flirt with both women and men. In love, he'll find himself in intriguing or difficult situations and will avoid people of his own age if he doesn't find them challenging enough. He's often found with an older lover, so long as they have power and money — the things he loves more than anything. Tuberose is ruthless — in business and in play.

Just as the Tuberose personality gets a kick out of being "close to the edge," they also enjoy putting people in that situation. They'll charm a cobra out of a tree, telling you it won't bite, and then as you approach and get closer to it, they'll suddenly "remember" that it does in fact bite and tell you a millisecond before you get

within attacking distance. No personality loves the dark side of the paranormal or mysterious more than Tuberose. The dark side of human nature may repel this floral type but at the same time, it holds an almost unhealthy fascination for them.

Shelly is a typical Tuberose personality. She married rather young, to a nice handsome man who was a kind father to their two daughters but — and this drove her crazy — he had no ambition. So when she started work as a secretary in the office of the chairman of a large manufacturer, and found that he was single, she set out to catch him. Being naturally charming and employing her feminine wiles to the fullest, Shelly became his lover within three months. She didn't stop there of course. Soon Shelly and her two daughters were living in her boss' luxurious mansion, divorce proceedings were in hand, and Shelly was enjoying her new life of designer clothes, expensive jewelry, health spas, and tennis clubs.

For the first few years Shelly was happy, sweet, charming, obliging, and attentive to her lover. Her children were now in private schools, vacations were spent at the villa in Spain, and Shelly thoroughly reveled in her new-found status. Then boredom set in. She started being ridiculously extravagant, treating her friends to endless expensive meals, evenings at the theater and nights out at the clubs, with Shelly lapping up the kudos that came with being lady bountiful. However, she still didn't love the man and gradually became bitter and vindictive towards him, "paying him back" by taking a stream of young lovers, who, in exchange for expensive gifts, told her they loved her. For several years this pattern continued, and eventually Shelly began taking any drugs she could lay her hands on.

Eventually, of course, the man became aware of what was going on and took a younger and prettier lover himself. Shelly found out and, at the same time, realized that because they didn't have any children together and weren't married, she wasn't actually in a very secure position. Still, she continued to lie and cheat on him and one day got caught *in flagrante*, as they say, and was promptly thrown out on the street. The man continued to house the

children and pay their school fees. The children, who were quite happy to stay where they were, were used by Shelly as tools for gaining sympathy. Her ploy didn't work, however, and Shelly was homeless, jobless, and broke — although still bejeweled.

At their best, Tuberoses are warm, seductive, and hypnotic. Their most challenging lesson in life is to learn to love genuinely, to forget the superficialities and appreciate people for their good qualities. They also need to learn to love themselves — without makeup. If they can do that, charm and warmth shines through.

VETIVER   ROOTIE
Vetiveria zizanoides

CHARACTER
Grounding, Centering, Visionary, Wisdom

USE FOR THESE POSITIVE ATTRIBUTES
Spiritual calmness, Growth, Integrity, Wisdom, Mind-body connection, Strength, Honorable, Protected, Self-esteem, Grounded

USE TO COUNTERACT THESE NEGATIVE ATTRIBUTES
Fear, Anxiety, Obsession, Overwork, Agitation, Intellectual fatigue, Hurt, Scattered thinking, Irritability, Anger, Emotional burnout, Mental exhaustion, Unworthiness, Loss of purpose, Emotional weakness, Addiction, Disconnection, Fantasizing, Emotional blockages, Neurotic behavior, Instability, Disoriented

VETIVER
Personality Profile

Vetivers are often strong and intellectual, with a strong sense of reality and awareness of what is happening around them, embodying the relationship between mind and body. The essential oil of vetiver is obtained from the root of the plant and has a vitality and energy associated with it that is earthy. This personality feels a connection with Gaia. This is an earthy kind of person, ready to laugh out loud at risqué jokes, not easily embarrassed. Vetivers are very comfortable with their sexuality, seeing sex very much as pure vitality and energy. They're also very likely to experiment, and their sensuality does have a deep, mysterious side.

Although the fragrance is often associated with the masculine, the Vetiver personality — whether male or female — will be perfectly balanced between their masculine and feminine sides. There is nothing delicate or ethereal about the Vetiver profile, it's very much of the here and now. Often gentle and wise in spirit, friends turn to Vetivers for advice, which will be blunt and straight.

The Vetiver type will be very interested in the esoteric side of life, particularly the journeys of the shamans and voyages to uncover the earth's mysteries, and may be visionaries. Green issues, such as pollution and the destruction of the rain forests concern them, and they'll very likely become disillusioned with the world as it is. Although not the best travelers, this personality will follow the quest for idealism and a place to be. They may travel with groups of people, but as they get older, will search for their roots. Vetivers are not exactly restless; they could settle down anywhere if they ignored the call of the wild. Remote villages in so-called "third world" countries hold an attraction for them — the raw elements of the earth and nature appeal to them.

Vetivers revel in the sensuality of life, very much the person who holds and touches things to appreciate fully all aspects of the object, but they are also often very academic and philosophical, sometimes teachers. However, Vetiver's academic associates, who may have lost touch with themselves through too much "living in the head," can't understand why, when there are intellectual problems to be solved, Vetiver should prefer to indulge his or her attraction to the opposite sex, or other earthly matters. At the same time, these people need Vetiver precisely because this personality helps them to be drawn into their own bodies.

Jan Kusmirek, MDDH, MED, LLFA, MIFA Reg., LCSP, DM, aromatherapist, medical herbalist and lecturer:

"It is a hidden oil to do with the dark recesses and the potential for life and energy. There is an earthy fragrance with spice overtones, warmth, and comfort as on a sun-drenched day. Tenacious, with a sense of belonging and grounding. Its personality is one of renewal, ripeness, and maturity, excellent for all those who have 'lost touch' with something."

YLANG YLANG   FLORAL
Canaga odorata

CHARACTER
Euphoric, Sensuous, Stimulating, Unifying

USE FOR THESE POSITIVE ATTRIBUTES
Self-confidence, Warmth, Awakened, Uplifted, Calm, Joyful, Enthusiastic, Meditative, Sensual, Soothed

USE TO COUNTERACT THESE NEGATIVE ATTRIBUTES
Depression, Anxiety, Tension, Stress, Frustration, Irritability, Emotional guilt, Resentment, Jealousy, Selfishness, Impatience, Irrationality, Stubbornness, Obstinacy, Shyness

YLANG YLANG
Personality Profile

The Ylang Ylang personality is intensely feminine. She has a passionate nature, tempered by a calm and balance many find unnerving. Ylang Ylangs are the femme fatales, the Casanovas, the mistresses, and the lovers. They are people who delight in the erotic and sensual. No shrinking violets here!

Neither male nor female, Ylang Ylangs are happy alone, flourishing best when they have an audience to applaud their achievements or commiserate with their failures. Ylangs are usually charismatic, bewitching, gracious, and delightful company, and their incredible fantasy life makes great entertainment for their friends. This type, however, rarely enters the world of entertainment themselves, much preferring to be friends or lovers of famous people, particularly people with power. Power is an aphrodisiac to these types, male or female, who are good companions in these relationships because they have a balancing quality about them, and will relieve the stress that often goes with powerful positions.

It's difficult to handle a true Ylang Ylang because they often live in a dream world where they are king or queen and nothing will ever harm them, where they always come out on top. Often these dreams are impossible to achieve, as is wealth for the majority of Ylang Ylangs. The female Ylang Ylang may resort to older men who indulge her image of herself, who enjoy her sexuality and power over younger men. She will be worn like a trophy until she leaves, bored and frustrated. This is not what Ylang Ylang women are intended for.

These passionate people live for love. As men, they love the thrill of the chase and conquest, and as women they delight in obtaining the unobtainable and having secret rendezvous. Ylang Ylang has a fiery, passionate nature, intensely sweet, and would sacrifice everything for love — and I mean *love* — at the time, at least, because this personality falls in and out of love easily.

Ylang Ylangs are found in jobs that give expression to the aesthetic side of life — those dealing with beautiful fabrics, cosmetics, hairdressing, and anything that entails love — a designer of bridal wear for example. They could also be involved in any profession involving exciting physical pursuits, such as racing cars.

Ylang Ylangs enjoy creating a mountain out of a mole hill and look for excitement continually. They scream and shout, and know how to "let rip" with anger if crossed, and of course, to get their own way. The daredevils of life are often Ylang Ylang types who will try anything once for the experience. There is insecurity in this type though, and this often manifests in their disliking their looks, or feeling any lack of money acutely. A male Ylang will need to have money to survive and may lose himself searching for it. He likes fast cars, expensive clothes, exotic locations, and beautiful women.

A negative Ylang Ylang will be neglectful of their appearance, not bothering with hair and clothes, careless of the impression they are making on others. As the neglect extends beyond themselves, Ylangs frequently lose interest in their work, so in the end they'll become depressed and downhearted, with no self-confidence. Barely living, they'll hide away from the world. Other Ylangs will become frustrated, extremely nervous and irritable, losing all interest in life and love. If in a partnership of any kind, this can lead to untold problems — just compounding the myth they have created about themselves being unlovable. Whatever relationship Ylangs may or may not be in when negative, they can be angry and jealous, and in need of rebalancing.

Love conquers all, so they say, and with Ylang Ylang that is certainly true. Love can brighten up the morning and dispel the darkest clouds, giving Ylangs a new lease on life. If empowered, Ylang Ylang can balance the two extremes of their character very well. They have a soft side to them and are joyful and fun, good friends who will never be dull company.

————

CHART 14.1–QUICK REFERENCE CHART
Essential Oils for Mind, Mood, and Emotion

BASIL	*Ocimum basilicum*	HERBIE/LEAFIE

CHARACTER
Uplifting, Awakening, Clarifying, Stimulating

USE FOR THESE POSITIVE ATTRIBUTES
Positivity, Purposefulness, Concentration, Assertiveness, Decisiveness, Straightforward-ness, Trust, Integrity, Enthusiasm, Clarity, Cheerfulness, Strength

USE TO COUNTERACT THESE NEGATIVE ATTRIBUTES
Indecision, Mental fatigue, Mental exhaustion, Negativity, Lack of direction, Fear, Burnout, Confusion, Intellectual fatigue, Apathy, Bitterness, Resentment, Addiction, Conflict, Fear of intimacy, Shame, Doubts, Melancholy, Sadness

---

BERGAMOT	*Citrus bergamia*	FRUITIE

CHARACTER
Joyous, Refreshing, Uplifting, Encouraging

USE FOR THESE POSITIVE ATTRIBUTES
Concentration, Confidence, Balance, Strength, Joy, Motivation, Good cheer, Harmony, Completeness

USE TO COUNTERACT THESE NEGATIVE ATTRIBUTES
Depression, Anxiety, Helplessness, Apathy, Bitterness, Burnout, Despondency, Emptiness, Exhaustion, Grief, Hopelessness, Sadness, Loneliness, Stress, Tension, Emotional imbalances

---

BLACK PEPPER	*Piper nigrum*	FRUITIE/SPICIE

CHARACTER
Security, Comforting, Directional, Endurance

USE FOR THESE POSITIVE ATTRIBUTES
Comfort, Stamina, Endurance, Motivation, Changeability

USE TO COUNTERACT THESE NEGATIVE ATTRIBUTES
Emotional Blockages, Compulsions, Confusion, Disorientation, Fatigue, Begrudging, Indecision, Irrationality, Anger, Frustration, Emotional coldness, Apathy, Mental exhaustion

---

CARDAMOM   *Elettaria cardamomum*   FRUITIE/SPICIE

CHARACTER
Clarifying, Stimulating, Encouraging, Enthusiastic

USE FOR THESE POSITIVE ATTRIBUTES
Clarity, Concentration, Direction, Motivation, Straightforwardness, Enthusiasm, Confidence, Courage, Fortitude, Purpose

USE TO COUNTERACT THESE NEGATIVE ATTRIBUTES
Mental stress, Apathy, Confusion, Inflexibility, Judgmental, Intolerance, Unreasonableness, Burnout, Suspicion, Sluggishness, Self-pity, Bewilderment, Rigidity

---

CARNATION   *Dianthus caryophyllus*   FLORAL

CHARACTER
Secretiveness, Stillness, Originality, Liberating

USE FOR THESE POSITIVE ATTRIBUTES
Self-worth, Communication, Radiating, Creativity, Independence, Tenderness, Nurturing, Encompassing, Cushioning, Openness, Releasing

USE TO COUNTERACT THESE NEGATIVE ATTRIBUTES
Disregard, Neglect, Detachment, Cynicism, Disorientation, Doubt, Mental loneliness, Aloneness, Emotional domination, Emotional solitude, Neglect, Self-criticism

---

CEDARWOOD   *Cedrus atlantica*   WOODIE

CHARACTER
Grounding, Strengthening, Dignified, Powerful

USE FOR THESE POSITIVE ATTRIBUTES
Focus, Concentration, Strength, Confidence, Balance, Stability, Comfort, Persistence, Fortitude, Nobility of spirit

USE TO COUNTERACT THESE NEGATIVE ATTRIBUTES
Scattered thoughts, Thoughtlessness, Fixation on past, Anxiety, Obsessions, Mental strain, Irrationality, Emotional sensitivity, Touchiness, Gloomy thoughts, Worry, Fear, Too analytical, Paranoia, Selfishness

---

CHAMOMILE GERMAN   *Matricaria chamomilla*   HERBIE/FLORAL

CHARACTER
Strong, Peaceful, Healing, Cooling

USE FOR THESE POSITIVE ATTRIBUTES
Communicative, Relaxed, Understanding, Organized, Soothing, Empathy, Patience, Calm

USE TO COUNTERACT THESE NEGATIVE ATTRIBUTES
Nervousness, Frayed nerves, Anger, Frustration, Emotional dramas, Emotional tension, Irritability, Temper, Tenseness, Overly sensitive, Moodiness, Stormy, Bitterness, Resentment, Indifference, Deep emotional baggage

---

CHAMOMILE ROMAN   *Anthemis nobilis*   HERBIE/FLORAL

CHARACTER
Harmonizing, Peaceful, Soothing, Spiritual

USE FOR THESE POSITIVE ATTRIBUTES
Stillness, Calm, Softness, Gentleness, Relaxed, Serene, Spiritually aware, Emotionally stable, Inner peace, Understanding, Cooperative

USE TO COUNTERACT THESE NEGATIVE ATTRIBUTES
Nervousness, Irritability, Temper, Anger, Depression, Hysteria, Fear, Anxiety, Exhaustion, Worry, Stress, Tension, Grief, Emotional imbalance, Broken heart, Grumpiness, Moroseness, Discontent, Impatience, Short temper, Oversensitivity, Melancholy, Spiritual disconnection

---

CINNAMON   *Cinnamomum zeylanicum*   LEAFIE/SPICIE

CHARACTER
Warming, Secular, Fair-minded

USE FOR THESE POSITIVE ATTRIBUTES
Invigorated, Steadfast, Benevolent, Strength, Practicality, Energized, Realistic, Direct

USE TO COUNTERACT THESE NEGATIVE ATTRIBUTES
Instability, Severity, Bleakness, Malice, Spitefulness, Coldness, Fear, Nervous exhaustion, Debility, Introversion, Superficiality

---

CLARY SAGE　　　*Slavia sclarea*　　　HERBIE/FLORAL

CHARACTER
Euphoric, Restoring, Harmonizing, Warming

USE FOR THESE POSITIVE ATTRIBUTES
Calm, Soothed, Confidence, Grounded, Regenerated, Inspired, Tranquil, Revitalized, Uplifted, Balanced, Strength, Relaxed, Restores equilibrium

USE TO COUNTERACT THESE NEGATIVE ATTRIBUTES
Nervousness, Stress, Tension, Changeability, Worried, Anxious, Claustrophobic, Compulsive, Depression, Nightmares, Hostility, Hyperactivity, Lethargy, Obsession, Panic, Mental strain, Fear, Paranoia, Melancholy, Burnout, Delusions, Emotional debility, Absentmindedness, Weepiness, Guilt

---

CORIANDER　　　*Coriandrum sativul*　　　SEEDIE/SPICIE

CHARACTER
Enlivening, Motivating, Encouraging

USE FOR THESE POSITIVE ATTRIBUTES
Creativity, Imagination, Good memory, Confidence, Motivation, Optimism, Sincerity, Expressiveness, Enthusiasm

USE TO COUNTERACT THESE NEGATIVE ATTRIBUTES
Emotional tiredness, Weariness, Irritability, Nervousness, Stress, Nervous debility, Doubt, Fear of failure, Sulkiness, Being uncooperative, Vulnerability

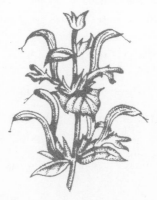

Clary Sage

CYPRESS   *Cupressus sempervirens*   LEAFIE/WOODIE

CHARACTER
Protective, Righteous, Wise, Direction

USE FOR THESE POSITIVE ATTRIBUTES
Strength, Comfort, Change, Direction, Assertion, Control, Understanding, Balance, Sensitivity, Generosity of spirit, Contentment, Stillness, Confidence, Inner peace, Wisdom, Purity of heart, Stability, Patience, Trust, Incorruptibility, Structured, Softly powerful, Direct, Willpower, Straightforward

USE TO COUNTERACT THESE NEGATIVE ATTRIBUTES
Grief, Sorrow, Self-loathing, Pressurised, Being dominated, Opinionated, Jealous, Lethargic, Weak-willed, Fearful, Timid, Emotional turmoil, Unbalanced, Isolated, Inconsolable, Frustrated, Unable to speak up for oneself, Emotionally tired, Emotionally unstable, Tearful, Loss, Regret, Distracted, Lack of concentration, Absentminded, Uncontrollable passions

---

EUCALYPTUS   *Eucalyptus globulas*   LEAFIE/WOODIE

CHARACTER
Energy, Stimulation, Balance, Sheltering

USE FOR THESE POSITIVE ATTRIBUTES
Emotional balancer, Energy balancer, Concentration, Logical thought, Centering, Rationality, Cooling, Predictability

USE TO COUNTERACT THESE NEGATIVE ATTRIBUTES
Exhaustion, Heated emotions, Mood swings, Lack of concentration, Cluttered thoughts, Temper tantrums, Irrational thoughts, Explosive nature, Argumentative

---

EUCALYPTUS CITRIODORA (Lemon)   *Eucalyptus citriodora*   LEAFIE/WOODIE

CHARACTER
Soundness, Trust, Vitality, Harmonious

USE FOR THESE POSITIVE ATTRIBUTES
Stimulant, Concentration, Enthusiastic, Uplifting, Vitality, Understanding, Creativity, Regeneration, Optimism, Letting go, Encouraging, Empathy, Positive change, Freedom, Expressiveness, Comforting

USE TO COUNTERACT THESE NEGATIVE ATTRIBUTES
Sluggishness, Emotional crisis, Emptiness, Confusion, Disillusionment, Restlessness, Fear, Despondency, Emptiness, Loneliness

---

FENNEL, SWEET   *Foeniculum vulgare dulce*   SEEDIE

CHARACTER
Clearing, Resolute, Enlightened

USE FOR THESE POSITIVE ATTRIBUTES
Enlivened, Motivated, Fortitude, Clarity, Forceful, Perseverance, Courageous, Reliable, Confident, Assertive

USE TO COUNTERACT THESE NEGATIVE ATTRIBUTES
Mental blockages, Emotional blockages, Boredom, Unable to adjust, Fear of failure, Hostile, Overburdened, Lack of creativity

---

FRANKINCENSE   *Boswellia carteri*   RESINI

CHARACTER
Elevating, Spiritual, Meditative, Wisdom

USE FOR THESE POSITIVE ATTRIBUTES
Comfort, Healing, Emotional stability, Enlightenment, Protective, Introspection, Courage, Resolution, Fortitude, Acceptance, Inspiration

USE TO COUNTERACT THESE NEGATIVE ATTRIBUTES
Fears, Grief, Blockages, Overattachment, Burnout, Exhaustion, Insincerity, Panic, Anxiety, Disconnection, Repression, Resistance, Self-destruction, Apprehension, Despair

---

GERANIUM   *Pelargonium graveolens*   FLORAL/HERBIE

CHARACTER
Balancing, Healing, Uplifting, Comforting

USE FOR THESE POSITIVE ATTRIBUTES
Consoling, Cushioning, Solace, Adjustment, Elevating, Regenerating, Humor, Friendliness, Stimulant, Balancing, Soothing, Security, Assuring, Shielding, Mothering, Stability, Tranquillity, Steadiness

USE TO COUNTERACT THESE NEGATIVE ATTRIBUTES
Anxiety, Depression, Acute fear, Extreme moods, Confusion, Rigidity, Instability, Abuse, Moodiness, Lack of self-esteem, Insecurity, Sensitivity, Tension, Stress, Hurt, Overly emotional, Crisis, Apprehension, Aggression, Irrationality, Discontent, Worry, Heartache

---

GINGER   *Zingiberaceae officinale*   ROOTIE/SPICIE

CHARACTER
Warming, Strengthening, Encouraging

USE FOR THESE POSITIVE ATTRIBUTES
Confidence, Warmth, Fortitude, Empathy, Courage

USE TO COUNTERACT THESE NEGATIVE ATTRIBUTES
Sexual anxieties, Lack of direction, Purposelessness, Unfocused, Apathy, Burnout, Confusion, Fatigue, Loneliness, Sadness, Resignation

---

GRAPEFRUIT   *Citrus paradisi*   FRUITIE

CHARACTER
Radiating, Cheering, Joyful, Liberating, Boosting,

USE FOR THESE POSITIVE ATTRIBUTES
Joyful, Positive, Confident, Clarity, Balanced, Attuned, Alert, Inspired, Generous, Uplifted, Emotionally purified, Spontaneous, Cooperative

USE TO COUNTERACT THESE NEGATIVE ATTRIBUTES
Depression, Dependency, Sadness, Grief, Apathy, Mental pressure, Mental exhaustion, Emotional violence, Self-doubt, Self-criticism, Aggravated, Frustration

---

HELICHRYSUM   *Helichrysum angustifolium, H italicum, H orientale*   FLORAL
(Immortelle or Italian Everlasting)

CHARACTER
Gentleness, Harmonizing, Caring, Warming, Meditative

USE FOR THESE POSITIVE ATTRIBUTES
Calm, Accepting of change, Buffered, Dreams, Energy, Patience, Idealism, Understanding, Perserverence, Inner strength, Acceptance, Awareness, Positive inner child

USE TO COUNTERACT THESE NEGATIVE ATTRIBUTES
Abuse, Stress, Tension, Emotional crisis, Depression, Lethargy, Mental exhaustion, Emotional exhaustion, Tiredness, Emotional blockages, Disorientation, Overwork, Loneliness, Insecurity, Hypersensitivity, Grief, Addiction, Negative inner child

HYACINTH	*Hyacinthus orientalis*	FLORAL

CHARACTER
Gentle, Trusting, Soothing, Enlightening

USE FOR THESE POSITIVE ATTRIBUTES
Calming, Forgiving, High self-esteem, Perseverance, Equilibrium, Trust, Faith, Courage

USE TO COUNTERACT THESE NEGATIVE ATTRIBUTES
Instability, Stress, Repression, Apathy, Lovesick, Dejection, Distress, Grieving, Sorrow, Powerlessness, Regret, Unforgiving, Naiveté, Dependency, Apprehension

JASMINE	*Jasminum officinale, J. grandiflorum, J. sam*	FLORAL

CHARACTER
Euphoric, Sensuality, Welcoming, Intuitive, Soothing,

USE FOR THESE POSITIVE ATTRIBUTES
Uplifted, Confident, Sexual, Assertive, Relaxed, Optimistic, Open, Sensitive, Harmonized, Aware, Profound, Inspired, Joyful

USE TO COUNTERACT THESE NEGATIVE ATTRIBUTES
Depression, Anxiety, Pessimism, Tension, Indifference, Repression, Bitterness, Jealousy, Low self-esteem, Guilt, Emotional frigidity, Emotional abuse, Emotional violence

JUNIPER	*Juniperus communis*	FRUITIE/WOODIE

CHARACTER
Cleansing, Purifying, Sacredness, Visionary

USE FOR THESE POSITIVE ATTRIBUTES
Self-worth, Spiritually supported, Peace, Inner vision, Uplifted, Strength, Vitality, Cleansed, Meditative, Conviction, Sincerity, Enlightened, Wisdom, Humility

USE TO COUNTERACT THESE NEGATIVE ATTRIBUTES
Nervous exhaustion, Emotional exhaustion, Guilt, Lack of self-worth, Dissatisfaction, Anxiety, Abused, Listlessness, Weakness, Transience, Emptiness, Conflict, Defensive

LAVENDER *Lavendula officinalis, L. angustifolia* FLORAL/HERBIE

CHARACTER
Harmonious, Calming, Healing, Caring, Compassionate, Embracing

USE FOR THESE POSITIVE ATTRIBUTES
Secure, Gentle, Compassionate, Balanced, Reconciled, Vital, Clarity, Comforted, Acceptance, Inner peace, Relaxed and alert, Rested, Aware, Emotionally balanced, Spiritual growth, Meditative, Visualization, Rejuvenated

USE TO COUNTERACT THESE NEGATIVE ATTRIBUTES
Anxiety, Irritability, Stress, Tension, Mental exhaustion, Panic, Hysteria, Shock, Apprehension, Fears, Nightmares, Insecurity, Lost inner child, Restlessness, Moodiness, Distracted, Addiction, Obsessional behavior, Trauma, Conflict, Emotional violence, Agitation, Jitteryness, Depression, Psychosomatic illness, Nervousness, Worry, Overexcitedness, Burnout

LEMON *Citrus limomum, C. medica* FRUITIE

CHARACTER
Purifying, Stimulating, Directional, Versatile

USE FOR THESE POSITIVE ATTRIBUTES
Joy, Emotional Clarity, Direction, Awareness, Calm, Concentration, Lively, Conscious, Strength, Clarity of thought, Memory, Emotionally invigorated

USE TO COUNTERACT THESE NEGATIVE ATTRIBUTES
Resentful, Depressed, Bitter, Touchy, Apathetic, Lethargic, Humorless, Indecisive, Bad attitudes, Distrust, Mental blocks, Stress, Mental fatigue, Turmoil, Irrationality, Fear

LINDEN BLOSSOM *Tilia vulgaris* FLORAL

CHARACTER
Consoling, Serenity, Security, Patience

USE FOR THESE POSITIVE ATTRIBUTES
Relaxed, Calm, Soothed, Self-confident, Secure, Balanced, Structured, Stable

USE TO COUNTERACT THESE NEGATIVE ATTRIBUTES
Nervousness, Anxiety, Nervous tension, Emotional debility, Hysteria, Overexcitement, Insecurity, Emotional blockages, Possessiveness, Jealousy, Anger, Stress, Irritability, Mood swings, Guilt, Lovelorn, Oversensitivity, Indecision

---

MANDARIN   *Citrus reticulata, C. nobilis*   FRUITIE

CHARACTER
Gentle, Peaceful, Revitalizing, Sympathetic

USE FOR THESE POSITIVE ATTRIBUTES
Calm, Uplifted, Refreshed, Inspired, Soothed, Sprightly, Integrity, Tranquil

USE TO COUNTERACT THESE NEGATIVE ATTRIBUTES
Anxiety, Depression, Grief, Inner child, Abuse, Dejection, Emptiness, Dwelling on the past, Overexcitable, Desolate, Emotional trauma

---

MARJORAM, SWEET   *Origanum marjorana*   HERBIE/LEAFIE

CHARACTER
Comforting, Soothing, Warming, Strengthening

USE FOR THESE POSITIVE ATTRIBUTES
Calm, Balanced, Direct, Self-assured, Integrity, Courage, Confidence, Focus, Perseverance, Restored, Sincere

USE TO COUNTERACT THESE NEGATIVE ATTRIBUTES
Anxiety, Hysteria, Hostility, Withdrawn, Mental strain, Tantrums, Anger, Irritability, Overactivity, Weak will

---

MELISSA   *Melissa officinalis*   HERBIE/LEAFIE

CHARACTER
Calming, Supportive, Sensitive, Fostering

USE FOR THESE POSITIVE ATTRIBUTES
Strength, Revitalized, Happy, Gentle, Spiritual growth, Relaxed, Peaceful, Positive, Progressive, Cheerful

USE TO COUNTERACT THESE NEGATIVE ATTRIBUTES
Nervous tension, Stress, Anxiety, Irritability, Overexcitement, Restlessness, Melancholy, Sadness, Grieving, Sorrow, Emotional crisis, Depression, Mental exhaustion, Lethargy, Negativity

---

NARCISSUS *Narcissus poeticus* FLORAL

CHARACTER
Hypnotic, Empowering, Mesmerizing, Sagacious

USE FOR THESE POSITIVE ATTRIBUTES
Inspired, Creative, Stillness, Meditative, Inner vision, Aspirations, Idealistic, Sensuous, Visionary, Discovery, Truthful

USE TO COUNTERACT THESE NEGATIVE ATTRIBUTES
Hysteria, Nervousness, Irritability, Tension, Grief, Addictions, Withdrawal, Loneliness, Illusions, Disillusionment, Longings, Hopelessness, Obsessions, Trauma, Emotional wounding, Misery, Anguish, Emotional analgesia

---

NEROLI *Citrus aurantium, C. brigaradia, C. vulgaris* FLORAL
(Orange Blossom)

CHARACTER
Spiritual, Pure, Loving, Peaceful

USE FOR THESE POSITIVE ATTRIBUTES
Lightness, Lifting of sorrows, Spiritual, Connected, Completeness, Joy, Understanding, Guided, Calm, Stable, Regenerated, Peaceful

USE TO COUNTERACT THESE NEGATIVE ATTRIBUTES
Anxiety, Stress, Tension, Shock, Emotional crisis, Sadness, Longing, Panic, Grief, Inner child, Abused as child, Abused as adult, Depression, Hopelessness, Fear

---

ORANGE *Citrus sinensis, C. aurantium* FRUITIE

CHARACTER
Warming, Happy, Resolute, Energizing

USE FOR THESE POSITIVE ATTRIBUTES
Joy, Uplifted, Sunny, Balanced, Light-hearted, Regenerated, Strong, Creative, Positive, Self-confident, Sympathetic, Courageous

USE TO COUNTERACT THESE NEGATIVE ATTRIBUTES
Depression, Hopelessness, Sadness, Apathy, Resignation, Withdrawn, Self-conscious-ness, Anxiety, Emotional violence, Emotional abuse, Worry, Selfishness, Obsessions, Addiction, Burnout

ORMENIS FLOWER *Ormenis multicaulis* HERBIE/FLORAL
(Chamomile Maroc)

CHARACTER
Unhurried, Composed, Mindful, Mystic

USE FOR THESE POSITIVE ATTRIBUTES
Calm, Empathetic, Courageous, Earthed, Relaxed, Mindful, Able to let go, Attentive, Meditative, Consoled, Soothing

USE TO COUNTERACT THESE NEGATIVE ATTRIBUTES
Stress, Tension, Anxiety, Dread, Overactive mind, Highly strung, Impulsive, Indecisive, Confused, Bad temper, Emotionally controlling, Emotional blockages, Abused, Fearful

PATCHOULI *Pogostemon cablin* LEAFIE

CHARACTER
Grounding, Soothing, Unruffled, Assured

USE FOR THESE POSITIVE ATTRIBUTES
Invigorated, Restored, Reasonable, Lucid, Astute, Stimulating, Persistent

USE TO COUNTERACT THESE NEGATIVE ATTRIBUTES
Depression, Anxiety, Indecision, Lethargy, Sluggishness, Egotistical, Tension, Stress, Mood-swings, Touchiness

PEPPERMINT *Mentha piperita* HERBIE/LEAFIE

CHARACTER
Clarifying, Awakening, Stimulating, Penetrating

USE FOR THESE POSITIVE ATTRIBUTES
Regenerating, Emotionally refreshed, Self-acceptance, Concentration, Vitality, Vibrancy

USE TO COUNTERACT THESE NEGATIVE ATTRIBUTES
Mental fatigue, Shock, Helplessness, Overwork, Sluggishness, Lethargy, Apathy

---

PETITGRAIN   *Citrus aurantium, C. brigaradier*   LEAFIE/WOODIE

CHARACTER
Revitalizing, Balancing, Restoring, Clarifying

USE FOR THESE POSITIVE ATTRIBUTES
Harmonized, Uplifted, Joyful, Relaxed, Inner vision, Strength, Self-confidence, Stability, Optimism, Expressiveness

USE TO COUNTERACT THESE NEGATIVE ATTRIBUTES
Disharmony, Confusion, Difficulties, Depression, Mental fatigue, Nervous exhaustion, Insomnia, Sadness, Disappointment, Rigidity, Betrayal, Anger, Irrationality, Introversion, Pessimism

---

PINE   *Pinus sylvestris*   WOODIE/LEAFIE

CHARACTER
Acceptance, Understanding, Patience, Self-forgiveness

USE FOR THESE POSITIVE ATTRIBUTES
Humility, Simplicity, Assured, Buffered, Forgiving, Perserverence, Sharing, Mindful, Trusting, Directness, Direction, Acceptance of love, Tenacity, Confident, Exhilarated

USE TO COUNTERACT THESE NEGATIVE ATTRIBUTES
Regrets, Guilt, Self-blame, Dissatisfaction, Self-critical, Worried, Overly responsible, Unconfrontational, Self-reproach, Unworthiness, Exhaustion, Masochistic, Shameful, Feeling rejected, Unsympathetic, Miserable, Feeling inadequate

---

ROSEMARY   *Rosemarinus officinalis*   HERBIE/LEAFIE

CHARACTER
Vigorous, Strengthening, Restorative, Centering

USE FOR THESE POSITIVE ATTRIBUTES
Energy, Upliftment, Confidence, Creativity, Clarity, Structured, Concentration, Stabilized, Fortified, Sincere, Purified, Aware

USE TO COUNTERACT THESE NEGATIVE ATTRIBUTES
Loss of memory, Learning difficulties, Lethargy, Disorientation, Fatigue, Indecision, Nervous exhaustion, Overburdened, Overworked, Strain, Emotional exhaustion, Sluggishness

ROSE MAROC   *Rosa centifolia*   FLORAL

CHARACTER
Passionate, Harmonious, Reassuring, Comforting

USE FOR THESE POSITIVE ATTRIBUTES
Motivated, Inner vitality, Revived, Confident, Passionate, Cooperative, Sense of freedom, Fulfilled, Forgiving, Sensual

USE TO COUNTERACT THESE NEGATIVE ATTRIBUTES
Grief, Bitterness, Fear of letting go, Fear of love, Fear of sexuality, Jealousy, Resignation, Passivity, Deception, Lack of ambition/motivation, Self-destruction, Vengefulness

ROSE OTTO   *Rosa damascena*   FLORAL

CHARACTER
Loving, Harmonizing, Comforting, Happy, Caring, Euphoric, Gentle, Peaceful

USE FOR THESE POSITIVE ATTRIBUTES
Comforted, Contentment, Devoted, Motivated, Inner vision, Revival, Joy, Happiness, Inner freedom, Acceptance, Completeness, Wisdom, Spirituality, Patience, Love, Sensuality, Purity

USE TO COUNTERACT THESE NEGATIVE ATTRIBUTES
Depression, Sadness, Grief, Anger, Anxiety, Bitterness, Emptiness, Fear of loving, Fear of not being loved, Broken heart, Guilt, Shyness, Jealousy, Touchiness, Emotional crisis, Resignation, Inexpression, Hopelessness, Despair, Abused, Emotional violence, Hurt inner child

SANDALWOOD   *Santalum album*   WOODIE

CHARACTER
Enlightenment, Meditative, Balancing, Connecting

USE FOR THESE POSITIVE ATTRIBUTES
Warm, Comforted, Sensitive, Serene, Trusting, Harmonized, Peaceful, Wise, Sensual, Expressive, Good self-esteem, Open, Insightful, Unity

USE TO COUNTERACT THESE NEGATIVE ATTRIBUTES
Anxiety, Nervous tension, Possessiveness, Manipulating, Unforgiving, Obsessive, Lonely, Accepting, Cynical, Insecurity, Recurrent nightmares, Selfishness, Distressed, Uneasy, Hasty, Aggressive, Irritable, Dwelling on the past

---

THYME LINALOL   *Thymus vulgaris, sp linalol*   HERBIE/LEAFIE

CHARACTER
Gently empowering, Invigorating, Assisting

USE FOR THESE POSITIVE ATTRIBUTES
Fortified, Balanced, Tolerant, Courageous, Supportive, Decisive, Alert, Focused, Concentration, Warming

USE TO COUNTERACT THESE NEGATIVE ATTRIBUTES
Lack of direction, Intellectual or physical exhaustion, Weakness, Overreactive, Nervous debility, Blockages

---

TUBEROSE   *Polianthes tuberosa*   FLORAL

CHARACTER
Transformative, Spontaneous, Extroverted, Centering

USE FOR THESE POSITIVE ATTRIBUTES
Motivated, Enthusiastic, Encouraged, Expansive, Sensuous, Sensitive, Spontaneous, Expressive, Frank

USE TO COUNTERACT THESE NEGATIVE ATTRIBUTES
Stress, Irritability, Emotional conflict, Oversensitivity, Jealousy, Bitterness, Anger, Confusion, Disorientation, Hostility, Insincerity, Resentment, Selfishness, Falsity

---

VETIVER   *Vetiveria zizanoides*   ROOTIE

CHARACTER
Grounding, Centering, Visionary, Wisdom

USE FOR THESE POSITIVE ATTRIBUTES
Spiritual calmness, Growth, Integrity, Wisdom, Mind-body connection, Strength, Honorable, Protected, Self-esteem, Grounded

USE TO COUNTERACT THESE NEGATIVE ATTRIBUTES
Fear, Anxiety, Obsession, Overwork, Agitation, Intellectual fatigue, Hurt, Scattered thinking, Irritability, Anger, Emotional burnout, Mental exhaustion, Unworthiness, Loss of purpose, Emotional weakness, Addiction, Disconnection, Fantasizing, Emotional blockages, Neurotic behavior, Instability, Disorientated

YLANG YLANG   *Canaga odorata*   FLORAL

CHARACTER
Euphoric, Sensuous, Stimulating, Unifying

USE FOR THESE POSITIVE ATTRIBUTES
Self-confidence, Warmth, Awakened, Uplifted, Calm, Joyful, Enthusiastic, Meditative, Sensual, Soothed

USE TO COUNTERACT THESE NEGATIVE ATTRIBUTES
Depression, Anxiety, Tension, Stress, Frustration, Irritability, Emotional guilt, Resentment, Jealousy, Selfishness, Impatience, Irrationality, Stubbornness, Obstinacy, Shyness

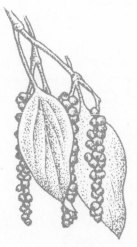

Black Pepper

CHART 14.2
QUICK REFERENCE CHART
Positive Emotional States

The following only lists those essential oils outlined in this book and by no means is it meant to be a comprehensive list of oils that could be used for the listed purposes. The essential oils in italics are those traditionally used in aromatherapy, the others have been adopted for these uses in more recent times.

Ablility to Let Go
Ormenis flower, *Coriander, Lemon, Peppermint, Pine, Tuberose*

Acceptance (general)
Frankincense, Grapefruit, Lavender, Pine, Rose Otto, Helichrysum

Acceptance (of love)
Pine, *Rose Otto, Chamomile Roman, Melissa*

Acceptance (self)
Peppermint, *Cypress, Helichrysum, Petitgrain*

Acceptance (of change)
Grapefruit, Helichrysum, *Geranium, Lemon*

Alertness
Grapefruit, lavender, Thyme, *Basil,* Bergamot, Black Pepper, Cardamon, Cinnamon, Coriander, Eucalyptus Citriodora (lemon), *Grapefruit,* Juniper, Lime, *Peppermint,* Petitgrain, Pine, *Rosemary,* Thyme Linalol

Assertion
Jasmine, Fennel, *Basil, Cedarwood,*
Cypress, Sweet Fennel, Frankincense, Ginger, Patchouli, *Ylang Ylang,* Black Pepper, Jasmine, *Ormenis Flower, Bergamot,* Coriander, Carnation, *Tuberose,* Pimento Berry, Lime, *Cardamon,* Cistus, *Litsea Cubeba*

Assisting
Thyme Linalol, *Lavender, Marjoram, Jasmine, Geranium*

Assuring
Geranium, Marjoram, Patchouli, Pine, *Ginger, Frankincense, Cederwood*

Astuteness
Patchouli, *Fennel, Rosemary, Coriander, Eucalyptus Citriodora (lemon)*

Attentive
Ormenis flower, *Lemon, Cypress, Clove, Litsea Cubeba*

Attuned
Grapefruit, *Frankincense, Sandalwood, Neroli, Chamomile Roman, Juniper*

Awakened
Ylang Ylang, *Jasmine, Juniper, Black Pepper*

Awakening
Basil, Peppermint, *Juniper, Frankincense, Petitgrain, Rosemary, Coriander, Neroli, Carnation*

Awareness (self)
Grapefruit, Lemon, Jasmine, Lavender, Rosemary, Helichrysum

Awareness (spiritual)
Chamomile Roman, *Neroli, Frankincense, Juniper, Rose Otto*

Balanced
Bergamot, Cedarwood, Clary Sage, *Cypress, Mandarin, Geranium, Benzoin,* Lavender, Linden Blossom, Marjoram, Orange, Grapefruit, Thyme Linalol, Eucalyptus Radiata

Balanced (emotionally)
Lavender, *Lemon, Rose Otto, Cedarwood, Cardamon, Orange, Mandarin*

Balancing
Petitgrain, Sandalwood, *Juniper, Lavender, Hyacinth, Neroli*

Benevolence
Cinnamon, *Benzoin, Vetiver, Patchouli, Linden Blossom, Lavender*

Boosting
Grapefruit, *Orange, Melissa, Bergamot, Myrtle, Pimento Berry*

Buffering
Helichrysum, Pine, *Benzoin, Vetiver, Patchouli, Sandalwood*

Calming (general)
Hyacinth, Lavender, Melissa

Calmness
Chamomile German, *Chamomile Roman, Clary Sage,* Helichrysum, Lemon, Linden Blossom, Mandarin, *Marjoram, Neroli, Ormenis Flower,* Ylang Ylang

Calmness (spiritual)
Vetiver, *Benzoin, Neroli, Chamomile Roman, Rose Otto, Spikenard, Frankincense*

Caring
Helichrysum, Lavender, Rose Otto, *Chamomile Roman, Sandalwood*

Centering
Rosemary, Tuberose, Vetiver, *Benzoin, Myrrh, Ginger*

Changeability
Black pepper, *Cinnamon, Clove, Hyacinth, Bay, Bergamot, Geranium*

Changes (going through)
Cypress, *Cedarwood, Eucalyptus Radiata, Rosemary, Lemon*

Cheerful
Melissa, Grapefruit, Orange, *Mandarin,* Basil, Bergamot

Clarifying
Basil, Cardamom, Peppermint, *Rosemary, Eucalyptus Radiata,* Petitgrain

Clarity
Basil, Cardamom, Fennel, *Grapefruit,* Lavender, *Lemon, Rosemary*

Clarity (of thought)
Lemon, Rosemary, Basil, Pimento Berry, Clove, Petitgrain

Cleansing
Juniper, *Cypress, Pine, Cedarwood, Frankincense, Neroli, Lemon*

Clearing
Fennel, *Juniper, Pine, Cypress*

Comforting
Black Pepper, Cedarwood, *Chamomile Roman,* Cypress, Eucalyptus Citriodora (lemon), *Frankincense, Geranium,* Marjoram, Rose Maroc, *Rose Otto,* Lavender, *Sandalwood, Benzoin, Melissa*

Communication
Carnation, Geranium, *Chamomile German, Grapefruit, Peppermint, Bay, Linden Blossom, Lemon*

Compassionate
Chamomile Roman, Lavender, Rose Otto, Neroli, *Nutmeg, Pine, Cypress, Melissa*

Completeness
Bergamot, Neroli, Rose Otto, *Cistus, Chamomile Roman*

Composed
Ormenis Flower, *Frankincense, Lavender, Rose Maroc, Jasmine, Cedarwood,* Eucalyptus Globulus

Concentration
Basil, Bergamot, Cardamom, Peppermint, Rosemary, Cedarwood, Eucalyptus Citriodora (lemon), Eucalyptus Globulus, Lemon, Thyme Linalol

Intellectual
Intellectual - *Lemon, Basil,* Lemongrass, *Litsea Cubeba,* Cardamom, Bergamot, Orange, Cedarwood, *Rosemary,* Eucalyptus Radiata, Peppermint, *Frankincense*
Spiritual - *Frankincense,* Neroli, Chamomile Roman, Rose Otto, Narcissus, Hyacinth

Confidence
Bergamot, *Cardamom,* Cedarwood, Clary Sage, Coriander, Cypress, Fennel, Ginger, Grapefruit, *Jasmine,* Ylang Ylang, Linden Blossom, Marjoram, Orange, Pine, Petitgrain, Rose Maroc, Rosemary, Tuberose

Confusion
Ginger, *Rosemary, Benzoin, Cinnamon, Clove, Marjoram, Lavender*

Connecting
Rose Otto, *Neroli, Petitgrain, Fennel, Coriander, Jasmine,* Sandalwood

Consoling
Ormenis Flower, *Chamomile Roman, Cypress,* Linden Blossom, *Benzoin, Melissa, Rose Maroc, Geranium*

Contentment
Cypress, *Rose Otto, Lavender,* Neroli, *Bergamot,* Orange, Sandalwood, Patchouli, Ylang Ylang, Chamomile Roman, Clove

Conscious
Lemon, *Rosemary, Bergamot, Basil, Lavender*

Control (being in)
Cypress, Cedarwood, Pine, Vetiver, Ginger, Clove

Conviction

Juniper, *Vetiver, Frankincense, Thyme Linalol, Cedarwood*

Cooling

Chamomile German, *Eucalyptus Citriodora (lemon), Eucalyptus Radiata, Peppermint*

Cooperation

Chamomile Roman, Grapefruit, *Rose Maroc, Jasmine, Ylang Ylang*

Courage

Cardamom, Frankincense, Ginger, Hyacinth, Marjoram, *Cedarwood, Benzoin*, Fennel, Orange, Ormenis Flower, Thyme

Creativity

Carnation, Coriander, Eucalyptus Citriodora (lemon), Bergamot, Cistus, Narcissus, Orange, Rosemary, *Frankincense*, Geranium, *Neroli*, Rose Maroc, Jasmine, Bay, Clove, Mimosa, Litsea Cubeba, Sandalwood, Cypress, *Juniper*

Cushioning

Carnation, Geranium, *Benzoin, Rose Otto, Lavender, Chamomile Roman*

Decisiveness

Basil, Thyme, *Cedarwood, Vetiver, Patchouli, Peppermint*

Devotion

Rose Otto, *Chamomile Roman*, Neroli

Dignified

Cedarwood, Cypress, *Frankincense, Vetiver*

Directness

Pine, *Cypress, Cedarwood, Clove, Pimento Berry*, Cinnamon, Cypress, Marjoram

Direction

Cardamom, Cypress, *Lemon*, Pine

Directional

Black Pepper, *Lemon, Ginger, Juniper*

Discovery

Narcissus, *Grapefruit, Black Pepper, Bay*

Dreams

Helichrysum, *Narcissus, Mimosa, Cedarwood*

Earthed

Ormenis Flower, *Vetiver, Ginger*

Elevating

Frankincense, *Juniper, Rose Otto, Neroli, Lindon Blossom, Geranium, Clary Sage, Spikenard*

Embracing

Lavender, *Benzoin, Geranium, Melissa*

Emotional Clarity

Lemon, *Petitgrain, Grapefruit, Melissa, Black Pepper*

Emotionally Invigorated

Lemon, *Grapefruit, Rosemary, Eucalyptus Citriodora (lemon)*

Emotionally Purified

Grapefruit, *Frankincense, Neroli, Helichrysum, Melissa*

Emotionally Refreshed
Peppermint, *Helichrysum, Lemon, Grapefruit*

Emotionally Stable
Chamomile Roman, Frankincense, *Vetiver, Sandalwood*

Empathetic
Ormenis Flower, Chamomile Roman, Lavender, *Melissa*

Empathy
Chamomile German, Eucalyptus Citriodora (lemon), Ginger, *Ormenis flower*

Empowering
Narcissus, Thyme, *Jasmine, Cedarwood, Frankincense*

Encompassing
Carnation, *Benzoin, Hyacinth, Rose Maroc*

Encouraging
Bergamot, Cardamom, Coriander, Ginger, *Cinnamon, Clove,* Eucalyptus Citriodora (lemon), Tuberose, *Jasmine*

Endurance
Black Pepper, *Ginger, Thyme, Nutmeg, Rosemary, Pine*

Energizing
Orange, *Rosemary, Thyme Linalol, Basil, Peppermint, Juniper, Pine,* Cinnamon, *Eucalyptus Globulus, Grapefruit, Helichrysum*

Energy
Helichrysum, Rosemary, *Orange, Peppermint*

Enlightening
Fennel, Frankincense, Hyacinth, Juniper, *Neroli, Chamomile Roman, Rose Otto, Cistus, Yarrow, Spikenard,* Sandalwood

Enlivening
Coriander, *Rosemary, Peppermint, Eucalyptus Citriodra (lemon),* Fennel, *Petitgrain, Litsea Cubeba, Melissa*

Enthusiasm
Cardamom, *Carnation, Orange, Jasmine, Lemon, Grapefruit,* Tuberose, *Bay,* Ylang Ylang, Basil, Coriander, Eucalyptus Citriodora (lemon), *Geranium, Melissa, Pimento Berry*

Equilibrium (restores)
Clary Sage, Hyacinth, *Cedarwood, Vetiver, Litsea Cubeba, Patchouli, Sandalwood*

Euphoria
Clary Sage, Jasmine, Rose Otto, *Rose Maroc, Tuberose, Narcissus,* Ylang Ylang

Exhilaration
Pine, *Cypress, Juniper, Mandarin, Coriander*

Expansive
Tuberose, *Benzoin, Clary Sage, Nutmeg, Spikenard, Geranium, Lavender*

Expressiveness
Coriander, Eucalyptus Citriodora (lemon), Petitgrain, *Neroli, Cardamon, Pimento Berry,* Sandalwood, Tuberose, Jasmine, *Cistus, Rose Maroc*

Extroverted
Tuberose, *Jasmine, Rose Maroc, Carnation, Cinnamon, Clove, Bay*

Fairminded

Cinnamon, *Cedarwood, Cistus, Cypress, Pine, Vetiver, Lavender,* Marjoram

Faith

Hyacinth, *Frankincense, Spikenard, Juniper,* Basil, Coriander, *Chamomile Roman,* Neroli, *Linden Blossom*

Flexibility

Geranium, *Lavender, Clary Sage, Lemon, Myrtle, Black Pepper, Ylang Ylang*

Focus

Cedarwood, Marjoram, *Thyme Linalol, Lemon,* Fennel, Bergamot, *Basil, Cypress,* Juniper, Lemongrass, *Litsea Cubeba,* Ginger, Cinnamom, Clove, Ylang Ylang, Linden Blossom, Nutmeg, *Rosemary*

Forceful

Fennel, *Peppermint, Cinnamon, Clove, Clary Sage*

Forgiving

Hyacinth, Pine, Rose Maroc, *Rose Otto, Neroli, Chamomile Roman*

Fortitude

Cardamom, Cedarwood, Fennel, Frankincense, Ginger, Rosemary, Thyme

Fostering

Melissa, *Chamomile Roman, Benzoin, Linden Blossom, Cardamon*

Frankness

Tuberose, *Jasmine, Ylang Ylang, Cedarwood, Cypress, Black Pepper*

Freedom

Eucalyptus Citriodora (lemon), Rose-Maroc, *Rose Otto, Neroli, Petitgrain, Sandalwood, Cistus*

Friendliness

Geranium, *Mandarin, Orange, Lavender, Marjoram, Clove, Cinnamon, Bergamot*

Fulfilled

Rose Maroc, *Jasmine, Clary Sage, Geranium, Lavender, Chamomile Roman, Ormenis Flower, Benzoin, Ylang Ylang*

Generosity

Grapefruit, *Benzoin, Nutmeg, Cinnamon, Sandalwood, Melissa, Lavender, Geranium*

Generosity (of spirit)

Cypress, *Frankincense, Lavender, Geranium, Chamomile Roman, Petitgrain, Coriander, Rose Otto, Neroli, Carnation*

Gentle

Lavender, Mandarin, Melissa, Rose Otto, Hyacinth

Gentleness

Chamomile Roman, Helichrysum, Mandarin, Melissa

Grounded

Clary Sage, Patchouli, Vetiver, *Spikenard, Ginger*

Grounding

Cedarwood, *Vetiver, Black Pepper, Ginger*

Growth

Vetiver, *Coriander, Fennel, Cardamon, Orange, Mimosa*

Guided

Neroli, Chamomile Roman, Frankincense, Juniper

Happiness

Rose Otto, *Orange,* Jasmine, Coriander, Ginger, Clove, Cinnamon, Benzoin, Carnation, *Pimento Berry*, *Geranium,* Melissa

Harmonizing

Chamomile Roman, Clary Sage, *Lavender,* Eucalyptus Citriodora (lemon), *Geranium,* Helichrysum, Rose Maroc, Rose Otto

Harmony (general)

Bergamot, Jasmine, Sandalwood, Petitgrain, Geranium, Ormenis Flower

Healers

All essential oils are healing —
the following have a healing character.

Chamomile German, Chamomile Roman, Lavender, Geranium, Frankincense

Honorable

Vetiver, *Spikenard, Lavender, Cedarwood, Cypress, Myrrh, Frankincense*

Humility

Juniper, Pine, *Chamomile Roman, Chamomile German, Ormenis Flower, Melissa,* Neroli

Humor

Geranium, *Orange*

Hypnotic

Narcissus, *Carnation, Tuberose*

Idealism

Helichrysum, *Bay, Petitgrain, Coriander, Chamomile Roman,* Neroli

Imagination

Coriander, *Ginger, Orange, Helichrysum, Pimento Berry,* Jasmine, Carnation

Incorruptibility

Cypress, *Cedarwood, Vetiver, Lavender, Frankincense, Lemon, Bay*

Independence

Carnation, *Tuberose, Geranium, Clary Sage, Lemon, Grapefruit, Peppermint*

Inner Child (for a positive)

Helichrysum, *Melissa, Mandarin, Lavender, Chamomile Roman*

Inner Freedom

Rose Otto, *Helichrysum, Neroli*

Inner Peace

Chamomile Roman, Cypress, Lavender, *Rose Otto*

Inner Strength

Helichrysum, *Geranium, Chamomile Roman, Melissa*

Inner Vision

Juniper, Rose Otto, *Petitgrain, Linden Blossom, Chamomile Roman, Sandalwood, Sage*

Inner Visionary

Narcissus, *Frankincense, Juniper, Sandalwood, Basil, Cypress, Sage*

Inner Vitality

Rose Maroc, *Lemon, Pine, Juniper, Litsea Cubeba*

Insightfulness

Sandalwood, *Juniper, Clary Sage, Sage, Pine, Lavender*

Inspiration

Frankincense, *Neroli, Rose Otto, Bergamot, Lemon, Benzoin, Hyacinth, Carnation, Jasmine, Bay*

Inspiring

Clary Sage, Grapefruit, Jasmine, Mandarin, Narcissus

Integrity

Basil, Mandarin, Marjoram, Vetiver, *Lavender, Cedarwood*

Introspection

Frankincense, *Chamomile Roman, Neroli, Rose Otto, Pine, Nutmeg*

Intuitiveness

Jasmine, *Neroli, Cistus*

Invigorating

Thyme, *Peppermint, Rosemary, Eucalyptus Radiata, Petitgrain, Pine, Cedarwood, Cypress,* Cinnamon, *Patchouli, Eucalyptus Citriodra (lemon)*

Joy

Bergamot, Lemon, *Neroli,* Orange, Rose Otto, Sandalwood, Frankincense, Petitgrain, Ylang Ylang, Chamomile Roman, Linden Blossom, *Mimosa,* Grapefruit, Jasmine, Helichrysum, Pimento Berry

Liberating

Carnation, Bergamot, *Tuberose, Grapefruit, Geranium, Lavender*

Lifting of Sorrow

Neroli, Chamomile Roman, *Cypress*

Light Hearted

Orange, Grapefruit, *Petitgrain*

Lightness

Neroli, Petitgrain, *Lemon, Linden Blossom, Lavender*

Liveliness

Lemon, *Grapefruit, Rosemary, Peppermint, Eucalyptus Radiata*

Love

Rose Otto, *Rose Maroc, Jasmine, Chamomile Roman, Melissa*

Loving

Rose Otto, Neroli, *Jasmine*

Lucidity

Patchouli, *Black Pepper, Cardamom, Litsea Cubeba, Coriander, Lemon, Rosemary*

Meditative

Frankincense, Helichrysum, Juniper, Lavender, Narcissus, Ormenis Flower, Sandalwood, Ylang Ylang, *Spikenard*

Memory (good)

Coriander, Lemon, *Rosemary, Eucalyptus Citriodora, Peppermint*

Mesmerizing

Narcissus, *Tuberose, Narcissus, Rose Maroc, Jasmine, Clary Sage, Cistus*

Mindful
Ormenis Flower, Pine, *Cypress, Lavender,*
Yarrow

Mind-body Connection
Vetiver, *Benzoin, Lavender, Geranium,*
Helichrysum

Mothering
Geranium, *Lavender, Marjoram*

Motivated
Fennel, Rose Maroc, Rose Otto

Motivating
Coriander, *Lavender, Clove, Rosemary,*
Grapefruit, Lemon, Pine, Cypress, Bay,
Bergamot, Black Pepper, Cardamom,
Tuberose

Mystic
Ormenis Flower, *Myrrh, Galbanham,*
Frankincense, Vetiver, Spikenard

Nobility of Spirit
This section could apply to all essential
oils; this list is therefore extremely limited.

Cedarwood, *Neroli, Chamomile Roman,*
Basil, Frankincense

Nurturing (feelings)
Carnation, *Lavender, Geranium, Mandarin,*
Ormenis Flower

Openness
Carnation, *Petitgrain, Ylang Ylang, Fennel,*
Mimosa, Jasmine, Sandalwood, *Palma*
Rosa, Helichrysum

Optimism
Coriander, Eucalyptus Citriodora
(lemon), Jasmine, Petitgrain

Organized
Chamomile German, *Cedarwood,*
Peppermint, Eucalyptus Radiata, Lemon

Originality
Carnation, *Tuberose, Hyacinth, Litsea*
Cubeba, Black Pepper, Clove

Passionate
Rose Maroc, *Jasmine, Ylang Ylang,*
Tuberose, Pimento Berry, Clove, Bay

Patience
Chamomile German, Cypress, Pine,
Helichrysum, Linden Blossom, Rose Otto

Peace
Each individual person has essential oils
they can attune to for peace; these are
only a guide.

Juniper, Chamomile Roman, Neroli,
Frankincense, Rose Otto, Melissa,
Angelica Seed, Spikenard, Yarrow,
Jasmine, Carnation

Peaceful
Chamomile German, Chamomile Roman,
Mandarin, Melissa, Sandalwood, Neroli

Penetrating
Peppermint, Thyme, Galbanham

Performance
Bay, Bergamot, Cistus, Eucayptus
Citriodora (lemon), *Frankincense, Lemon,*
Lavender, *Grapefruit, Helichrysum,* Rose
Maroc, Jasmine, Geranium, Ormenis
Flower, Cypress, Tuberose

Persistence
Cedarwood, Patchouli, Vetiver

Perseverance
Fennel, Helichrysum, *Hyacinth,* Marjoram, *Pine*

Positivity
All essential oils used in aromatherapy can have a positive effect.

Basil, Bay, Lemon, Cedarwood, *Grapefruit,* Pine, Vetiver, *Patchouli,* Juniper, Melissa, Myrrh, Cypress, Cardamom, Orange, Petitgrain, *Geranium, Frankincense*, Rosemary, Hyssop, Pimento Berry

Powerful (self)
Cedarwood, *Cypress, Thyme, Sandalwood, Patchouli, Cinnamon*

Practicality
Cinnamon, *Pine, Lemon, Thyme, Black Pepper, Peppermint, Rosemary, Lavender*

Profoundness
Jasmine, *Narcissus, Spikenard, Frankincense, Juniper, Chamomile Roman*

Progressiveness
Melissa, *Cistus, Helichrysum*

Protected
Vetiver, *Myrrh, Spikenard, Yarrow, Chamomile German, Chamomile Roman, Frankincense, Rose Otto, Sandalwood*

Protective
Cypress, Frankincense, *Cedarwood, Chamomile Roman, Geranium, Lavender,* Rose Otto, *Sandalwood*

Purifying
Juniper, Lemon, *Pine, Sage, Lavender, Cypress,* Rosemary

Purity of Heart
Cypress, *Neroli, Rose Otto, Chamomile Roman, Melissa, Helichrysum*

Purpose
Cardamom, *Cinnamon, Vetiver, Patchouli, Cedarwood, Cypress, Black Pepper, Ormenis Flower, Carnation, Jasmine*

Purposefulness
Basil, *Cedarwood, Peppermint, Eucalyptus Radiata, Bay, Pimento Berry*

Radiating
Carnation, *Grapefruit, Tuberose, Jasmine, Ylang Ylang, Rose Maroc, Rose Otto*

Realistic
Cinnamon, *Lavender, Peppermint, Black Pepper, Marjoram, Pine*

Reasonable
Patchouli, *Lavender, Peppermint, Lemon, Thyme, Clary Sage*

Reassuring
Rose Maroc, *Benzoin, Chamomile Roman, Bay, Helichrysum, Sandalwood*

Reconciled
Lavender, *Geranium, Bergamot, Sandalwood, Clary Sage, Helichrysum*

Refreshing
Mandarin, *Lemon, Bergamot, Lavender, Lime, Juniper, Eucalyptus Citriodora (lemon)*

Regenerating

Clary Sage, Geranium, Neroli, Orange, Eucalyptus Citriodora (lemon), *Melissa, Lavender, Rose Otto*, Lavender, Peppermint

Relaxed

Chamomile German, Chamomile Roman, Clary Sage, Jasmine, Lavender, Linden Blossom, Melissa, Ormenis Flower, Petitgrain

Releasing

Carnation, *Palma Rosa, Hyacinth, Rose Maroc, Linden Blossom, Lavender*

Reliable

Fennel, *Vetiver, Cedarwood, Frankincense, Myrrh, Pine*

Resolution

Frankincense, *Myrrh, Lavender, Cistus*

Restfullness

Lavender, Geranium, Rose Maroc, Clary Sage, *Linden Blossom, Neroli, Marjoram,* Petitgrain, *Sandalwood,* Mimosa

Restorative

Rosemary, *Eucalyptus Radiata, Peppermint, Pine, Cinnamon, Cardamon, Clary Sage, Petitgrain, Lavender, Cypress, Bergamot*

Restored

Marjoram, Patchouli, *Ginger, Pine, Lavender*

Revitalizing

Mandarin, Petitgrain, *Orange, Grapefruit, Melissa, Rosemary,* Clary Sage, Melissa, *Lavender, Neroli, Lemon*

Reviving

Rose Otto, *Eucalyptus Citriodora (lemon), Lavender, Rosemary, Melissa, Linden Blossom,* Rose Maroc, *Bergamot, Geranium, Mandarin, Palma Rosa*

Sacredness

Juniper, *Neroli, Chamomile Roman, Sandalwood, Basil,* Frankincense

Sagacious

Narcissus, Frankincense

Secretiveness

Carnation, *Bay, Hyacinth, Rose Otto, Lavender*

Secular

Chamomile Roman, Cinnamon

Secure

Geranium, *Lavender, Benzoin, Linden Blossom. Chamomile Roman*

Security

Black Pepper, *Frankincense, Cedarwood, Cinnamon, Clove, Clary Sage*

Security

Linden Blossom, *Geranium, Benzoin,* Sandalwood

Self-awareness

Clary sage, Ylang Ylang, Cypress, Geranium, Pine, *Sandalwood,* Bay, Ormenis Fower, *Jasmine,* Clove, Pimento Berry, Mandarin, Coriander, Angelica Seed, Sage, Cistus, *Myrtle,* Rosemary

Self-esteem

Hyacinth, Sandalwood, Vetiver, *Ylang Ylang,* Rose Maroc, *Jasmine,* Carnation, *Bergamot,* Geranium, Ormenis Flower, *Cedarwood,* Tuberose

Self-forgiveness

Pine, Chamomile Roman, Frankincense, Geranium, Lemon

Self-image

Orange, Lavender, Melissa, Neroli, Chamomile Roman, Ylang Ylang, Rose Maroc, Jasmine, Sandalwood, Cypress, Juniper, Cedarwood, Pine, Black Pepper, Frankincense, Mandarin, Nutmeg, Myrtle, Bay

Self-worth

Carnation, Juniper, Rose Otto, Mandarin, Orange, Patchouli, Bay

Sensitivity

Cypress, Jasmine, *Hyacinth, Rose Otto, Neroli,* Linden Blossom, Marjoram, Sandalwood, Tuberose, Carnation, Melissa

Sensuality

Jasmine, Rose Otto, Rose Maroc, Sandalwood, Ylang Ylang, Tuberose

Sensuous

Tuberose, Ylang Ylang

Serene

Chamomile Roman, Sandalwood

Serenity

Chamomile Roman, Linden Blossom

Sharing

Pine, Lavender, Ormenis Flower, Hyacinth

Shielding

Geranium, Lavender, Marjoram, Bergamot, Cedarwood, Benzoin

Simplicity

Pine, Chamomile Roman, Chamomile German, Ormenis Flower

Sincere

Marjoram, Rosemary, Cypress, *Cedarwood*

Sincerity

Coriander, Juniper, *Chamomile Roman, Clary Sage*

Softly

Cypress, *Chamomile Roman, Mandarin, Rose Otto, Melissa*

Softness

Chamomile Roman, *Mandarin, Rose Otto, Melissa*

Soothed

Clary Sage, Geranium, Linden Blossom, Mandarin, Ylang Ylang, *Benzoin*

Soothing

Chamomile German, Chamomile Roman, Hyacinth, Jasmine, Marjoram, Ormenis Flower, Patchouli

Soundness

Eucalyptus Citriodora (lemon), Petit-grain, Black Pepper, Mimosa

Spontaneous
Grapefruit, Tuberose, Lemon, *Coriander,* *Orange,* Neroli, Chamomile Roman

Stability
Chamomile Roman, Geranium, Linden Blossom, Neroli, Rosemary, Cedarwood, Cypress, Petitgrain

Stamina
Black Pepper, *Cinnamon*

Steadfast
Cinnamon, *Vetiver, Patchouli*

Steadiness
Geranium, *Lavender, Pine, Fennel,* *Cedarwood*

Stillness
Carnation, Chamomile Roman, Cypress, Narcissus

Stimulating
Basil, Cardamom, Eucalyptus Citriodora (lemon), Eucalyptus Radiata, Lemon, Patchouli, *Peppermint,* Ylang Ylang, *Rosemary*

Straightforwardness
Black Pepper, Peppermint, Frankincense, Cedarwood, Basil, Cardamom, Cypress

Strength
Basil, Bergamot, *Cedarwood, Cinnamon,* Clary Sage, *Cypress,* Juniper, Lemon, Melissa, Petitgrain, *Vetiver*

Strengthening
Cedarwood, *Ginger,* Marjoram, Rosemary

Strong
Chamomile German, Orange

Structured
Cypress, Linden Blossom, Rosemary

Supportive
Melissa, Thyme

Sympathetic
Mandarin, Orange, Lavender, Geranium

Tenacity
Pine

Tenderness
Carnation, *Rose Otto, Mandarin, Benzoin*

Tolerant
Thyme, *Peppermint, Frankincense, Clary Sage, Lavender, Marjoram*

Tranquil
Geranium, Mandarin, *Clary Sage, Chamomile Roman*

Transformation
Tuberose, Carnation, *Patchouli, Sandalwood*

Trust
Basil, Hyacinth, Cypress, *Lavender*

Trusting
Hyacinth, *Pine,* Sandalwood, Eucalyptus Citriodora (lemon), Cypress

Truthful
Narcissus, *Frankincense*

Understanding
Chamomile German, *Chamomile Roman,
Cypress,* Eucalyptus Citriodora (lemon),
Helichrysum, *Neroli, Pine*

Unhurried
Ormenis Flower, *Marjoram, Vetiver*

Unifying
Ylang Ylang, Carnation

Unity
Sandalwood

Uplifted
Clary Sage, *Grapefruit,* Jasmine, Juniper,
Mandarin, Orange, *Petitgrain,* Ylang Ylang

Upliftment
Eucalyptus Citriodora (lemon), *Rosemary,
Basil,* Bergamot

Unruffled
Patchouli

Versatile
Lemon, *Lavender*

Vibrancy
Peppermint

Vigorous
Rosemary

Visionary
Juniper

Visualization (relaxing)
Lavender, Neroli, Rose Otto, Chamomile
Roman, Clary Sage

Visualization (stimulating)
Rosemary, Ginger, Black Pepper, Thyme

Vitality
Eucalyptus Citriodora (lemon), Juniper,
Peppermint

Warming
Cinnamon, Clary Sage, Ginger,
Helichrysum, Marjoram, Orange, Thyme

Warmth
Ginger, Ylang Ylang, Sandalwood

Welcoming
Jasmine

Willpower
Cypress

Wisdom
Frankincense, Juniper, Rose Otto,
Vetiver, Cypress

Wise
Cypress, Sandalwood

Part 4

Appendixes I–IV

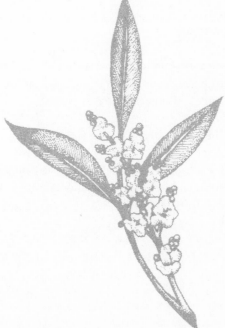

Author's Note:

Valerie Ann Worwood is always grateful to receive feedback and readers' comments but regrets that she is unable to reply personally to all letters. Please write to:

P.O. Box 210
Romford
Essex RM7 7DW
United Kingdom

Workshops in Aroma-Genera are conducted in Britain, Canada, the United States, and New Zealand. For information please send a large, stamped, self-addressed envelope or International Response Coupon, if applicable, to:

UK: P.O. Box 210, Romford, Essex RM7 7DW

Canada: Anahata Centre, P.O. Box 149, 185-9040 Blundell Road, Richmond, British Columbia, V6Y 1K3, Telephone: (604) 473-6097

USA: Global Essence, P.O. Box 332 82, San Diego, California 92136-3282, Telephone: (888)-WORWOOD

New Zealand: P.O. Box 8083, New Plymouth, New Zealand, Telephone: 06758 5859, FAX: 06758 1566

APPENDIX I

SAFETY DATA

Not all natural plants or plant products are beneficial to health. Deadly Nightshade can be poisonous and stinging nettles sting. The following essential oils should NOT be used under any circumstances:

Bitter Almond	Sassafras
Boldo leaf	Savin
Calamus	Southernwood
Horseradish	Tansy
Jaborandi leaf	Thuja
Mugwort	Wintergreen
Mustard	Wormseed
Pennyroyal	Wormwood
Rue	Yellow Camphor

This list is as recommended by the International Federation of Aromatherapists' code of practice. See also *Safety Data Manual* by Robert Tisserand.

Essential oils are highly concentrated plant essences and should not be taken orally unless under medical supervision.

People with sensitive skin or allergic reactions to aromatic materials should always do a skin test 24 hours before use.

Some essential oils have been documented to create photosensitivity and should not be applied to the skin before exposure to the sun. Of those mentioned in this book, those that may fall into this category are among the citrus oils – especially Bergamot, and Angelica.

PREGNANCY

In pregnancy, the usual quantities should be reduced by at least half volumes of essential oils. Certain essential oils should be avoided altogether during pregnancy or when breastfeeding. These are:

Basil	Cinnamon	Aniseed
Fennel	Juniper	Marjoram
Peppermint	Rosemary	Thyme
Clary Sage	Oregano	Clove
Nutmeg	Bay	Pimento Berry
Cistus	Hops	Sage
Valerian	Spikenard	Black Pepper
Tarragon	Cedarwood	

APPENDIX II

THERAPEUTIC COMPONENTS OF ESSENTIAL OILS AND ABSOLUTES

Principal chemical components of essential oils relevant to *The Fragrant Mind*.

Most scientists and researchers have attributed the therapeutic action of essential oils on the brain/mind to several identified groups of naturally occurring botanical chemicals. It is evident that there are other components, albeit traces, that are as yet unidentifiable but which may play a significant part in the action of essential oils on the brain.

Although these identified components account for some of the therapeutic effects, it cannot be said that they account for all the properties ascribed to many of the essential oils. In fact, in aromatherapy some essential oils that are used for emotional conditions contain no known compound that would explain their efficacy — Frankincense being among them (Lunny V N). Essential oils extracted by methods other than steam distillation, such as flower absolutes, contain other heavier compounds that cannot be obtained by steam distillation. CO_2 extraction yields even more compounds that would have been lost using either of the other methods. Therefore the process by which essential oils are obtained defines which chemical compounds they may contain.

Many essential oils are known to have an adaptogenic character — having either a stimulant or sedative action, depending upon the physiological and pathological condition of the body/brain it is applied to. Another level of complexity occurs when essential oils are combined in formulations; it is possible that they form new synergistic compounds that are unidentifiable by scientific procedures. New methods of analysis are also identifying components not previously known to be part of certain essential oils' make-ups and with the advance of technology, undoubtedly more will come to light. Whether for home use or for use in a clinical setting, these essential oils have a long and successful history of safe therapeutic use.

Several researchers, including Louis-Claude Vincent, Jean Mar, and most recently

Pierre Franchomme and Daniel Penoel, have shown that essential oils have positive and negative charges, which at present are attributed to the major chemical groups. For example, Phenols, which are known to be warming and potentially strong, have been attributed with a positive charge; alderhydes are thought to be cooling and calming with a negative charge, and so on. Only certain individual components have been tested, however, rather than complete essential oils, which may in their entire synergistic form give an entirely different picture. One must suspect that overall the story is far more complex (see Part 1).

The chemical components listed are only some of those contained in essential oils, those that are particularly relevant to the subject material of *The Fragrant Mind*. The list is by no means conclusive, and has been included for those who need foundational evidence for the aromatherapeutic use of essential oils and absolutes.

Basically, chemicals affect receptors in the body by sedating or stimulating.

ACIDS: Stimulant
ALCOHOLS: Stimulant, Sedative
ALDERHYDES: Calming
COUMARINS Sedative, Hypnotic
ETHERS: Calming, Analgesic

ESTERS: Sedative, Calming
HYDROCARBONS: Calming
TERPENES: Stimulant, Tonic
PHENOLS: Stimulant, Tonic

ANTI-SPASMODIC
Ethers, Esters, Phenols, Sesquiterpenes

CALMING
Alderhydes, Coumarines, Ethers Esters, Sesquiterpenes

ENERGIZING
Alcohols

TONING
Alcohols

SEDATIVE
Alderhydes, Coumarines, Ethers

STIMULATING
Alcohols, Ethers, Ketones, Monoterpenes, Monoterpenols, Oxides, Phenols, Terpenes

BALANCING:
Ethers, Esters, Alcohols

COOLING
Aldehydes, Esters

HYPNOTIC
Esters, Lactones,

RELAXING
Alderhydes, Coumarines, Ethers, Esters, Lactones, Sequiterpenes

SOOTHING
Alderhydes, Ethers, Esters

WARMING
Phenols, Oxides, Terpenes

APPENDIX III

SUPPLIERS

ESSENTIAL OILS

Britain:

Valerie Ann Worwood Aromatherapy Products & Essential Oils
Mail order service with fully comprehensive aromatherapy product list, including all essential oils mentioned in this book, essential oil body products, Landel portable diffusers, and other related items — for both public and professionals. For catalog and other information, send large self-addressed envelope or International Response Coupon, to the value of UK£5, refundable against first order, to:

P.O. Box 2256, Romford RM7 7BU, England

Earthway Aromatherapy
For catalog and other information send a large self-addressed envelope and International Response Coupon, to the value of UK£5, refundable against first order, to:

P.O. Box 5278, Westcliff-on-Sea, Essex SSO 7TT, England

North America:

The Anahata Centre
Essential oils including Aroma-Genera personality oils:

6240 Constable Drive, Richmond, British Columbia V7E 3Y2 (Tel: 604 241 9774)

Aroma Vera Inc.
PO Box 3609, Culver City, California 90231, USA

Original Swiss Aromatics
Pacific Institute of Aromatherapy
PO Box 606, San Rafael, California 94915, USA

Australasia:

Auroma-Australian Botanical Products
54 Stawell Street, Richmond, Melbourne, Victoria, Australia (428 4192)

Essentially Yours New Zealand
225 Coronation Avenue, New Plymouth, New Zealand (6-758-9599)

COMMERCIAL DIFFUSER SYSTEMS

Britain:

Dale Air Products
23 Arkwright Court, Blackpool and Fylde Industrial Estate, Lancashire FY4 5DR
(Tel: 01253 698687)

North America:

AromaSys Inc.
3208 West Lake Street, Minneapolis, Minnesota 55416, USA (Tel: (612) 924-0336)

APPENDIX IV

USEFUL ADDRESSES

Please send a large, stamped, self-addressed envelope to these addresses if you require a reply. Overseas correspondents should send an International Response Coupon.

AROMATHERAPY

The Aroma-Genera Association of North America
For information and list of professional Aroma-Generists:
1917 West 4th, Vancouver, British Columbia V6S 1M7, Canada

International Federation of Aromatherapists
Information on aromatherapy and list of registered aromatherapists; information on professional courses and training:
Stamford House, 2-4 Chiswick High Road, London W4 1TH,
Telephone 0181 742 2605, Fax: 0181 742 2606

International Society of Professional Aromatherapists
Hinkley and District Hospital and Health Centre, The Annexe, Mount Road, Hinkley, Leicestershire LE10 1AG

National Association for Holistic Aromatherapy
P.O. Box 17622, Boulder, Colorado 80308-7622

American Alliance of Aromatherapy
P.O. Box 750428, Petaluma, California 94975

The American Phytotherapy and Aromatherapy Association
P.O. Box 3679, South Pasadena, California 91031

Canadian federation of Aromatherapists
868 Markham Rd, Suite #109, Scarborough, Ontario, MIH-2Y2

Global Essence
P.O. Box 33282, San Diego, California 92136-3282
Telephone 1-888-WORWOOD

NOTES TO CHAPTERS 1-14

CHAPTER 1
[1] Dr. Varro E. Tyler, *Natural Products and Medicines*, in Herbalgram, No 28, 1993.
[2] Peter Gorman, "Making Magic," *Omni*, July 1993, 86.
[3] Ibid., 86.
[4] Richard Evans Schultes and Albert Hofmann, *Plants of The Gods* (Rochester: Healing Arts Press), 1992, 173.
[5] Ibid.

CHAPTER 2
[1] Richard Thompson, *The Brain: A Neuroscience Primer* (New York: W. H. Freeman and Company), 1993, 4.
[2] Ibid., 5.
[3] Ibid., 3.
[4] Peter Tompkins and Christopher Bird, *Secrets of the Soil* (London Penguin/Arkana, 1992), 126.
[5] Pierre Francomme and Daniel Pénoël, *Aromatherapie Exactement* (Limoges: Rogor Jollois), 1990.
[6] Tompkins and Bird, *Secrets of the Soil.*
[7] Craig Warren and Stephen Warrenburg, "Mood Benefits of Fragrance," *The International Journal of Aromatherapy*, Summer 1993, Vol. 5 No. 2.
[8] Thompson, *The Brain*, 121.
[9] Ibid., 151.
[10] Ibid., 150.
[11] Ibid., 175.

[12] Ibid., 159.

[13] Rob McCaleb, *Herbalgram*, Vol. 29, 1993, 20.

[14] Buchbauer, *International Journal of Aromatherapy*, Spring 1993, 13.

[15] Ibid., 12.

[16] Tompkins and Bird, *Secrets of the Soil*, 103.

[17] After Dark, Channel 4 TV, Open Media Productions.

[18] Tompkins and Bird, *Secrets of the Soil*, 101.

[19] Christopher Bird, *The Persecution and Trial of Gaston Naessens — The True Story of The Effort to Suppress an Alternative Treatment for Cancer, AIDS, And Other Immunologically Based Diseases* (Tiburon, California: H J Kramer Inc.), 1991, 15.

[20] Ibid., 300-301.

[21] Ibid., 304.

[22] Michael Talbot, *The Holographic Universe* (New York: HarperCollins), 1991.

[23] Johnson and Goldfinger, *Health Letter Book*, 418.

[24] Prozac (fluoxetine hydrochloride) Data Sheet IFDO2MAR93, Dista Products Ltd., Basingstoke, Hants RG21 2XA.

[25] *Chemical Marketing Reporter*, June 4, 1990.

[26] Brendan O'Regan, "Healing, Remission, and Miracle Cures," Institute of Noetic Sciences Special Report, May 1987, 3.

[27] Ibid.

[28] Thomas J Hurley III, "Placebo Effects: Unmapped Territory of Mind/Body Interactions," *Investigations* 2, no 1, 1985, 9.

[29] *A Prescription for Improvement*, Audit Commission, London HMSO, March 1994, 18.

[30] Ibid., 23.

CHAPTER 3

[1] Jane Butterworth, "The Day I Went Insane...," *Practical Health*, 82.

[2] William Lowther, "Beaming up...a human computer," *The Mail on Sunday*, February 13, 1994.

[3] Bill Moyers, *Healing and the Mind* (London: Thorsons/HarperCollins), 1993, 182.

[4] Jeanne Achterberg, "Mind and Medicine: The Role of Imagery in Healing," *ASPR Newsletter* 14, no 3, June 1988, 20.

[5] Talbot, *The Holographic Universe*, 105.

[6] Ibid.

[7] *The British Medical Association Complete Family Health Encyclopedia* (London: Dorling Kindersley), 1990.

[8] *A Prescription for Improvement*, Audit Commission Report, 1994, HMSO, 21.

[9] Russell Murray, Donna Hurle and Anthony Grant, *Tranquilizers, The MIND Guide to Where to get Help*, MIND/Bradford University, 1991 (available from MIND, Granta House,15-19 Broadway, Stratford, London E15, £5).

[10] Moyers, *Healing and the Mind*, 97.

[11] P. Goldberg, *The Intuitive Edge* (Wellingborough: Turnstone Press), 1985.

CHAPTER 4

[1] James A. Duke, PhD, "Father Nature's Farmacy," *HerbalGram*, No 12, Spring 1987, 6.

[2] Erin P. Reed, "Environmental Fragrancing Technology Makes Dollars & Scents," *The AromaChology Review*, September 1993, 6.

[3] Ibid., p5

[4] *Crains Chicago Business*, Dec. 2-8, 1991, 1.

[5] See *The Anahata Centre* in the list of suppliers on page 405.

[6] *Daily Express*, February 12, 1994.

[7] Georgia Persinos, PhD, *Herbalgram*, No 26, 1992, 14.

[8] *Washington Insight*, June 15, 1989 & September 15, 1991.

[9] A. R. Hirsch, P. M. Piecinski and K. M. Rankin, "Trichloroethylene Exposure and Headache," *Headache*, 275.

CHAPTER 7

[1] Dr. Seymour Epstein, *Sunday Express*, January 10, 1993, 34.

CHAPTER 8

[1] Debbie Taylor, "Women: An Analysis," *Women: A World Report* (London: New Internationalist/Methuen), 1985, 65.

[2] J. Kleijnen and P. Knipschild "Gingko biloba" *The Lancet*, 1992, 340(7):1136-39, see also Kleijnen & Knipschild "Gingko biloba for cerebral insufficiency," *British Journal of Clinical Pharmacology,* 1992, 34, 352-58.

[3] Glyn Jones, "A Shrinking of The Spirit," *The Guardian*, March 8, 1994, 21.

[4] I am grateful to *Herbalgram* for this information: No. 14, *Fall* 1987, page 3, referring to a report in *Planta Medica*, 53 (1), 5-8.

[5] "Femail," *Daily Mail*, March 1, 1993.

[6] *Los Angeles Times*, October 1, 1991.

[7] Tony Buzan, *The Mind-Map Book* (London, BBC Books), 1993.

[8] NSF Information sheet What is Schizophrenia? NSF, Kingston upon Thames, Surrey.

CHAPTER 10

[1] Dr Roger J. Woolger, *Other Lives, Other Selves* (New York: Doubleday), 1987.

CHAPTER 12

[1] Woolger, *Other Lives, Other Selves*, 16.

[2] Truddi Chase, *When Rabbit Howls* (New York: EP Dutton), 1987.

[3] Dr. Ronald Livingston, "Natrum muriaticum," *Health and Homeopathy* The Hahnemann Society of Great Britain, Summer 1992.

BIBLIOGRAPHY

Adams, R.B. and Victor, M. *Principles of Neurology*. New York: McGraw-Hill, 1991.

Aikman, Lonnelle. "Nature's Gifts to Medicine." *National Geographic*, September 1974.

Alexander, F.M. *The Use of Self*. New York: Dutton, 1932.

Anholt, R.R.H. "Primary Events in Olfactory Reception." *Trends in Biochemical Science*, 12, 1987, p. 58.

Anholt, R.R.H. "Odor Recognition and Olfactory Transduction." *Chem, Senses*, 16, 1991, p. 421.

Argyle, M. *The Psychology of Interpersonal Behavior*. London: London, 1967.

Atanassova-Shopova, S. and Roussinov, K. "Effects of Salvia Sclarea Essential Oil on the Central Nervous System." *Bulletin of the Institute of Physiology*, Bulgarian Academy of Sciences, 13, 1970, p. 89-95.

Badia, P. "Olfaction Sensitivity in Sleep: The Effects of Fragrance on the Quality of Sleep." *Perfumer and Flavorist*, 16, 1991, p. 33-34.

Badia, P. Wesensten N., Lammers W., Culpepper J. and Harsh J. "Responsiveness to Olfactory Stimuli Presented in Sleep." *Physiology & Behavior*, 48, 1990, p. 87-90.

Baerheim, Svendsen A. and Scheffer, J.J.C. (eds). *Essential Oils and Aromatic Plants*. The Netherlands: Dr. W. Junk Publications, 1984.

Balz, R. *Les Huiles Essentielles: Et Comment Les Utiliser*. Crest: Balz publication, 1986.

Bardeau, F. *La Medicine Aromatique*. Paris: Robert Laffont, 1976.

Baron, R.A. "Environmentally-Induced Positive Effect: Its Impact on Self-efficacy, Task Performance, Negotiation, and Conflict." *Journal of Applied Social Psychology*, 20, 1990, p. 368-384.

Baron, R. and Byrne, D. *Social Psychology: Understanding Human Interaction*. Fifth Edition, Allyn and Bacon Inc., 1974.

Beck, A.T. *Cognitive Therapy and the Emotional Disorders*. New York: Penguin, 1991.

Benson, D.F. "Treatable Dementias" in Benson, D.F., Blumer, D. (eds), *Psychiatric Aspects of Neurologic Disease*. New York: Grune & Stratton, 11, 1992, p. 139.

Bernadet, M. *La Phyto-Aromatherapie Practique*. Paris: Editions Dangles, 1983.

Blakeslee, T. *The Right Brain: A New Understanding of the Unconscious Mind and Its Powers*. London: Macmillan.

Bromberg, J.J. *Fasting Girls*. Cambridge, MA: Harvard University Press, 1988.

Brown, G.W. and Harris, T. *Social Origins of Depression*. London: Tavistock Publications, 1979.

Buchbauer, G., Jirovetz, L., Jager, W., Dietrich, H. and Plack, C. "Aromatherapy: Evidence for Sedative Effects of the Essential Oil of Lavender after Inhalation." Zeitschrift fur Natuforschung. Section C. *Journal of Biosciences*. 46 Nov-Dec 1991, p. 11-12; p. 1067-72.

Buchbauer, G. "Biological Effects of Fragrance and Essential Oils," *Perfumer & Flavorist*. 18, 1993, p. 19-23.

Buchbauer, G., Jirovetz, I., and Jager, W. "Aromatherapy: Evidence for Sedative Effects of the Essential Oil of Lavender After Inhalation." Institute of Pharmaceutical Chemistry, University of Vienna, 1991.

Buchbauer, G., Jirovetz, L. and Jager, W. "Kurzmitteilungen: Passiflora and Lime Blossoms: Motility Effects after Inhalation of the Essential Oils and of Some of the Main Constituents in Animal Experiment," *Aech. Pharm. (Weinheim)*, 325, 1992, p. 247-248.

Budlong, Ware T. *Performing Plants*. New York: Simon & Schuster, 1969.

Burbank, L. *The Training of the Human Plant*. New York: Century Co, 1907.

Burbank, L. *How Plants Are Trained to Work for Man*. New York: P.F. Collier & Son, 1921.

Capeland, I. and Gurnsey, J. *Managing Stress*. London: Constable & Company, Ltd., 1987.

Chase, T. *When Rabbits Howl*. London: Pan Books, 1987.

Chopra, Deepak, M.D. *Perfect Health*. London: Bantam Books, 1990.

Cousins, N. *Anatomy of an Illness as Perceived by the Patient : Reflections on healing and regeneration*. London/New York: Bantam, 1981.

Dally, P. and Watkins, M.J. *Psychology and Psychiatry*. Stevenoaks: Hodders & Stoughton, 1986.

Dimoff, T. and Carper, S. *How to Tell if Your Kids Are on Drugs*. New York: Facts and File, Inc., 1992.

Dossetor, D.R., Couryer, S., and Nicol, A.R. "Massage for Very Severe Self-injurious Behavior in a Girl with Cornelia de Lange Syndrome," *Developmental Medicine & Child Neurology*. 33 (7), 1991, p. 636-40.

Doty, R., Reyes, P. and Gregor, T. "Presence of Both Odor Identification and Detection in Alzheimer's Disease." *Brain Res. Bulletin*, 18, 1987, p. 598.

Dowden, A.O. *The Secret Life of Flowers*. New York: Odyssey Press, 1964.

Drydon, W. *Rational-Emotive Counseling in Action*. London: Sage Publications, 1990.

Durafound, P. *The Best of Health: Thanks to Essential Oils*. Perigny: La Vie Clair, 1984.

Dywer, J. *The Body at War*. London: Unwin Hyman, 1988.

Ehrlichman, H. and Bastone, L. "Odor Experience as an Affective State: Effects of Odor Pleasantness on Cognition. *Perfumer & Flavorist*, 16, 1991, p. 11-12

Ehrlichman, H. and Bastone, L. "Olfaction and Emotion." In Serby, M.J. and Chobor, K. L.

(eds). *Science of Olfaction*. New York: Springer-Verlag, 1992, p. 410-417.

Ehrlichman, H. and Halpern, J.N. "Affect and Memory: Effects of Pleasant and Unpleasant Odors on Retrieval of Happy and Unhappy Memories." *Journal of Personality and Social Psychology*, 55, 1988, p. 769-779.

England, Marjorie A. and Wakely, Jennifer. *A Color Atlas of the Brain and Spinal Cord*. London: Wolfe Publishing, 1991.

Fakouri, C. and Joners, P. "Relaxation RX: Slow Stroke Back Rub." *Journal of Gerontological Nursing*, Feb. 13, 1987, 2, p. 32-5.

Field, T., *et al*. "Massage Reduces Anxiety in Child and Adolescent Psychiatric Patients." *Journal of American Academy Child Adolescent Psychiatry*, 31(1), 1992, p. 125-31.

Forward, S. *Toxic Parents*. London: Bantam Press, 1990.

Franchomme, P., and Penoel, Dr. D. *L'aromatherapie Exactement*. Limoges: Roger Jollois Editeur, 1990.

Fraser, J., and Kerr, J. R. "Psychophysiological Effects of Back Massage on Elderly Institutionalized Patients." *Journal of Advanced Nursing*, 18 (2), 1993, p. 238-45.

Fredrickson, R. *Repressed Memories*. New York: Fireside Publications, 1992.

Gardner, H. *The Shattered Mind*. London: Routledge and Kegan P., 1977.

Gattefosse, R.M. *Aromatherapy*. Saffron Waldon: C. W. Daniel, 1993.

Gatti, G. Cayola. "L'azione Delle Essenze Sul Sistema Nervosa." *Rivista Italiana Essenza e perfumi*, 5 (12), 1923.

Giannitrapani, D. "*The Electrophysiology of Intellectual Functions*." Basel: Karger, 1985.

Gilling, D. and Brightwell, R. *The Human Brain*. London: Orbis Publishing, Ltd., 1982.

Graham, H. *Time Energy and Psychology of Healing*. London: Jessica Kingly, 1990.

Grieve, M. *A Modern Herbal*. London: Jonathon Cape, 1979.

Grof, Stanislav, M.D. *The Holotropic Mind*. San Francisco: HarperSanFrancisco, 1990.

Grof, Stanislav, M.D. *The Adventure of Self-Discovery*. New York: State University Press, 1988.

Guenther, E. *The Essential Oils*. 4 vols, 1948-1952.

Guillemain, J., Rousseau, A. and Delaveau, P. "Neurodepressive Effects of the Essential Oils of Lavendula Angustifolia Mill." *Annales Pharmaceutiques Francaises*, 6, 1989, p. 337-43.

Hall, M. P. *The Mystical and Medical Philosophy of Paracelsus*. Los Angeles: Philosophical Research Society, 1969.

Harris, B. and Lewis, R. "Psychophysiological Effects of Odor, Part 1-2." *IJACM*, Jan - March, 1994.

Hassett, James and White, Kathleen M. *Psychology in Perspective*. New York: Harper and Row, 1989.

Hernandez-Peon, R., Lavin, A., Alcocer-Cuaro, C., and Marcelin, J.P. "Electrical Activity of the Olfactory Bulb During Wakefulness and Sleep." *EEG Clinical Neurophysiology*, 12, 1960, p. 41-58.

Hirsch, A.R. and Trannel, T.J. *Depression and Chemosensory Dysfunction*. Chicago: Smell & Taste Treatment and Research Foundation, Ltd.

Hirsch, A.R. "*Olfaction and Psychiatry*." 144th Annual Meeting, American Psychiatric

Association, New Orleans, LA, May 16, 1991.

Hirsch, A.R. "Nostalgia, the Odors of Childhood and Society." *The Psychiatric Times. Medicine and Behavior*, August, 1992, p. 29.

Hirsch, A.R. "Olfaction and Anxiety." *Clinical Psychiatry*, 16, 1993, p. 4.

Hirsch, A.R. and Gay, S.E. "Effect of Ambient Olfactory Stimuli on the Evaluation of a Common Consumer Product," *Chem. Senses*, 5, 1991, p. 535.

Hope, M. *The Psychology of Healing*. London: Element books, 1989.

Hopkins, S.J. *Principle Drugs*. London: Faber & Faber, 1988.

Jacobsen, C.F. "Electrical Measurements of Neuromuscular Styates During Mental Activities: Imagination Involving Skeletal muscle." *American Journal of Physiology*, 91, p. 597-608.

Jager, W., Buckbaur, Jirovetz L., and Fritzer, M. "Percutaneous Absorption of Lavender Oil from a Massage Oil." *J Soc Cosm*, 43, 1992, p. 49-54.

Jori, A. and Bianchetti, Prestini P.E. "Effects of Essential Oils on Drug Metabolism" *Biochemical Pharmacology*, 1969, p. 2081-2085.

Kaada, B. and Torsteinbo, O. "Increase of Plasma Beta-Endorphins in Connective Tissue." *General Pharmacology*, 20 (4), 1989, p. 487-9.

Keeny, B.P. *Aesthetics of Change*. London: Guilford Press, 1983.

Kirk-Smith, M.D., Van Toller, S. and Dodd, G.H. "Unconscious Odor Conditioning in Human Subjects." *Biological Psychology*, 17, 1983, p. 221-231.

Klemm, W.R., Lutes, S.D., Hendrix, D.V. and Warrenburg, S. "Topographical EEG Maps of Human Responses to Odors." *Chemical Senses*, 17 (3), 1992, p. 347-361.

Kline, N. and Rausch, J. "Olfactory Precipitants of Flashbacks in Post-Traumatic Stress Disorders: Case Reports." *Journal of Clinical Psychiatry*, 46, 1985, p. 383-384.

Knasko, S.C., Gilbert, A.N. and Sabini, J. "Emotional State, Physical Well-being, and Performance in the Presence of Feigned Ambient Odor." *Journal of Applied Social Psychology*, 20, 1990, p. 1345-1357.

Knasko, S.C. "Ambient Odor and Shopping Behavior." *A Chem*, S-XI, 1989.

Knasko, S.C. "Ambient Odor's Effect on Creativity, Mood and Perceived Health," *Chemical Senses*, 17 (1), 1992, p. 27-35.

Kobal, G. and Hummal, T. "Olfactory Evoked Potentials." In Getchell, T.V. *et al* (eds) *Smell and Taste in Health and Disease*. New York: Raven Press, p. 255-275.

Koob, G.F. "Neuropeptides and Memory" In Iversen, L.L., Iversen, S.D., Snyder, S.H. (eds). *Handbook of Psychopharmacology*, New York: Plenum Press, 1987, p. 532.

Kreig, M.B. *Green Medicine*. London: George Harrap, 1964, (New York: Rand McNally, 1964.)

Kuipeis, L. and Bebbington, P. *Living with Mental Illness*. London: Souvenir Press Ltd., 1987.

Landis, C. and Hunt, A.W. *The Startle Pattern*. New York: Farrar & Rinehart, 1939.

Landis, C., and Hunt, A.W. *Perceptual and Motor skills*." 19, 1964, p. 21-22.

Langland, R.M., and Panicucci, E. "Effects of Touch on Communication with Elderly Confused Patients." *Journal of Gerontology and Nursing*, 8 (3), 1982, p. 152-5.

Lautie, R. and Passebecq, A. *Aromatherapy*. Wellingborough: Thorsons Publishers, 1979.

Lavabre, M. *Aromatherapy Workbook*. Rochester: Healing Arts Press, 1990.

Lawrence, B. *Essential Oils*. 3 Vols, 1976-1987.

Lee, C. *Safety Guide on the Use of Essential Oils*. London: Nature by Nature, Ltd., 1993.

Lele, R. *Ayurveda and Modern Science*. Bombay: Brharatiya Vida Bhavan, 1986.

Lewis, D. *Fight Your Phobia and Win*. London: Sheldon Press, 1984.

Linskens, H.F. and Jackson, J.F. (eds). *Essential Oils and Waxes*. Vol. 2, New York: Springer Verlag, 1991.

Loehr, Rev. Franklin. *The Powers of Prayer on Plants*. New York: Signet books, 1969.

Long, T.S., Huffman, E., Demartino, A.B. and Demarco, J. "EEG and Behavioral Responses to Low-level Galaxolide Administration, *Association Chemoreception Science Annual Meeting*, Sarasota, FL, 1989.

Lorenzetti, B.B., Souza, G.E., Sarti, S.J., Santos Filho, D. and Ferreira, S.H. "Myrcene Mimics the Peripheral Analgesic Activity of Lemongrass tea." *Journal of Enthnopharmacology*, 34 (1), Aug. 1991, p. 43-8.

Lorig, T. S., Schwartch, G.E. "Brain and Odor 11: EEG Alpha Activity During Administration of Perceptually Similar Odors." *Psychophysiology*, 24, 1987, p. 599.

Lowen, A., M.D. *Bioenergetics*. London: Penguin Books, 1976.

Ludvigson, H.W. and Rottman, T.R. "Effects of Ambient Odors of Lavender and Cloves on Cognition, Memory, Affect and Mood," *Chem Senses*, 14, 1989, p. 525-536.

Luscher, Dr. Max. *Luscher Color Test*. (Trans. Ian Scott), London: Pan Books, 1971.

MacLean, P.D. "The Limbic System, (Visceral Brain) Incidence of Interdependent and Emotional Processes," *Psychosomatic Medicine*, 42.

Mair, R.G. and Harrison, L.M. "Influence of Drugs on Smell Function," In Laing, D.C., Doty, R.L., Preipohl, W. (eds), *Human Sense of Smell*. Berlin: Springer-Verlag, 1991.

Manley, C.H. "Psychophysiological Effect of Odor." *Critical Reviews in Food and Sciences and Nutrition*, 33 (1), 1993, p. 57-62.

Maslow, A. *Towards a Psychology of Being*. New York: Van Nostrand Reinhold, 1966.

Maury, M. *The Secret of Life and Youth*. London: MacDonald & Co., 1964.

McCaffery, M. and Wolff, M. "Pain Relief Using Cutaneous Modalities, Positioning, and Movement," *Hospice Journal*, 8 (1-2), 1992, p. 121-53.

McKechnie, A.A., Wilson, F., Watson, N. and Scott, D. "Anxiety States: A Preliminary Report on the Value of Connective Tissue Massage," *Journal of Psychosomatic Research*, 27 (2), 1983, p. 125-9.

Meek, S. S. "Effects of Slow Stroke Back Massage on Relaxation in Hospice Patients." *Image — the Journal of Nursing Scholarship*, 25 (1), 1993, p. 17-21.

Melody, P., Miller, A.W. and Miller, J.K. *Facing Codependence*. San Francisco: Perennial Library, Harper and Row, 1989.

Melville, A. and Johnson, C. *Cured to Death*. London: Martin Secker & Warburg, Ltd., 1982.

Melzig, M. and Teucsher, E. "Investigations of the Influence of Essential Oils and their Main Components on the Adenosine Uptake by Cultivated Endothelial Cells," *Planta Med.*, Feb. 1991, 57 (1), p. 41-2.

Milne, L. and Milne, M. *The Nature of Plants*. Philadelphia: B. Lippincott, 1971.

Morton, I., Hall, J. and Halliday, J. *Tranquilizers*. London: Bloomsbury, 1991.

Moyers, Bill. *Healing and the Mind*. London: Thorsons, 1993.

Naranjo, Claudio, M.D. *Ennea-Type Structures*. Nevada City: Gateways/IDHHB, 1990.

Nwaiwu, J.L. and Akah, P.A. "Anticonvulsant Activity of the Volatile Oil from the Fruit of Tetrapleura Tetraptera." *Journal of Ethnopharmacology*, Nov. 1986, 18 (2), p. 103-7.

Oldfield, Harry and Coghill, Roger. *The Dark Side of the Brain*. Shaftesbury: Element Books, 1988.

Ornstien, R. and Sobel, D. *The Healing Brain*. London: Macmillan, 1988.

Ortiz de Urbina, A.V., Martin, M.L., Montero, M.J., Moran, A. and San Roman, L. "Sedating and Antipyretic Activity of the Essential Oil of Calamintha Sylvatica Subsp. Ascendens." *Journal of Ethnopharmacology*, 25 (2), April 1989, p. 165-71.

Pelletier, K. *Mind as Slayer, Mind as Healer*. London: Allen & Unwin, 1987.

Penoel, D. and Penoel, R. *Pratique Aromatique Familial*. Aouste-sur-sye: Osmobiose, 1992.

Perls, F.S. *The Gestalt Approach and Eyewitness to Therapy*, London: Bantam, 1976.

Pustjarvi, K., Airaksinen, O. and Pontinen, P.J. "The Effects of Massage in Patients with Chronic Tension Headache," *Acupuncture & Electro-Therapeutics Research*, 15 (2), 1990, p. 159-62.

Ratsch, C. *Sacred and Magical Plants*. translated by Hofmann, A. Dorset: Prism Press, 1992.

Redd, W.H. and Mann, S.L. *Fragrance Administration to Reduce Patient Anxiety During Magnet Resonance Imaging in Cancer Diagnosis Work-Up*, Sloane-Kettering Memorial Cancer Center, New York.

Reed, B.V. and Held. J.M. "Effects of Sequential Connective Tissue Massage on Autonomic Nervous System of Middle-aged and Elderly Adults." *Physical Therapy*. Aug, 1988, 68 (8), p. 1231-4.

Reese, A.J.M. *The Principles of Pathology*. London & Boston: Wright PSG, 1987.

Rhoades, Robert E. "The World's Food Supply at Risk." *National Geographic*, April 1991.

Ridley, H.N. *Spices*. London: Macmillan & Co., 1983.

Riordan, J. and Whitmore, B. *Living with Dementia*. New York: Manchester University Press, 1990.

Riso, Don Richard. *Personality Types*. London: Aquarian/HarperCollins, 1987.

Riso, Don Richard. *The Practical Guide to Personality Types*. London: Aquarian/Harper Collins, 1991.

Roberts, A. "Alzheimer's Disease May Begin in the Nose and May Be Caused by Aluminosicates" *Neuro-biological Aging*, 7, 1986, p. 561-567.

Rovesti, P. *In Search of Perfumes Lost*. Venice, 1980.

Royal, D. *The Human Side to Plants*. New York: Frederick A. Stokes Co., 1914.

Royal, D. and Fitch, F.E. *Personality of Plants*. New York: Bouilon-Biggs, 1923.

Russell, P. *The Brain Book*. London: Routledge & Kegan, 1990.

Sacks, O. *Migraine*. London: Faber & Faber, 1991.

Schaef, Anne Wilson. *Beyond Therapy, Beyond Science*. San Francisco: HarperSanFrancisco, 1994.

Schilcher, H. "Effects and Side-effects of Essential Oils," Baerheim Svenden, Scheffer (eds) *Essential Oils and Aromatic Plants,* The Netherlands: Dr. Junk Publishers, 1985.

Schultes, Richard Evans and Hofmann, Albert. *Plants of the Gods*. Rochester: Healing Arts Press, 1992.

Schwing, G. *A Way to the Souls of the Mentally Ill*. New York: International Press, 1954.

Selgman, M.E.P. *Helplessness*. San Francisco: Freeman & Company, 1975.

Serby, M., Corwin, J., Novatt, A., Conrad, P. and Rotrosen, J. "Olfaction in Dementia," *Journal Neurol-neurosurg Psychiatry*, 1985, 48, p. 849.

Sharma, Pandit Shiv, ed. *Realms of Ayurveda*. New Delhi: Arnold-Heinemann, 1979.

Sheldrake, R.A. *A New Lease of Life*. London: Granada, 1988.

Siegal, Bernie, M.D. *Love, Medicine and Miracles*. London: Rider, 1986.

Silverman, A.F., Pressman, M.E. and Bartel, H.W. "Self-esteem and Tactile Communication." *Journal of Humanistic Psychology*, 13, 1973, p. 73-7.

Springer, S.P. and Deusch, G. *Left Brain, Right Brain*. New York, 1989.

Stanford, T.L. *Strong at the Broken Places*. London: Virago Press Ltd., 1991.

Stern, J.A., Brown, M., Ulet, G.H. and Stellen, I. "A Comparison of Hypnosis, Acupuncture, Morphine, Valium, Aspirin and Placebo in the Management of Expression of Experimentally Induced Pain," *Annuals of New York Academy of Science*, 296, 1987, p. 175-193.

Stoddart, Michael D. *The Scented Ape*. Cambridge: Cambridge University Press, 1990.

Stone, H. and Winkelman, S. *Embracing Ourselves: The Voice Dialogue Manual*. Novato, CA: New World Library, 1989.

Sugano, H. "Effects of Odors on Mental Function (Abstract)," JASTS, 1988, XX11, p. 8.

Synge, Patrick. *Plants with Personality*. London: Lindsay Drummond, Ltd., 1939.

Talbot, Michael. *The Holographic Universe*. New York: HarperCollins, 1991.

Taylor, J.E. *The Sagacity and Morality of Plants*. London: Chatto & Windus, 1884.

Tecces, J.J. and Scheff, N.M. "Attention Reduction and Suppressed Direct Current Potentials in the Human Brain," *Science*, 164, 1969, p. 331.

Thompson, Richard F. *The Brain*. New York: W.H. Freeman and Co., 1993.

Tisserand, R. *Aromatherapy for Everyone*. London: Arkana, 1988.

Tisserand, R. *The Safety Data Manual*. Brighton: Association of Tisserand Aromatherapists, 1985.

Torri, S., Fukuda, H., Kanemoto, H., Miyanchi, R., Hamauzu, Y. and Kawasaki, M., "Contingent Negative Variation (CNV) and the Psychological Effects of Odor." In Van Toller, S., Dodd, G.H., (eds). *Perfumery: Psychology and Biology of Fragrance*. New York: Chapman and Hall, p. 107-120.

Turner, P., Richens, A. and Routledge, P. *Clinical Pharmacology*. London: Churchill Livingstone, 1986.

Uphof, J.C. *Dictionary of Economic Plants*. New York: Verlag Von J. Cramer, 1968.

Valnet, J., Duraffourd, C. and Lapraz, J.C. *Phytotherapy & Aromatherapy*. Paris Presse de la Renaissance, 1978.

Valnet, J. *The Practice of Aromatherapy*. Saffron Walden: C.W. Daniel Company, Ltd., 1982.

Van Toller, S. "Odors, emotion and psychophysiology." *International Journal of Cosmetic Science*, 10, p. 171-197.

Van Toller, Steve and Dodd, George H. *Perfumery: The Psychology and Biology of Fragrance*.

London: Chapman and Hall, 1988.

Van Toller, Steve and Dodd, George H. *Fragrance: The Psychology and Biology of Perfume*, London: Elsevier Science Publishers, 1992.

Viaud, H. and Dufour, D. *Huiles Essentielles — Hydrolats: Distillation Qualite Controle de la Purete Indications Majeures*. Sisteron: Editions Presence, 1983.

Walker, J.T. "The Anxious Patient." *Journal of Family Practitioners*, 12, 1981, p. 733-738.

Walker, M., *Dirty Medicine*, London: Slingshot publications, 1993.

Warm, J.S., Dember, W.N. and Parasuraman, R. "Effect of Olfactory Stimulation on Performance and Stress in a Visual Sustained Attention Task." *Journal of Cosmetic Chem.*, 42, 1991, p. 199-210.

Watson, Lyall. *Supernature*. London: Coronet/Hodder Paperbacks, 1974.

Watt, M. *Plant Aromatics Data & Reference Manual*. Essex: Watt, 1991.

Weinrich, S.P. and Weinrich, M.C. "The Effect of Massage on Pain in Cancer Patients." *Applied Nursing Research*, 3 (4), 1990, p. 140-5.

Weisskopf-Joelsov, E. *Father I Have Kept My Promise*. Purdue Research Foundation, 1988.

West, M. "Meditation." *British Journal of Psychiatry*, 135, 1979, p. 457-69.

Wilson, Dr. Glen. *Your Personality and Potential*. Topsfield, MA: Salem House Publishers, 1989.

Wilson, M. *Crossing the Boundaries*. London: Virago Press, 1993.

Woolger, Roger J., Ph.D. *Other Lives, Other Selves*. New York: Dolphin/Doubleday, 1987.

Worwood, V.A. *Aromantics*. London: Bantam Books, 1987.

Worwood, V. A. *The Complete Book of Essential Oils & Aromatherapy*. Novato, CA: New World Library, 1991.

Wren, R.C., Williamson and Evens, F. J. *Potters New Cyclopedia of Botanical Drugs and Preparations*. Saffron Walden: C.W. Daniel Company Ltd., 1989.

Yamaguchi, H. "Effect of Odor on Heart Rate," *The Psychophysiological Effects of Odor, Aromachology*, Indo, M., Ed, Koryo, 1990, p. 168.

Youngken, *Pharmaceutical Botany*. Dehra: R.P. Singh, 1986.

INDEX

About the Author

VALERIE ANN WORWOOD has been a leading aromatherapist for over twenty years. She is an active member of the International Federation of Aromatherapists and runs her own clinic in England, where she conducts research on aromatherapy and its effects on endometriosis and infertility. She works as a consultant for natural beauty clinics, health clinics, and celebrities, and lectures throughout the world on the benefits of aromatherapy and essential oils. *The Fragrant Mind* is her third book.

NEW WORLD LIBRARY is dedicated to publishing books and audios that help improve the quality of our lives. If you enjoyed *The Fragrant Mind*, we highly recommend the following books:

The Complete Book of Essential Oils & Aromatherapy, by Valerie Ann Worwood. A classic aromatherapy reference. An encyclopedic book that includes easy recipes for beauty products, health remedies, household cleaners, and more.

Essential Aromatherapy, by Susan Worwood. A lively A-to-Z pocket reference that shows how to prepare and use essential oils as holistic healing agents.

If you would like a catalog of our fine books and audios, contact:

NEW WORLD LIBRARY
14 Pamaron Way
Novato, CA 94949
(415) 884-2100 • Fax (415) 884-2199
Or call toll free: (800) 972-6657
Catalog requests: Ext. 50
Ordering: Ext. 52
E-Mail: escort@nwlib.com
NEWWORLDLIBRARY.COM